Customized Corneal Ablation
The Quest for SuperVision

Customized Corneal Ablation
The Quest for SuperVision

Scott M. MacRae, MD
University of Rochester Medical Center
Rochester, New York

Ronald R. Krueger, MD, MSE
Cole Eye Institute
Cleveland Clinic Foundation
Cleveland, Ohio

Raymond A. Applegate, OD, PhD
University of Texas Health Science Center
San Antonio, Texas

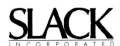

an innovative information, education and management company
6900 Grove Road • Thorofare, NJ 08086

Publisher: John H. Bond
Editorial Director: Amy E. Drummond
Senior Associate Editor: Jennifer Stewart

Customized corneal ablation : the quest for supervision / [edited by] Scott M. MacRae, Ronald R. Krueger, Raymond A. Applegate.
    p. ; cm.
    Includes bibliographical references and index.
    ISBN 1-55642-488-4 (alk. paper)
    1. LASIK (eye surgery) I. Title: Quest for supervision. II. MacRae, Scott. III. Krueger, Ronald R.
IV. Applegate, Raymond A.
    [DNLM: 1. Cornea--surgery. 2. Keratectomy, Photorefractive, Excimer Laser--methods. 3. Corneal Topography. WW 220 C987 2001]
RE336 .C87 2001
617.7'19059--dc21

                                                     00-053825

Printed in the United States.

Published by: SLACK Incorporated
                      6900 Grove Road
                      Thorofare, NJ 08086 USA
                      Telephone: 856-848-1000
                      Fax: 856-853-5991
                      www.slackbooks.com

Contact SLACK Incorporated for more information about other books in this field or about the availability of our books from distributors outside the United States.
Authorization to photocopy items for internal or personal use, or the internal or personal use of specific clients, is granted by SLACK Incorporated, provided that the appropriate fee is paid directly to Copyright Clearance Center, 222 Rosewood Drive, Danvers, MA 01923 USA, 978-750-8400. Prior to photocopying items for educational classroom use, please contact the CCC at the address above. Please reference Account Number 9106324 for SLACK Incorporated's Professional Book Division.
For further information on CCC, check CCC Online at the following address: http://www.copyright.com.

Last digit is print number: 10 9 8 7 6 5 4 3 2 1

DEDICATION

This book is dedicated to my father, Pete, and mother, Betty,
who loved and guided me in my long journey to become a physician.
To my curious 2-year-old daughter, Morgan,
whose sparkling eyes teach me the truly important lessons in life.
To my wife, Abby, my love and inspiration, whose poetry in life fills my spirit.
To the dedicated men and women in science who ask why.
Scott M. MacRae, MD

To my late father, Arthur M. Krueger, and loving mother, Lucie Krueger,
who raised me to follow biblical principles in life and aspire to achieve excellence
with integrity in my work. Their support and encouragement inspired me to become
an electrical engineer and ophthalmologist, leading to my interest in excimer laser photoablation
and wavefront customization. To all those who might visually benefit from the clinical application of the
science contained in this book. I, for one, look forward to participating in the process.
Ronald R. Krueger, MD, MSE

To Rachel, Aaron, Ryan, Camille, and Olivia.
Raymond A. Applegate, OD, PhD

CONTENTS

Section IV. Surgeon-Guided Customized Ablation

Section V. The Future of Customization

Appendices

ACKNOWLEDGMENTS

There are many who have supported, guided, and inspired me. The following are just a few of the treasured many to whom I am indebted. I wish to thank my early teachers and mentors, Dick Appen, MD, and Fred Brightbill, MD. I thank Matthew Davis, MD for inspiring me with his wonderful analytical mind and selfless dedication to medicine. To Hank Edelhauser, PhD, who nurtured my creativity and curiosity and taught me that science can be a source of great satisfaction and joy. To Bob Hyndiuk, MD and Dick Schultz, MD, who introduced me to the complexity and beauty of the cornea and to the world of science, which probes it. I am grateful to Fritz Fraundfelder, MD, for his enthusiastic support, thoughtful career guidance, and wonderful sense of humor. I am greatly indebted to my professional partner of 16 years, Larry Rich, MD, who inspired me with the highest standards of patient care and professional integrity. There are few physicians who are so lucky to have such a supportive colleague and friend.

Over the years, I have been truly fortunate to have journeyed with many exceptional individuals, including Doug Koch, MD; Dan Durrie, MD; George Waring, MD; Ross Pfister, MD; the late Lou Wilson, MD; Al Sommer, MD; Hugh Taylor, MD; Dennis O'Day, MD; Marguerite McDonald, MD; Roberto Zaldivar, MD; Arturo Chayet, MD; Paolo Vinciguerra, MD; and Howard Gimbel, MD. I am indebted to the wonderful professionals and friends at the Casey Eye Institute, including John Samples, MD; Joe Robertson, MD; Rachael Garrett, OD; Mark Andre; and Pat Caroline.

I am grateful to have partnered with two truly exceptional individuals—Ron Krueger, MD and Ray Applegate, OD, PhD—whose tireless energies and strong intellects made this book a reality. Ron brought his powerful intellect, creative talents, and endless drive for improving refractive surgical techniques. Ray brought us his unique knowledge of the world of vision as well as his passion for scientific inquiry and high-quality visual science. Ron and Ray brought together a world class group of vision scientists and refractive surgeons who give this book its unique flavor. Ron and Ray juggled their extremely busy lives to make this book a reality.

I greatly appreciate Peter Slack, whose strong early support allowed us to transform an idea into a book much larger than any of us had envisioned. I wish to give a very special thanks to Vikki Kristiansson, John Bond, and Jennifer Stewart, whose persistence, discipline, and patience was invaluable to the creation of this book. Without her professionalism, this book would not have materialized. Jennifer Anstey provided her invaluable thoughtfulness, dedication, and considerable editorial skills to weave each chapter into a solid text. She sculpted the book with her powerful intellect.

I cannot end without high accolades to the authors of this book. I am highly indebted to the very talented authors whose hard work and thoughtful insights have helped drive the world of refractive surgery to a higher plane. We live in a wonderful age when miracles can happen. The men and women who helped write this book are helping to create such a wondrous event.

Scott M. MacRae, MD

Although I have many colleagues and friends in the field whom I wish to acknowledge, I cannot possibly include them all. Rather, I would like to pay a special tribute to my mentors, those with whom I had the opportunity to professionally train or work over the years:

Stephen Trokel (my first mentor while I was still a medical student, who got me started with excimer laser photoablation).

George Florakis (my residency mentor, the person who trained me to be a corneal surgeon while I was still a resident).

Theo Seiler (my scientific mentor, the one who inspires me more than anyone regarding new insights and scientific projects in refractive surgery, including wavefront technology).

J. James Rowsey (my corneal fellowship mentor, who taught me much about the cornea, topography, how to mentor others, and how to honor God while being a great doctor).

Peter McDonnell (my refractive surgery fellowship mentor, who taught me how to incorporate academics and research into a refractive surgery practice).

David Schanzlin (my academic faculty mentor, who hired me into my first faculty position and taught me how to think independently as a refractive surgery subspecialist).

George Waring (my editorial mentor, who recruited me to be an associate editor for the *Journal of Refractive Surgery* and challenged me to write and editorialize with a rigorous scientific standard).

Bill Conrad (my medical missions mentor, who invited me to participate in a volunteer eye care project in Western China and instilled in me the desire to use my skill to help others less fortunate than me).

Hilel Lewis (my chairman mentor, who recruited me to a world class institution to be the medical director of the department of refractive surgery under his leadership).

To each of these, I formally thank you for your role in my professional development.

Ronald R. Krueger, MD, MSE

I wish to acknowledge and thank my co-editors, colleagues, parents, and family. Ron Krueger and Scott MacRae for their tolerance with my bluntness, and for their friendship. Larry Thibos, Howard Howland, Gene Hilmantel, Steve Burns, Austin Roorda, Jim Schwiegerling, Cindy Roberts, David Williams, George Pettit, and David Huang for their scientific talent, dedication to this project, and most of all for their friendship and comraderie. From my heart, I thank my parents and family for their love, support, and faith in my abilities.

Raymond A. Applegate, OD, PhD

ABOUT THE EDITORS

Scott M. MacRae, MD

Scott M. MacRae, MD has been a practicing clinician since 1983. He received his bachelor of science degree from the University of Wisconsin, Madison Biocore Honors Curriculum in 1974 and his medical degree from the University of Wisconsin Medical School in 1977. He completed internship and residency programs at the Tucson Medical Center in Tucson, Ariz, Stanford University in Palo Alto, Calif, and the University of Wisconsin Hospitals in Madison, followed by a cornea/external disease fellowship; a National Eye Institute corneal physiology research training fellowship, both at the Eye Institute of the Medical College of Wisconsin, and a corneal disease and a brief contact lens fellowship at Emory University in Atlanta, Ga. He was certified by the American Board of Ophthalmology in 1983.

Dr. MacRae entered the faculty of Oregon Health Sciences University in 1983, where he was director of the Oregon Eye Bank, 1986 to 2000. He has been a panel member or consultant for the US Food and Drug Administration Ophthalmic Devices Panel from 1986 to the present. He was chairman of the American Academy of Ophthalmology Public Health Committee from 1991 to 1994. He currently serves on the American Academy of Ophthalmology Research and Regulatory Committee.

Author of more than 60 published articles and book chapters, Dr. MacRae increasingly turned his attention to refractive corneal surgery and has performed more than 3000 refractive surgery procedures. He has a special interest in ablation design and interface keratitis. He has trained more than 300 clinicians in the practice of refractive surgery and has participated and helped lead several FDA clinical trials in the United States.

An editor for three ophthalmic journals, he is currently North American associate editor for the *Journal of Refractive Surgery*, has co-edited three special editions of the *Journal of Refractive Surgery*, and has chaired numerous international refractive symposiums.

In 2000, Dr. MacRae accepted an appointment as professor of ophthalmology at the University of Rochester, NY, where with the university's Center for Vision Science, he promotes research and development of new refractive surgery techniques and technology.

Ronald R. Krueger, MD, MSE

Dr. Ronald R. Krueger received his MD from the University of Medicine and Dentistry of New Jersey (1987). Prior to this, he received a BS in electrical engineering from Rutgers University and an MSE in biomedical engineering from the University of Washington, Seattle. He completed his ophthalmology residency at the Columbia-Presbyterian Medical Center of New York. He also completed two fellowships in cornea and refractive surgery from the University of Oklahoma and the University of Southern California, Los Angeles. Dr. Krueger is the medical director of the Department of Refractive Surgery at the Cleveland Clinic Foundation. He is the education committee chairman of the International Society of Refractive Surgery, and a board member of the LASIK Institute. He currently serves as associate editor of the *Journal of Refractive Surgery*, and is cofounder of the International Congress on Wavefront Sensing and Aberration-Free Refractive Correction. He has 16 years of experience in excimer laser research and is currently involved in research investigating the cause(s) of presbyopia and restoration of accommodation, as well as wavefront imaging of the eye for customized laser vision correction.

Raymond A. Applegate, OD, PhD

Raymond A. Applegate, OD, PhD is the second of four children born to K. Edwin Applegate and Elizabeth Dilts Applegate. He was born in Bloomington, Ind in 1949 and attended Indiana University from kindergarten through his bachelor of arts degree (1971), doctor of optometry (1975), and his master of science in physiological optics (1976). He practiced optometry in Galesburg, Ill before continuing his graduate education in physiological optics at the University of California, Berkeley, where he received his PhD (1983). Dr. Applegate joined the University of Texas Health Science Center faculty in 1988 from the School of Optometry, University of Missouri—St. Louis, where he served as an assistant professor of optometry. He rose through the faculty ranks quickly to become a tenured professor of ophthalmology in 1993. He has served as a feature editor of the *Journal of the Optical Society of America, Applied Optics,* and *Optometry and Vision Science* on several occasions. Dr. Applegate has served on the editorial board of *Optometry and Visual Science* and currently serves on the editorial board of the *Journal of Refractive Surgery.* He is a cofounder of the International Congress on Wavefront Sensing and Aberration-Free Refractive Correction, is widely published in leading journals, and is a sought-after consultant and international lecturer whose research interests center on the optics of the eye and early ocular disease detection and prevention.

CONTRIBUTING AUTHORS

Giovanni Alessio, MD
Department of Ophthalmology
University of Bari
Bari, Italy

Raymond A. Applegate, OD, PhD
Department of Ophthalmology
University of Texas
Health Sciences Center
San Antonio, Texas

Josef F. Bille, PhD
Kirchhoff Institute of Physics
University of Heidelburg
Heidelburg, Germany

Jean Brandau, MBA
Tracey Technologies
Bellaire, Texas

Joana Buechler Costa, Dipl Phys
Kirchhoff Institute of Physics
University of Heidelburg
Heidelburg, Germany

Stephen A. Burns, PhD
Schepens Eye Research Institute
Boston, Massachusetts

Fabrizio I. Camesasca, MD
Instituto Clinico Humanitas
Rozzano-Milano, Italy

Charles Campbell, PhD
Sola Optical USA
Petaluma, California

John A. Campin, BSc
Autonomous Technologies Corporation
Orlando, Florida

Arturo S. Chayet, MD
Chula Vista, California

Klaus Ditzen, MD
Eye Surgery Center
Weinheim, Germany

William J. Dupps, Jr, MD, PhD
College of Medicine
Ohio State University
Columbus, Ohio

Masano Fujieda, MA
Nidek Company, Ltd.
Gamagori, Japan

Antonio Guirao, PhD
Center for Visual Science
University of Rochester
Rochester, New York

Weldon W. Haw, MD
Stanford Health Services
Palo Alto, California

Gene Hilmantel, OD, MS
Department of Ophthalmology
University of Texas
Health Science Center
San Antonio, Texas

Heidi Hofer, BS
Center for Visual Science
University of Rochester
Rochester, New York

Howard C. Howland, PhD
Department of Neurobiology and Behavior
Cornell University
Ithaca, New York

David Huang, MD, PhD
Division of Ophthalmology
Cleveland Clinic Foundation
Cleveland, Ohio

Michael Huppertz
SensoMotoric Instruments
GmbH, Teltow/Berlin, Germany

Maik Kaemmerer, PhD
University of Dresden
Department of Ophthalmology
Dresden, Germany

Vikentia J. Katsanevaki, MD
Department of Ophthalmology
University of Crete Medical Center
Heraklion Crete, Greece

Stephen D. Klyce, PhD
Department of Ophthalmology
Louisiana State Health Science Center
New Orleans, Louisiana

Michael Knorz, MD
Department of Ophthalmology
Klinikum Mannheim
Mannheim, Germany

Ronald R. Krueger, MD, MSE
Cole Eye Institute
Cleveland Clinic Foundation
Cleveland, Ohio

M. Gabriella LaTegola, MD
Department of Ophthalmology
University of Bari
Bari, Italy

Scott M. MacRae, MD
Department of Ophthalmology
University of Rochester Medical Center
Rochester, New York

Edward E. Manche, MD
Stanford University School of Medicine
Stanford, California

Susana Marcos, PhD
Instituto de Optica
Madrid, Spain

Peter Mierdel, PhD
Department of Ophthalmology
University of Dresden
Dresden, Germany

Vasyl V. Molebny, DSc
Tracey Technologies
Bellaire, Texas

Michael Mrochen, PhD
University of Zurich
Department of Ophthalmology
Zurich, Switzerland

Frank Mueller, Dipl Phys
20/10 Perfect Vision Opticsche Geraete GmbH
Heidelburg, Germany

Ioannis G. Pallikaris, MD
Department of Ophthalmology
University of Crete Medical School
Heraklion Crete, Greece

Sophia I. Panagopoulou, PhD
Department of Ophthalmology
University of Crete Medical School
Heraklion Crete, Greece

George H. Pettit, MD, PhD
Autonomous Technologies Corporation
Orlando, Florida

Stefan Pieger, Dipl Ing
Wendelstein, Germany

Jason Porter, MS
Center for Visual Science
University of Rochester
Rochester, New York

Cynthia Roberts, PhD
Department of Ophthalmology and Biomedical
Engineering Center
Ohio State University
Columbus, Ohio

Austin Roorda, PhD
University of Houston College of Optometry
Houston, Texas

Carlo Sborgia, MD
Department of Ophthalmology
University of Bari
Bari, Italy

Eberhard Schmidt, MBA
SensoMotoric Instruments
GmbH, Teltow/Berlin, Germany

Jim Schwiegerling, PhD
Ophthalmology and Optical Sciences
University of Arizona
Tucson, Arizona

Theo Seiler, MD, PhD
Department of Ophthalmology
University of Zurich
Zurich, Switzerland

Mario G. Serrano, MD
Bogota Laser Refractive Institute
Bogota, Colombia

Robert W. Snyder, MD, PhD
Department of Ophthalmology
University of Arizona
Tucson, Arizona

Barrie D. Soloway, MD, FACS
New York Eye and Ear Infirmary
New York, New York

Gustavo E. Tamayo, MD
Bogota Laser Refractive Institute
Bogota, Colombia

Winfried Teiwes, PhD
SensoMotoric Instruments
GmbH, Teltow/Berlin, Germany

Larry N. Thibos, PhD
School of Optometry
Indiana University
Bloomington, Indiana

Tim N. Turner, PhD
Orbtek/Bausch & Lomb Surgical
Salt Lake City, Utah

Paolo Vinciguerra, MD
Instituto Clinico Humanitas
Rozzano-Milano, Italy

Joe S. Wakil, MD
Tracey Technologies
Bellaire, Texas

David R. Williams, PhD
Center for Visual Science
University of Rochester
Rochester, New York

Geun-Young Yoon, PhD
Center for Visual Science
University of Rochester
Rochester, New York

FOREWORD

Periodically in ophthalmology, a single meeting has an electric excitement and intrinsic power that simply by being in the room causes you to realize that you are witnessing an inflection point in the history of eye surgery. I have been present at four such meetings in the past 25 years.

1. The meeting of the Intraocular Implant Society in Santa Monica, Calif, in the late 1970s, where European colleagues presented their concept of implanting an artificial lens in the eye at the time of cataract extraction, a topic of such enormous interest that the entire meeting had to be moved from the auditorium to the cafeteria, with speakers standing on dinner tables to be seen and heard.

2. The evening meeting during the American Academy of Ophthalmology meeting held by the Keratorefractive Society that filled a ballroom and propelled itself far beyond midnight, as attendees savored the possibility of using a surgical technique developed in Japan and refined in Russia to eliminate myopia.

3. The first special interest group meeting of the American Academy of Ophthalmology in the early 1990s on refractive surgery—including excimer laser surgery, which filled all seats, all aisles, and all access points to the meeting room, spurring the fire marshall to disperse the crowd.

4. The First International Congress on Wavefront Sensing and Aberration-Free Refractive Correction in Santa Fe, NM, on February 12-13, 2000—the exciting interface of optical science, ophthalmic research, and clinical applications that produced this book.

The practical results of the first three of these meetings are now a matter of a historical yawn: aphakic IOLs are routine, refractive keratotomy has come and gone, and excimer laser corneal surgery has the appearance of a pop retail product. So where is the excitement about something that sounds as arcane as wavefront-guided corneal ablation? It is the excitement of giving individuals better vision than they can attain with conventional optical correction of glasses or contact lenses. The authors and editors of this book have assembled the scientific and clinical basis for this next major ophthalmic advance.

The book's broad scope contains something for everyone interested in this subject. For the novice who may ask, "What's this wavefront stuff?" there are superb chapters defining the basics of spherical and cylindrical defocus, higher-order optical aberrations, and the optical science that might apply this information to the cornea. Most striking in this area is the fact that many of these insights and techniques are more than a century old, a fact that will help keep us all humble amidst our excitement of new innovation.

One thesis that emerges from the book is the true complexity of this present understanding. My analogy—the historical inflection points I mentioned above—may appear simple. The task now is to take an aspheric axially asymmetric biological system (the eye) and measure not only its optics, but understand its psychophysics as part of the whole visual system, utilize optical and anatomic (topographic) information to direct a complex ultraviolet laser to perform with submicron accuracy (in the face of considerable biological variability from one eye to another), and modify the results in an iterative process that takes into consideration not only optical results, but also alterations in corneal biomechanics, hydration, and epithelial and stromal wound healing to come out with a visual circumstance that allows the individual to see near the limits of practical visual resolution—20/10 to 20/05. In this context, the authors and editors provide the groundwork for understanding, but it certainly is not a conclusive guide.

One of the problems alluded to but not fully addressed in detail in this book is what are the ideal optical conditions of the eye. Certainly, they are not the elimination of all optical aberrations. Preservation of some asphericity is required for good function of the eye. When one factors in the dynamic problems of the crystalline lens (accommodation and progressive changes in lens density), one sees that there is a temporal component to be overcome.

The title of the book limits itself to customized corneal ablations, but such customization for an individual eye could, of course, be applied to IOL implantation—especially in phakic eyes. If it is possible to create an individualized shape in a cornea, with all of its biological variability, it should be possible to create an individualized phakic IOL in which the shaping of the synthetic material should be easier. There would be an additional advantage: it would be removable and replaceable.

The reader fortunate enough to access this book and savor its contents will stand with the authors on the threshold of another giant leap in ophthalmology.

George O. Waring III, MD, FACS, FRCOphth
Emory Vision Correction Group
Atlanta, Georgia

INTRODUCTION

Customized Corneal Ablation is, to my knowledge, the first textbook dedicated to this important scientific advance in excimer laser surgery. It is a watershed moment in the development of refractive surgery, on par with the development of excimer laser surgery itself.

Why is customization so important? For the first time in history, we are able to eliminate the higher-order optical aberrations caused by current laser surgery (which decreases night vision for many of our patients). We are also able to improve on Mother Nature by routinely obtaining acuities that are better than 20/20. The experts in physiological optics and retinal neurobiology argue over the precise limit to human vision (somewhere between 20/10 and 20/5), though everyone agrees that human vision can be much improved when our optical system is perfected. With the detection and elimination of higher-order aberrations, new vistas will open for our patients.

We had the honor of performing the first wavefront-based excimer laser surgeries in the United States on October 12, 1999. Recently, one of my patients in the study (who sees 20/10 after wavefront-based LASIK) said to me," It's so wonderful to see fine details on the leaves at 500 yards away."

It is a great honor for me to write the Introduction for such an important book edited by three leaders in the field: Doctors Scott MacRae, Ronald Krueger, and Ray Applegate. Their international reputations allowed them to entice other experts in the field to contribute chapters.

Last but not least, the editors selected a publishing house with a long and wonderful track record in ophthalmic publications, known for their timelessness, easy readability, and great visual appeal.

I know you will enjoy this beautifully written and illustrated textbook; I am sure it will become a collector's item.

Marguerite B. McDonald, MD, FACS
Director, Southern Vision Institute
New Orleans, Louisiana

Introduction

Chapter One

What is Customization?
An Introduction to Customized Ablation

Scott M. MacRae, MD
Raymond A. Applegate, OD, PhD
Ronald R. Krueger, MD, MSE

Webster's Dictionary defines customize as: "to build, fit, or alter according to individual specifications or needs."[1]

We all customize. In a sense, our lives are customized based on our genetics, background, and environment. In a similar way, customized corneal ablation is based on our patients' underlying genetics, which largely determines their anatomy and, in turn, their refractive error. Corneal customization is based on our ability to detect significant optical abnormalities or wavefront errors and correct them. This chapter will outline the various ways we as clinicians and surgeons can customize treatment to optimize our patient's vision while maximizing safety.

ONE SIZE DOES NOT FIT ALL

Customized ablation attempts to optimize the eye's optical system using a variety of spherical, cylindrical, aspheric, and asymmetrical treatments based on an individual eye's optics and anatomy, as well as patient needs and preferences. Customization can be used to improve optical quality in normal eyes as well as eyes with atypical optical aberrations caused by corneal scarring, penetrating keratoplasty, central islands, decentered ablations, and lenticular abnormalities.

WAYS TO CUSTOMIZE

Vision is a complex process and can be divided into at least two broad subsections: optics and neural processing. Customization of corneal laser treatment to correct the refractive errors of the eye falls under the optics section. Translating the retinal image into a neural percept is neural processing. The focus of this book is on new methods to create an optimal retinal image. Creating an optimal retinal image requires consideration of several interactive factors. These factors can be broken into three classes (Table 1-1):
- Functional
- Anatomical
- Optical

Functional factors require an understanding of the patient's individual needs and circumstances. Anatomical factors require the consideration of individual structural variation of each eye. Optical factors require an understanding of unique refraction and aberration profile of the eye... all three factors must be considered when contemplating a customized corneal ablation.

Table 1-1

Interactive Factors to Consider for Customized Ablation

FUNCTIONAL CUSTOMIZATION FACTORS BASED ON PATIENT'S NEED

- Age
- Presbyopia
- Patient's occupational and recreational needs
- Refraction
- Psychological tolerance

ANATOMICAL FACTORS TO CONSIDER FOR CUSTOMIZED ABLATION

- Corneal diameter and thickness
- Pupil size (also important for optical customization)
- Anterior chamber depth
- Anterior and posterior lens shape
- Axial length

OPTICAL FACTORS TO CONSIDER FOR CUSTOMIZED ABLATION

- Customization based on corneal topography
- Customization based on wavefront measurements
    --Hartmann-Shack (Shack-Hartmann) wavefront sensor
    --Cross cylinder aberrometer (Howland and Howland)
    --Tscherning aberrometer
    --Tracey system
    --Slit-light bundle
    --Spatially resolved refractometer
    --Others

Functional Factors in Customization

Functional factors require an understanding of the patient's individual needs and circumstances, including the patient's age, refraction, occupation, and personal optical requirements (eg, monovision), as well as adaptability. Let us explore some of these areas in more detail.

> Functional customization includes considering under-correcting older myopes, which can provide functional near vision for many near tasks.

Age Considerations

Experience has taught us that age is an important consideration when treating patients with laser refractive surgery. A number of studies have shown that myopic patients over the age of 40 to 45 are more susceptible to hyperopic overcorrection.[2-4] Further, in

our experience, treating younger patients with myopia more aggressively and hyperopia less aggressively than recommended with current age-adjusted nomograms results in higher patient satisfaction. The reason is that young eyes generally have a large range of accommodation, and a slight overcorrection is not devastating. Conversely, we tend to treat older patients more aggressively for hyperopia and less aggressively for myopia, the reasons being that older hyperopic eyes need a full correction to see at distance, and surgical regression. On the other hand, older myopic eyes that are overcorrected would be blurred at both distance and near. Further, a slight undercorrection for the older myope can provide functional near vision for many near tasks.

Monovision

In addition to appropriate age adjustments, presbyopic patients may also benefit with monovision.

There are many factors affecting whether or not monovision is appropriate for a particular patient, including his or her occupational and recreation needs and perhaps most importantly, motivation. If they have never experienced monovision, fitting patients with disposable contact lenses to simulate monovision is very helpful in guiding them in their decision for or against monovision.[5,6]

Anatomical Factors in Customization

Anatomical factors require the consideration of individual structural variation of each eye, including the patient's pupil size in bright and dim light conditions,[7-12] the corneal diameter, and thickness prior to surgery.

> Anatomic factors such as the patient's pupil size, corneal diamter, and thickness are important considerations prior to surgery.

LASIK Flap Considerations

LASIK flaps are often customized depending on ablation design,[13-15] thickness,[13] diameter,[14] and whether one is treating myopia, hyperopia, or astigmatism. One of the authors (MacRae) prefers a flap size of 0.5 to 1.0 mm larger than the diameter of the ablation. Studies done on flap thickness and diameter indicate there is considerable variation in flap thickness, as well as diameter, with commonly used microkeratomes.[16-20] For instance, patients with thin corneas with high refractive error require special consideration. These eyes may require the surgeon to use a thinner flap (160 as opposed to 180 microns) and may require reducing the ablation optical zone based on the patient's scotoptic pupil size, age, and functional needs. Intraoperative pachymetry may also be more accurate in defining the amount of residual bed after the flap is created with the microkeratome (personal observation, Scott MacRae). One study evaluated the Chiron 160-micron microkeratome fixed plate and found that the mean corneal cap thickness measured 124.8 ± 18.5 microns, indicating the corneal flaps were thinner than predicted by the manufacturer's plate depth measurements.[17] Another study showed progressive thinning/thickening of the flap in the direction toward the hinge, as well as variation in flap diameter depending on the microkeratome used.[18]

Ablation Diameter Considerations

Hyperopic eyes require larger diameter ablations (8.5 to 10 mm) compared to myopic eyes (8.5 to 9.5 mm).[15-19] Individuals with higher astigmatism (> 1.50 diopters [D]) require larger flaps if they are to have round effective optical zones with minimal aberrations. Ablation optical zones that encompass the entire pupil under scotopic conditions are preferable to ablation optical zones that do not encompass the pupil under all physiological pupil diameters.[8-12,20] Larger astigmatic errors require larger transition zones to ensure a smooth transition and avoid regression.[21] Individuals with large amounts of myopic or mixed astigmatism may also benefit from cross cylinder ablation that reduces by 50% the amount of cylinder to be corrected in each meridian. This is because one can reduce tissue removal by 20% to 30%, minimize coupling effects, and perhaps improve the optics of the ablation.[22] In short, one should consider the ablation design before determining the optimal flap design.

Corneal Thickness Considerations

In corneas that are too thin to safely leave at least a 250-micron bed after LASIK, some surgeons recommend photorefractive keratectomy (PRK), the use of a phakic intraocular lens, or a combination of refractive surgery and intraocular lens (IOL) (bioptics) procedure.

We anticipate that the ocular anatomy (eg, posterior cornea shape, anterior chamber depth, the anterior and posterior lens shape, and thickness) will be interactive and a relevant factor in determining which optical designs are optimal for each patient. For instance, an 18 D myope may be a better candidate for a bioptics procedure, which combines a posterior chamber phakic IOL with LASIK, rather than having LASIK.[23,24]

Corneal Topography-Guided Ablation

Corneal first surface aberrations and/or shape can be calculated from corneal elevation data derived from corneal topography measurements[12,25-35] and used along with a standard refraction to design ablative corrections. Using such an approach should reduce aberrations in highly aberrated corneas but may be detrimental (induce more aberrations) in normal eyes. That is, the potential for visual enhancement beyond the 20/20 level is unknown because formulating the ideal shape for the cornea is not dependent on corneal first surface aberrations alone. Instead, an optimal compensating optic (one that reduces the aberrations in normal eyes [see Chapter Twenty]) must be designed to negate the aberrations of the whole eye. Corneal topography-guided ablation has the greatest potential in patients with visual loss known to be related to large corneal topographic abnormalities.

Corneal topography-guided ablation has been attempted on patients with regular and irregular astigmatism, decentered ablations, and central islands.[36-38] The results have been encouraging with regular astigmatism and decentered ablations but require refinement with irregular astigmatism.[38] The irregular astigmatism group is more challenging but may ultimately benefit most from corneal topography-guided ablation as the systems become more refined.

In a large study on quality of life,[39] it was noted that the second strongest indicator (after visual acuity) of improved quality of life after penetrating keratoplasty was the amount of postoperative astigmatism. Many patients after corneal transplantation complain of not being able to see despite 20/25 to 20/40 vision with spectacle correction. On closer scrutiny, many of these patients are found to have irregular astigmatism that produces poor vision. These groups of patients could benefit greatly if we could predictably treat those who have large amounts of corneal surface irregularity with post-trauma or surgical astigmatism. As one of the remaining frontiers in corneal surgery, correcting very irregular corneal surfaces is explored in detail in the chapters on topography-guided ablation in Section III of this book.

It is important to stress that corneal topography-guided ablations will probably be helpful in individuals with topographic abnormalities but have yet to demonstrate their usefulness in patients with relatively normal corneas with regular astigmatism. Most experienced refractive surgeons use corneal topography to confirm that the astigmatism is regular and that there is reasonable consistency between the refraction astigmatism and that noted on corneal topography, but their astigmatic treatment is based on the refraction and not the corneal topography. The refraction accounts for the entire optics of the eye, not just the cornea. Algorithms that utilize both refraction and corneal topography are worthy of further exploration.

Wavefront-Guided Corneal Ablation

Wavefront-guided corneal ablation is designed to correct the traditional sphere and cylindrical error of the eye and reduce the eye's higher-order optical aberration. Ablative corrections that reduce the optical aberrations of the eye will increase retinal image resolution (eg, acuity) and contrast, which in turn should allow one to see the world with finer detail and higher contrast (see Chapters Two, Three, Six, and Seven). When perfected, such corrections could well lead to providing our patients with better than normal vision and an era in which the expected outcome is evolving toward "supervision."

Measurement of the ocular aberrations can be accomplished in several ways, including using an objective aberroscope,[40] a Shack-Hartmann (Hartmann-Shack) wavefront sensor,[41] a Tscherning wavefront sensor,[42] a spatially resolved refractometer,[43] or one of many other new approaches beginning to appear on the market. These techniques measure all the eye's wavefront aberrations, including prism (first order), sphere and cylindrical (second order), asymmetric or coma-like (third, fifth, …order), and symmetric or spherical-like aberrations (fourth, sixth, … order). While all the systems utilize ray tracing in one form or another, each system has a unique way of measuring the displacement of a ray of light from its ideal position, which in turn defines the slope of the wavefront and then, by integration, the actual wavefront. The difference between the actual wavefront and an ideal wavefront defines the aberrations of the eye. In turn, the aberrations of the eye define the form of an ideal or customized laser treatment. Such technology is already improving refractive surgery outcomes.[42]

Laboratory studies by Liang and Williams[41,44] using wavefront sensing and adaptive optics on humans indicate that polychromatic vision may improve twofold, especially in low light conditions

---

Ablative corrections that reduce the optical aberrations of the eye will increase retinal image resolution (eg, acuity) and contrast, which in turn should allow one to see the world with finer detail and higher contrast.

While all the systems utilize ray tracing in one form or another, each system has a unique way of measuring the displacement of a ray of light from its ideal position.

Wavefront-guided ablations may allow us to treat all of the eye's aberrations, including sphere, cylinder, and higher-order aberrations.

when the pupil is more dilated. Such an improvement would aid a wavefront-enhanced normal driver on a wet, rainy night in seeing a cyclist at a much greater distance and with more confidence. In real world terms, objects would have sharper borders and higher contrast (see Chapter Seven).

Quantifying the optical aberrations of the eye will not only allow us to design corrections for subtle aberrations but also look into the eye to see retinal detail in vivo with unprecedented resolution and contrast (see Chapter Four). One can measure the optical aberrations of the eye with a wavefront sensor and correct for the wavefront error with a technique called adaptive optics, typically a deformable mirror. Such a combination has been built and can be thought of as an adaptive optic ophthalmoscope. The adaptive optic ophthalmoscope has already resulted in our ability to observe live human photoreceptors as small as 2 to 3 microns in diameter and human capillaries as small as 6 microns in diameter. This technology has allowed investigators to further characterize the three types of photoreceptors—S, M, and L—in living subjects.[44] As technology matures and becomes clinically viable, such devices will help us to detect subtle abnormalities of the retina, better understand their pathophysiology, and allow for earlier intervention and monitoring of therapeutic interventions (see Chapter Four).

SURGEON-GUIDED CUSTOMIZED ABLATION

Surgeon-guided ablation utilizes conventional treatments in unconventional ways. One can attempt to improve vision in patients with a variety of problems (eg, central islands, decentered ablations, or small optical zones) using modifications of conventional techniques.

These techniques are not recommended for the beginning or intermediate surgeon and are often deferred even by the most experienced surgeons. Nonetheless, challenging problems in well-selected cases can be helped without wavefront sensing technology. Wavefront sensing and the ability to locally customize with flying small spot technology over small areas of the cornea may revolutionize treatment of difficult problems. We will explore these topics in more detail in Section IV.

SUMMARY

As we review the many new and evolving techniques for treating our patients with customized ablation, it is obvious that there is a rapid evolution of technology and thought. Newly refined diagnostic technology, such as wavefront sensing, and more sophisticated spot laser delivery systems with eye tracking give the refractive surgical team much greater flexibility to tackle the often challenging optical abnormalities we encounter. The next decade in refractive surgery has the promise of providing tremendous gains in visual function by increasing retinal image contrast and to a more limited extent resolution. In this book we explore the concepts and methods on which the promise of improved unaided vision is based. This next decade promises even more remarkable gains in the quest for supervision!

REFERENCES

1. *Webster's Ninth New Collegiate Dictionary.* Springfield, Mass: Merriam Webster, Inc, Publishers; 1983:318.

2. Seiler T, Wollensak J. Myopic photorefractive keratectomy with the excimer laser: one-year follow-up. *Ophthalmology.* 1991;98:1156-1163.

3. Tengroth B, Epstein D, Fagerholm P, et al. Excimer laser photorefractive keratectomy for myopia: clinical results in sighted eye. *Ophthalmology.* 1993;100:739-745.

4. Chatterjee A, Shah S, Doyle SJ. Effect of age on final refractive outcome for 2342 patients following photorefractive keratectomy. *Invest Ophthalmol Vis Sci.* 1996;37(Suppl):S57.

5. DePaolis M, Aquavella J. Refractive surgery update: how to respond to common questions. *Contact Lens Spectrum.* 1993;8(12):48.

6. Aquavella J, Shovlin J, Pascucci S, DePaolis M. How contact lenses fit into refractive surgery. *Review of Ophthalmology.* 1994;1(12):36.

7. Applegate RA, Gansel KA. The importance of pupil size in optical quality measurements following radial keratotomy. *J Corneal Refract Surg.* 1990;6:47-54.

8. Maloney RK. Corneal topography and optical zone location in PRK. *J Corneal Refract Surg.* 1990;6:363-371.

9. Applegate RA. Acuities through annular and central pupils following radial keratotomy. *Optom Vis Sci.* 1991;68:584-590.

10. Roberts CW, Koester CJ. Optical zone diameters for

photorefractive corneal surgery. *Invest Ophthalmol Vis Sci.* 1993;34:2275-2281.

11. Diamond S. Excimer laser photorefractive keratectomy (PRK) for myopia present status: aerospace considerations. *Aviation Space Environmental Medicine.* 1995;66:690-693.

12. Martínez CE, Applegate RA, Klyce SD, McDonald MB, Medina JP, Howland HC. Effect of pupil dilation on corneal optical aberrations after photorefractive keratectomy. *Arch Ophthalmol.* 1998;116:1053-1062.

13. Machat JJ, Slade SG, Probst LE, eds. *The Art of LASIK.* 2nd ed. Thorofare, NJ: SLACK Incorporated; 1998:50-53.

14. Gimbel HV, Anderson Penno EE. *LASIK Complications.* Thorofare, NJ: SLACK Incorporated; 1998:60-61.

15. MacRae SM. Excimer ablation design and elliptical transition zones. *J Cataract Refract Surg.* 1999;25:1191-1197.

16. Sutton HF, Reinstein DZ, Holland S, et al. Anatomy of the flap in LASIK by very high frequency ultrasound scanning. *Invest Ophthalmol Vis Sci.* 1998;39 (Suppl):S244.

17. Maldonado MJ, Ruiz-Oblitas L, Mununera JM, Aliseda D, Garcia-Layana A, Moreno-Montanes J. Optical coherence tomography evaluation of the corneal cap and stromal bed features after laser in situ keratomileusis for high myopia and astigmatism. *Ophthalmology.* 2000;107(1):81-7.

18. Behrens A, Langenbucher A, Kus MM, Rummelt C, Seitz B. Experimental evaluation of two current-generation automated microkeratomes: the Hansatome and the Supratome. *Am J Ophthalmol.* 2000;129(1):59-67.

19. Dierick HG, Missotten L. Corneal ablation profiles for correction of hyperopia with the excimer laser. *J Refract Surg.* 1996;12:767-773.

20. Machat JJ. *Excimer Laser Refractive Surgery: Practice and Principles.* Thorofare, NJ: SLACK Incorporated; 1996:248-249.

21. Vinceguerra P. Special issue. *J Refract Surg.* 1999.

22. Chayet A. Special issue. *J Refract Surg.* 1998.

23. Zaldivar R, Davidorf JM, Oscherow S, Ricur G, Piezzi V. Combined posterior chamber phakic intraocular lens and laser in situ keratomileusis: bioptics for extreme myopia. *J Refract Surg.* 1999;15(3):299-308.

24. Moser C, Kampmeier J, McDonnell P, Psaltis D. Feasibility of intraoperative corneal topography monitoring during photorefractive keratectomy. *J Refract Surg.* 2000;16:148-154.

25. Hemenger P, Tomlinson A, Caroline PJ. Role of spherical aberration in contrast sensitivity loss with radial keratomtomy. *Invest Ophthalmol Vis Sci.* 1989;30:1997-2001.

26. Howland HC, Glasser A, Applegate RA. Polynomial approximations of corneal surfaces and corneal curvature topography. Noninvasive assessment of the visual system. *Technical Digest, Optical Society of America.* 1992;3:34-37.

27. Applegate RA, Howland HC, Buettner J, Yee RW, Cottingham Jr AJ, Sharp RP. Corneal aberrations before and after radial keratotomy (RK) calculated from videokeratometric measurements. Vision science and its applications. *Technical Digest, Optical Society of America.* 1994;2:58-61.

28. Howland HC, Buettner J, Applegate RA. Computation of the shapes of normal corneas and their monochromatic aberrations from videokeratometric measurements. Vision science and its applications. *Technical Digest, Optical Society of America.* 1994;2:54-57.

29. Hemenger P, Tomlinson A, Oliver K. Corneal optics form videokeratographs. *Ophthalmic and Physiological Optics.* 1995;1:63-68.

30. Applegate RA, Howland HC, Hilmantel G. Corneal aberrations increase with the magnitude of the RK refractive correction. *Optom Vis Sci.* 1996;73:585-589.

31. Applegate RA, Howland HC. Refractive surgery, optical aberrations, and visual performance. *J Refract Surg.* 1997;13:295-299.

32. Applegate RA, Howland HC, Sharp RP, Cottingham AJ, Yee RW. Corneal aberrations, visual performance and refractive keratectomy. *J Refract Surg.* 1998;14:397-407.

33. Oshika T, Klyce SD, Applegate RA, Howland HC, El Danasoury MA. Comparison of corneal wavefront aberrations after photorefractive keratectomy and laser in situ keratomileusis. *Am J Ophthalmol.* 1999;127:1-7.

34. Oshika T, Klyce SD, Applegate RA, Howland HC. Changes in corneal wavefront aberrations with aging. *Invest Ophthalmol Vis Sci.* 1999;40:1351-1355.

35. Applegate RA, Hilmantel G, Howland HC, Tu EY, Starck T, Zayac EJ. Corneal first surface optical aberrations and visual performance. *J Refract Surg.* In press.

36. Lafond G, Solomon L. Retreatment of central islands after photorefractive keratectomy. *J Cataract Refract Surg.* 1999;25:188-196.

37. Manche EE, Maloney RK, Smith RJ. Treatment of topographic central islands following refractive surgery. *J Cataract Refract Surg.* 1998;24:464-470.

38. Buzard KA, Fundingsland BR. Treatment of irregular astigmatism with a broad beam excimer laser. *J Refract Surg.* 1997;13:624-636.

39. Musch DC, Farjo AA, Meyer RF, et al. Assessment of health-related quality of life after corneal transplantation. *Am J Ophthalmol.* 1997;124:1-8.

40. Howland HC, Howland B. A subjective method for the measurement of monochromatic aberrations of the eye. *J Opt Soc Am.* 1977;67:1508-1518.

41. Liang J, Williams DR. Aberrations and retinal image quality of the normal human eye. *J Opt Soc Am A.* 1997;14(11):2873-2883.

42. Mrochen M, Kaemmerer M, Seiler T. Wavefront-guided laser in situ keratomileusis: early results in three eyes. *J Refract Surg.* 2000;16:116-121.

43. Webb, RH, Penney CM, Thompson KP. Measurement of ocular wavefront distortion with a spatially resolved refractometer. *Applied Optics.* 1992;31:3678-3686.

44. Liang J, Williams DR, Miller D. Supernormal vision and high-resolution retinal imaging through adaptive optics. *J Opt Soc Am A.* 1997;14(11):2884-2892.

45. Roorda A, Williams DR. Objective identification of M and L cones in the living human eye. *Invest Ophthalmol Vis Sci.* 1998;39(4):957.

46. Buzard KA, Fundingsland BR. Treatment of irregular astigmatism with a broad beam excimer laser. *J Refract Surg.* 1997;13:624-636.

47. Liang J, Williams DR. Aberrations and retinal image quality of the normal human eye. *J Opt Soc Am A.* 1997;14(11):2873-2883.

48. Mrochen M, Kaemmerer M, Seiler T. Wavefront-guided laser in situ keratomileusis: early results in three eyes. *J Refract Surg.* 2000;16:116-121.

Chapter Two

How Far Can We Extend the Limits of Human Vision?

David R. Williams, PhD
Geun-Young Yoon, PhD
Antonio Guirao, PhD
Heidi Hofer, BS
Jason Porter, MS

INTRODUCTION

Methods to correct the optics of the human eye are at least 700 years old. Spectacles have been used to correct defocus at least as early as the 13th century[1,2] and to correct astigmatism since the 19th century.[3] Though it is well established that the eye suffers from many more monochromatic aberrations than defocus and astigmatism—we will refer to these aberrations as *higher-order aberrations*—there has been relatively little work on correcting them until recently. In 1962, Smirnov, an early pioneer in the

> In 1962, Smirnov, an early pioneer in the characterization of the eye's higher-order aberrations, suggested that it would be possible with customized lenses to compensate for aberrations in individual eyes.

characterization of the eye's higher-order aberrations, suggested that it would be possible with customized lenses to compensate for aberrations in individual eyes. Recent developments increase the probability that Smirnov's suggestion may soon be realized. More rapid and accurate instruments for measuring the ocular aberrations are available, most notably the Hartmann-Shack wavefront sensor, first applied to the eye by Liang, et al.[4] Moreover, there are new techniques to correct higher-order aberrations. Liang, et al[5] showed that a deformable mirror

in an adaptive optics system can correct the eye's higher-order aberrations. This study was the first to demonstrate that the correction of higher-order aberrations can lead to supernormal visual performance in normal eyes. Presently, the visual benefits of adaptive optics can only be obtained in the laboratory, but the success of the technique encourages the implementation of higher-order correction in everyday vision through customized contact lenses, intraocular lenses (IOLs), or laser refractive surgery. Lathing and laser ablative technologies now exist that can create arbitrary surfaces on contact lenses, offering the possibility of truly customized contact lenses. There is a major ongoing effort to refine laser refractive surgery to correct other defects besides conventional refractive errors.[6]

Ultimately, the visual benefit of attempts to correct higher-order aberrations depends on two things. First, it depends on the relative importance of these aberrations in limiting human vision and, second, it depends on the finesse with which these aberrations can be corrected in everyday vision. The emphasis of this chapter is on the first of these issues: How large are the visual benefits that will accrue from correcting higher-order aberrations, and under what conditions will they be realized? We review what is known about the fundamental limits on visual acuity and

> There are optical, cone mosaic, and neural factors that limit the finest detail we can see.

provide theoretical and empirical evidence concerning the visual significance of higher-order aberrations. There are optical, cone mosaic, and neural factors that limit the finest detail we can see, and an understanding of all three is required to appreciate how much vision can be improved by correcting higher-order aberrations in addition to defocus and astigmatism. For example, as we will see later, improving the eye's optics is not always a good thing. Due to the nature of the limits on visual resolution set by the cone mosaic, improving the optical quality of the eye too much can actually lead to a decline in visual performance on some tasks. Before tackling this apparent paradox, however, we need to review some fundamental aspects of the optical quality of the retinal image.

OPTICAL LIMITS ON VISION

An understanding of the limits that the eye's optics place on vision requires a succinct description of the optical quality of the eye, independent of neural factors. In this chapter, we will use the modulation transfer function (MTF) to characterize the ability of the eye's optics to create a sharp image on the retina. The curves of Figure 2-1 show the MTFs for eyes at two pupil sizes—3 and 7.3 mm. These curves reveal how faithfully the eye's optics can form an image of sine waves of different spatial frequency. Sine waves describe the variation in intensity across simple patterns of light and dark bars used as visual stimuli. The x-axis of the MTF represents sine waves with spatial frequency varying from low, corresponding to a large angular spacing between adjacent white bars, to high spatial frequency (ie, fine gratings). Though not as familiar to the clinician as Snellen letters, sine wave gratings produce a response not only from the optics, but also from the photoreceptor mosaic and the neural visual system, which provide a much richer characterization of how well each stage in the visual system performs. Sine waves can be added together to create any visual scene at which the eye might care to look. The crucial implication of this fact is that if you know how well the eye images sine waves of different spatial frequency, it is possible to predict the retinal image for any visual scene. Intuitively, the eye's MTF at low

> If you know how well the eye images sine waves of different spatial frequency, it is possible to predict the retinal image for any visual scene.

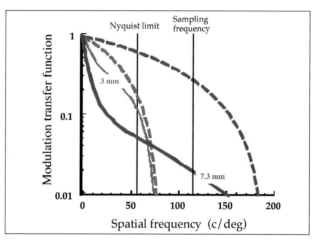

Figure 2-1. Solid curves show MTF of the eye (averaged across 14 subjects) for two pupil sizes (3- and 7.3-mm diameter), with the correction of astigmatism and defocus calculated from wavefront sensor measurements of the eye's wave aberration. Dotted curves show the MTF for the same pupil sizes in hypothetical eyes that are free from aberrations and scatter so that the only source of image blur is diffraction. The wavelength was 670 nm. The vertical line at 57 c/deg corresponds to the Nyquist limit for the average human foveal cone mosaic. The vertical line at 114 c/deg indicates the mosaic sampling frequency.

spatial frequencies reveals how well the eye images large features in visual scenes, whereas the response to high frequencies tells us how well the eye images fine detail, closer to the limits of visual acuity. The y-axis of the MTF is the modulation transferred by the eye's optics and corresponds to the ratio of the contrast of the sine wave image on the retina to that of the original sine wave pattern viewed by the eye. The more blurring by the eye's optics, the more the modulation transfer departs from one and approaches zero.

There are three sources of image blur in the human eye: diffraction, aberrations, and scatter. We will not discuss scatter here because it is generally a minor source of image blur in young, normal eyes. Diffraction at the eye's pupil is an important source of image blur when the pupil is small, becoming less important with increasing pupil size. The dashed lines in Figure 2-1 show the MTF of eyes that suffer only from diffraction and are free of aberrations. The MTF extends to much higher spatial frequencies (ie, there is less blur from diffraction) for the 7.3-mm pupil than the 3-mm pupil. The highest spatial frequency that can be imaged on the retina of an aberration-free eye is $\pi p/180\lambda$, where p is the diameter of

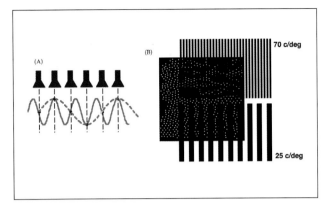

Figure 2-2. A: Two sinusoidal stimuli sampled by an array of cones. The spatial frequency of one stimulus (solid line) is three times the frequency of the other (dashed line). The cone response is identical for the two patterns, illustrating aliasing and the ambiguity introduced by sampling. B: Two square wave patterns are seen through a sampling array resembling the cone mosaic. After sampling, the high-frequency pattern appears as a distorted, low-frequency pattern, though the sampling rate is adequate for the low-frequency pattern. The Nyquist limit in this example is 62 c/deg.

the pupil and λ is the wavelength. Thus, for a 3-mm pupil and a wavelength of 670 nm, the highest spatial frequency is 78 c/deg (190 c/deg for a dilated pupil of 7.3 mm). Blurring by diffraction is unavoidable, quite unlike aberrations, which can be corrected.

The solid curves show the MTFs of normal human eyes for the same 3- and 7.3-mm pupil sizes, including the blurring effects of the eye's higher-order aberrations as well as diffraction. We have not included blur due to defocus and astigmatism, which conventional spectacles can correct. At low spatial frequencies, the 7.3-mm curve lies below the 3-mm curve because the blurring from aberrations increases strongly with increasing pupil diameter. The central area in the dilated pupil typically has better optical performance than the pupil margin. The aberration-free MTFs lie above the MTFs that include higher-order aberrations, especially for the larger pupil. These results suggest that a rather large increase in retinal image contrast could be achieved by correcting higher-order aberrations when the pupil is large. However, this analysis overestimates the benefit of correcting higher-order aberrations for at least two reasons. First, it does not take account of the limitations on visual acuity imposed by the photoreceptor mosaic and subsequent neural processing,

a topic we will address next. Second, this analysis is valid only in monochromatic light, whereas vision normally involves broadband, polychromatic light. As we will see later, in addition to suffering from higher-order monochromatic aberrations, the eye suffers from chromatic aberration that also blurs the retinal image in polychromatic illumination.

LIMITS IMPOSED BY THE PHOTORECEPTOR MOSAIC ON VISION

The retinal image is a spatially continuous distribution of light intensity, but the cone mosaic is made of photoreceptors that discretely sample the image. This sampling process results in the loss of information about the retinal image because the brain can never know about the behavior of the retinal image between the sample locations defined by the cone mosaic. The information loss caused by sampling superficially resembles that by optical blurring in that it is high spatial frequencies (ie, fine details in the retinal image) that are affected most. However, the similarity ends there. Optical blurring is a reduction in contrast in the retinal image, whereas sampling does not generally reduce contrast but rather causes errors in the brain's interpretation of the retinal image.

The term used to describe errors due to sampling is *aliasing*. This is because sampling causes high spatial frequencies in the image to masquerade or alias

> The term used to describe errors due to sampling is aliasing.

as low spatial frequencies. Figure 2-2A shows this effect for a one-dimensional array of photoreceptors that is sampling two sinusoidal gratings with different spatial frequencies. Notice that the light intensity is identical at each of the sample locations. The cone mosaic is blind to the fact that the retinal images differ between the sample locations defined by the photoreceptors. Since the photoreceptor mosaic does not retain any information that these two images are in fact different, the brain cannot distinguish them. The brain interprets the pattern as the low frequency alternative whether the low or high spatial frequency is in fact present. Figure 2-2B shows aliasing for an array of sample locations taken from an image of the human cone mosaic. When the fundamental spatial frequency of a grating is low, the mosaic has an ade-

Table 2-1

Spatial Sampling by the Human Foveal Cone Mosaic

SOURCE	DENSITY (CONES/MM²)	SPACING (MICRONS)	SPACING (MIN/ARC)	NYQUIST (C/DEG)
Østerberg (1935)	147×10^3	2.43	0.50	60
Miller (1979)	128×10^3	2.6	0.54	55.9
Yuodelis and Hendrikson (1986)	208×10^3	2.04	0.42	71.4
Curcio, et al (1987)	162×10^3	2.57 ± 0.71	0.53 ± 0.15	56.6
Curcio, et al (1990)	197×10^3	2.55 ± 0.52	0.53 ± 0.11	56.6
Williams (1985)	126×10^3	2.62 ± 0.17	0.54 ± 0.04	55.6
Williams (1988)	129×10^3	2.59 ± 0.12	0.54 ± 0.02	55.6
Average	**157×10^3**	**2.49**	**0.51**	**58.8**

quate number of samples to represent it. However, when the spatial frequency is high, a low frequency pattern emerges. The irregularity of the low frequency alias is a result of the disorder in the cone mosaic.

How can we quantify the limits imposed by the spacing of cones on vision? Helmholtz[3] knew that the finest grating the eye could resolve required at least one sample for each light and each dark bar of the grating. This simple intuition is captured in modern terms by the sampling theorem,[7] which states that the highest frequency that can be recovered without aliasing from a sampling array is one-half the sampling frequency of the array. The sampling frequency of the array is the reciprocal of the spacing between samples, which in this case is the spacing between rows of cones at the fovea. Half the sampling frequency is the so-called Nyquist limit. Anatomical and psychophysical estimates of the spacing between rows of foveal cones indicate an average of about 0.51 minutes of arc, which makes the average sampling rate 118 c/deg and the average Nyquist limit half that, or about 59 c/deg. Table 2-1 compares the results of several studies. The conversion between columns in Table 2-1 has been made assuming triangular packing of cones.[8] The Nyquist limit indicates the finest grating patterns that human foveal vision can reasonably expect to resolve in the sense of being able to see the regular stripes of the grating imaged on the retina. Indeed estimates of the foveal visual acuity for gratings generally agree with the Nyquist limit. In some circumstances, subjects can obtain correct information about, for example, the orientation of a grating at spatial frequencies slightly above the Nyquist limit,[9] but the perception of a distinct grating pattern ends at spatial frequencies very near the Nyquist limit.

At spatial frequencies above the Nyquist limit, gratings appear more like wavy zebra stripes and appear coarser than the actual gratings on the retina, as shown in Figure 2-3. Williams[8,10] studied these perceptual effects with a laser interferometer, extending earlier reports by Bergmann,[11] Byram,[12] and Campbell and Green,[13] showing conclusively that they result from aliasing by the cone mosaic. Laser interferometry is a method to image gratings in the form of interference fringes on the retina that are immune to blurring by the eye's optics. Gratings with spatial frequencies over 200 c/deg can be imaged on the retina at essentially unity contrast. In the range between 0 and 45 c/deg, interference fringes can be seen across the central foveal region. As the spatial frequency increases toward 60 c/deg, the bars of the fringe can be seen only in a progressively smaller region of the fovea. At about 60 c/deg, the fine, regular bars are lost, and most subjects report the appearance of an annulus of fine wavy lines (see Figure 2-3). The annulus corresponds to aliasing by cones just outside the foveal center, which are more widely spaced and alias at a lower spatial frequency than in the foveal center. As spatial frequency increases, this annulus collapses to a circular patch at a frequency of 90 to 100 c/deg. Subjects describe this patch as resembling a fingerprint or a pattern of zebra stripes. Between 150 and 160 c/deg, the zebra stripe pattern disappears. Due to the sampling limits imposed by the cone mosaic, no matter

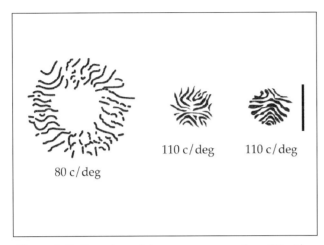

Figure 2-3. Drawing of the appearance of an 80 c/deg and an 110 c/deg (two subjects) interference fringe. Scale bar corresponds to 1 degree of visual angle. The zebra stripe appearance results from aliasing by the cone mosaic.

how much one could improve the eye's optics, one could never expect an increase in visual acuity beyond about 60 c/deg in the average human eye.

Aliasing can potentially distort the appearance of not only grating stimuli but of any visual scene that contains spatial frequencies above the Nyquist limit. For example, sharp edges would be expected to take on a jagged appearance. There are also errors in the color appearance of fine details—referred to as chromatic aliasing—caused by the fact that the retina contains three cone submosaics for color vision, each sampling the visual scene even more coarsely than the combined mosaic.[14] Aliasing errors are not generally visible in everyday viewing conditions, partly because the blurring of the retinal image by the eye's optics plays a protective role. This is illustrated in Figure 2-1, which compares the optical MTF with the foveal cone Nyquist limit. At the Nyquist limit, the retinal image contrast cannot be greater than about 10% for any pupil size, and it is usually far less than this since the contrast in the original scene is usually much less than 100%. For aliasing to disrupt vision in ordinary scenes, the optical quality of the eye would have to be considerably better than it is. An indication that this must be true comes from the observation that aliasing errors are not seen in ordinary vision outside the fovea. At a eccentricity of about 4 degrees, the optical quality of the eye is essentially the same as that at the foveal center, yet the Nyquist limit has declined by a factor of about three. The fact that aliasing is not visible at this eccentricity suggests

that the MTF of the eye could be extended by at least a factor of three at the fovea without running the risk of incurring aliasing errors. This realization runs counter to the prevailing view that evolution has matched the optics of the eye and the spacing of foveal cones. Instead, it appears that the optics could afford to be substantially better in the average eye without introducing an important loss of image fidelity due to foveal aliasing. Even in controlled laboratory conditions, it is difficult to produce aliasing effects without the use of interference fringe stimuli. This is true even in extrafoveal vision, which is less protected from aliasing by the eye's optics. Increasing the optical quality of the eye runs a greater risk of causing aliasing outside the fovea. But even there, unusually high contrast stimuli are required and careful attention must be paid to the eye's refractive state. This is good news for attempts to correct higher-order aberrations in the eye, because it suggests that the deleterious effects of sampling will not interfere with vision and will not reduce the visual benefit of improving retinal image contrast.

NEURAL LIMITS ON VISION

Are the postreceptoral retina and the brain equipped to take advantage of the improved optical quality that customized correction can provide? There would be little point in improving the eye's optics if the brain were incapable of resolving the high spatial frequencies deblurred by a customized correction. Experimentally, this question has been explored by measuring the contrast sensitivity function (CSF) with laser interference fringe stimuli. The CSF is a measure of how sensitive subjects are to gratings of different spatial frequencies. The CSF is determined by finding the threshold contrast at which the subject can detect a sinusoidal grating at each of a number of spatial frequencies. The reciprocal of the threshold is the contrast sensitivity. At high spatial frequencies, the CSF monotonically decreases with spatial frequency, which means that the subject needs higher contrast to detect finer details. This is true even when interference fringes are used to eliminate optical blurring in the eye, as shown in Figure 2-4. This shows that, just as the optics blur the retinal image, the postreceptoral visual system blurs the neural image. The important point is that, despite the neural blur, the nervous system is equipped with the machinery to resolve spatial frequencies as high as

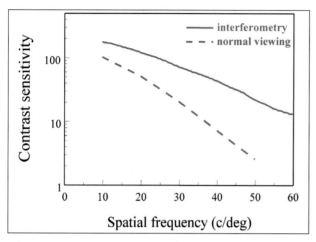

Figure 2-4. CSF measured with interferometry (neural CSF) and CSF for normal viewing conditions for a pupil of 3 mm.[55]

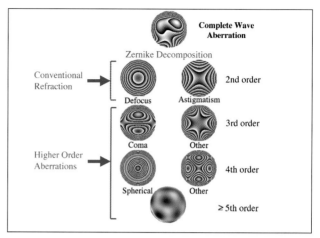

Figure 2-5. Zernike decomposition. An arbitrary wave aberration can be decomposed into individual Zernike modes. The second-order Zernike modes, which are defocus and two astigmatism terms, can be corrected with a conventional refraction. Note: some modes (eg, the two for astigmatism) have been combined for simplicity.

the foveal cone Nyquist limit. This makes it quite likely that it can take advantage of improvements in retinal image contrast for spatial frequencies up to the limits set by the photoreceptor mosaic. Indeed, we will show direct empirical evidence for this later.

VISUAL BENEFIT OF HIGHER-ORDER CORRECTION BASED ON WAVE ABERRATION MEASUREMENTS

This section describes an analysis of the visual benefit of correcting higher-order aberrations based on measurements of the aberrations found in a large population of eyes. Based on subjective observations of a point source of light, Helmholtz argued that the eye suffered from a host of aberrations that are not found in conventional, manmade optical systems.[15] There have been a number of methods developed to quantify these aberrations.[16-22] Recently, Liang, et al[4] developed a technique based on the Hartmann-Shack principle[23] that provides a rapid, automated, and objective measure of the wave aberration simultaneously at a large number of sample points across

> Helmholtz argued that the eye suffered from a host of aberrations that are not found in conventional, manmade optical systems.[15]

the eye's pupil. Using this technique, Liang and Williams[24] provided what is arguably the most complete description to date of the wave aberration of the eye. They measured the eye's aberrations up to 10 radial orders, quantifying the irregular aberrations predicted by Helmholtz and subsequent investigators.[17,18,25]

The wave aberration can be described as the sum of a number of component aberrations such as defocus, astigmatism, coma, spherical aberration, as well as other higher-order aberrations. The wave aberration can be decomposed into these constituent aberrations in much the same way that Fourier analysis can decompose an image into spatial frequency components. For an optical system such as the eye, it is convenient to use Zernike polynomials as the basic functions because of their desirable mathematical properties for circular pupils. Figure 2-5 shows the wave aberration for a typical eye and its decomposition into its constituent Zernike modes. Each mode has a value that indicates its magnitude, usually expressed in microns, corresponding to its root mean square or standard deviation across the pupil (see Appendix Two).

Defocus is one of the simplest Zernike modes. Clinicians are familiar with defocus expressed in diopters, which corresponds to the reciprocal of the focal length in meters. In an eye that suffers from defocus alone, the relationship between diopters and the root mean square wavefront error is

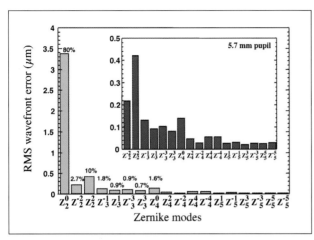

Figure 2-6. Mean absolute RMS values for 18 Zernike modes as measured from a population of 109 normal human subjects for a 5.7-mm pupil. The inset excludes the first Zernike mode corresponding to defocus (Z_2^0) and has an expanded ordinate to illustrate the magnitudes of the higher-order aberrations. Percentages labeled above the first eight modes designate the percent of the variance accounted for by each mode.

$$\text{Diopter (D)} = \frac{-4\sqrt{3}\ Z_2^0}{(\text{pupil radius})^2}$$

where Z_2^0 is the magnitude of Zernike defocus mode in microns and the pupil radius is in millimeters.

From the wave aberration, we can easily calculate the eye's modulation (and phase) transfer functions, which provide a complete description of retinal image quality. The modulation and phase transfer functions can be obtained from the complex autocorrelation of the pupil function, where the pupil function includes the pupil aperture and the wave aberration.[7] Alternatively, the point spread function (PSF) captures the same information as the modulation and phase transfer functions. The PSF is the Fourier transform of the modulation and phase transfer functions. Intuitively, it is the image on the retina of a single point of light. We can calculate any retinal image by the convolution of the object with the PSF.

The beauty of this is that we can compute from the aberrations, which are defined in the eye's pupil, the impact they will have on the quality of the image formed on the retina. Both diffraction and aberrations are taken into account and it is only light scatter that is ignored, as it is usually small in young, normal eyes. This computational link between pupil and retina is very valuable because we can use it to deduce the relative importance of different aberra-

tions on image quality. This is critical for deciding which aberrations are worth correcting and which are not.

An important feature of the eye's wave aberration is that it is a single function that captures all the optical defects in both the cornea and the lens. The final retinal image quality depends on the combined effects of the cornea and the lens rather than on the optical quality of each isolated component. For example, in young eyes, the spherical aberration introduced by the cornea is usually reduced by the lens.[26] Other corneal aberrations may also be compensated by the lens[27,28] in younger subjects. These results have important implications for customized correction because they emphasize the necessity to capture the total wave aberration. For example, if the ablation profile in customized laser refractive surgery is computed solely from corneal topography, the final aberrations of the eye could be larger in some eyes than before ablation.

Population Statistics of the Wave Aberration

A conventional refraction (sphere, cylinder, and axis) typically corrects for only three components of the wave aberration (one defocus and two astigmatic modes), while wave aberrations have been meas-

> A conventional refraction (sphere, cylinder, and axis) typically corrects for only three components of the wave aberration (one defocus and two astigmatic modes).

ured, even in normal eyes, that incorporate as many as 65 individual Zernike modes. The average magnitudes of the lowest 18 monochromatic aberrations are presented in Figure 2-6 for 109 normal subjects between the ages of 21 and 65 years (mean age of 41 years) with natural accommodation. Each adult had a spherical refraction between 6.00 D and -12.00 D and a refractive astigmatism no larger than -3.00 D, and no pathological patients were included in this study.[29] In general, there is a tendency for the magnitude of the aberrations to decrease with increasing order. The aberration with the largest magnitude is defocus, Z_2^0, followed by the two Zernike modes representing astigmatism, Z_2^{-2} and Z_2^2. Defocus is expected to be the largest aberration, but it is especially large in this population because the majority of the subjects were patients at a local clinic and tended to be myopic. Higher-order aberrations in this figure

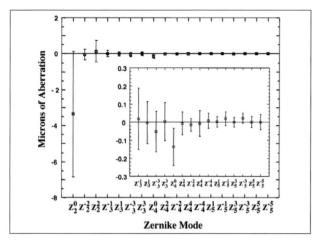

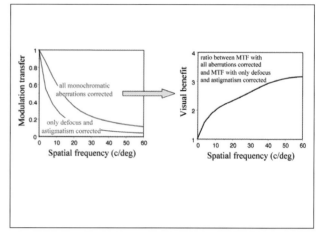

Figure 2-7. Mean values of the first 18 Zernike modes in the population of 109 human subjects for a 5.7-mm pupil. The error bars indicate plus and minus one standard deviation. The inset excludes the first three Zernike modes corresponding to defocus and astigmatism (Z_2^0, Z_2^{-2}, and Z_2^2) and has an expanded ordinate to illustrate the variability of the higher-order aberrations.

Figure 2-8. The visual benefit is obtained as the ratio between the MTF in white light with no monochromatic aberrations and the eye's MTF in white light with only astigmatism and defocus corrected. The MTF in white light was calculated from the polychromatic PSF determined by integrating the monochromatic PSF affected by the eye's chromatic aberration across the spectrum and weighted with the ocular spectral sensitivity. The baseline MTF corresponding to a conventional correction was calculated by finding the amount of defocus and astigmatism required to maximize the volume of the CSF obtained as the product of the MTF and the neural contrast sensitivity function.

correspond to all those beyond the first three. The 15 higher-order aberrations shown here in aggregate account for about two-thirds as much of the variance of the wave aberration as the two modes associated with astigmatism.

In addition to examining the magnitude of each mode, we can also look at the distribution of each Zernike coefficient in the same population. These results, displayed in Figure 2-7, show that each Zernike coefficient, with the exception of spherical aberration, has a mean value that is approximately zero. The mean value for spherical aberration in this population was -0.138 ± 0.103 μm.

Population Statistics of the Visual Benefit of Higher-Order Correction

The distribution and magnitude of monochromatic aberrations in the population of human eyes shown above does not inform us directly about the visual improvement from correcting higher-order aberrations. For this purpose, we define a quantity we call the *visual benefit*. It is the increase in retinal image contrast at each spatial frequency that would occur if one were to correct all the eye's monochromatic aberrations instead of just correcting defocus and astigmatism as one does with a conventional refraction. More specifically, the visual benefit is the ratio of the eye's polychromatic MTF when all the monochromatic aberrations are corrected to that

when only defocus and astigmatism are corrected, as shown in Figure 2-8.

Because customized correction with contact lenses, IOLs, and laser refractive surgery would involve everyday viewing conditions in which the spectra of objects are broadband or polychromatic, we chose to calculate the visual benefit for white light instead of monochromatic light of a single wavelength. The eye suffers from chromatic aberration of two kinds, axial and transverse. The axial chromatic aberration is the chromatic difference of focus on the optical axis of the eye. Short wavelength light is brought to a focus nearer to the cornea and lens than the long wavelength light so that only one wavelength in a broadband stimulus can be in focus on the retina at any one time. Wald and Griffin[30] and many other researchers have measured the axial chromatic aberration of the eye. There is almost no variation from observer to observer because all eyes are made of essentially the same materials with the same chromatic dispersion. The total chromatic difference of focus is approximately 2 D over the entire visual range. We have included axial chromatic aberration in the calculation because, as we will see later, it can

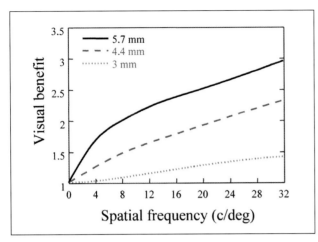

Figure 2-9. Visual benefit at each spatial frequency for three pupil diameters averaged across a normal population of 109 subjects.

have large effects on retinal image quality when one is trying to eliminate all monochromatic aberrations in the eye.

The transverse chromatic aberration (TCA) is the wavelength-dependent displacement of the image position on the retina. The image of a point lies closer to the achromatic axis in short wavelength light than it does in long wavelength light. The amount of TCA at the fovea is relatively small since the natural pupil is usually well aligned with respect to the achromatic axis. In our experience, foveal TCA does not typically reduce retinal image quality much, and we have ignored it in the following calculations.

The white light MTF was computed by summing the monochromatic MTF defocused by axial chromatic aberration and weighted by the spectral sensitivity of the eye at each wavelength. A visual benefit of one corresponds to no benefit of correcting higher-order aberrations. A value of two would indicate a two-fold increase in retinal image contrast provided by correcting higher-order aberrations in addition to defocus and astigmatism. Though the visual benefit is calculated from retinal image quality, the visual benefit is directly applicable to visual performance as assessed with contrast sensitivity measurements. That is, a visual benefit of two will lead to a two-fold increase in contrast sensitivity as well as a two-fold increase in retinal image contrast.

Figure 2-9 shows the mean values of the visual benefit across a population of 109 normal subjects for three different pupil sizes as a function of the spatial frequency. For a pupil of 3 mm, the visual benefit is modest. For small pupils, diffraction dominates and

aberrations beyond defocus and astigmatism are relatively unimportant. A small visual improvement might be realized for the 3-mm pupil at high spatial frequencies (about 1.5 at 32 c/deg). In bright daylight conditions, the natural pupil of most normal eyes is sufficiently small (~3 mm) that the retinal image would not be greatly affected by aberrations. However, for mid and large pupils, because of the well-known fact that the aberrations grow with increasing pupil size,[24,31] an important visual benefit can be obtained across all spatial frequencies by correcting the monochromatic higher-order aberrations. For example, with a 5.7-mm pupil, the average visual benefit across the population is about 2.5 at 16 c/deg and about 3 at 32 c/deg. This would correspond to a distinct improvement in the sharpness of the retinal image. Thus, for the normal population the visual benefit of a customized ablation would be largest in younger patients in which the pupil is large and in situations such as night driving.

What fraction of the population could benefit by correcting the higher-order aberrations? Just as there is large variability in the population as to the amount of astigmatism present, so there is variability in the amount of higher-order aberrations. Some people will derive much more visual benefit from higher-order correction than others. The frequency histograms in Figure 2-10 show how much the visual

> Some people will derive much more visual benefit from higher-order correction than others.

benefit for a 5.7-mm pupil varies among eyes in the normal population of 109 normal subjects and in a small population of four keratoconic patients. The distributions of visual benefit at spatial frequencies of 16 c/deg and 32 c/deg are shown because they correspond roughly to the highest frequencies that are detectable by normal subjects viewing natural scenes. Some normal eyes have a visual benefit close to one (ie, show almost no benefit of correcting higher-order aberrations). At the other extreme, some normal eyes show a benefit of more than a factor of five.

To provide a better indication of the typical visual benefits that subjects would incur with customized correction, Figure 2-11 shows the effect on the retinal image in white light of correcting higher-order aberrations for four subjects over a 5.7-mm pupil. In each case, the PSF computed from the wave aberration is convolved with a letter E subtending 30 minutes of arc, roughly corresponding to the 20/100 line on the Snellen chart. The letters are substantially more blurred than that in the diffraction-limited case. We emphasize that these are the retinal images expected from these eyes and do not represent the perceptual experience these subjects would have of the retinal images.

The visual benefit in keratoconic patients is much larger. One of the subjects of the sample, who is in the early stages of keratoconus, presents a visual benefit similar to the normal population. But the other three show larger benefits than any subject does in the normal population (one of them as high as a factor of 25). Figure 2-12 shows the average visual benefit in the sample of four keratoconics for the three pupil sizes. These patients can expect a large benefit at all pupil sizes. Clearly, the development of technologies to correct the idiosyncratic higher-order aberrations of such patients would be an especially valuable outcome of wavefront sensing. The wavefront sensor coupled with calculations such as these can efficiently screen those patients who stand to gain the largest benefit from customized correction.

THE VISUAL BENEFIT OF HIGHER-ORDER CORRECTION MEASURED WITH ADAPTIVE OPTICS

The analysis so far has been based on calculation and theory. It would be greatly reassuring if a reliable, noninvasive method existed that allowed higher-order aberrations to be quickly corrected in normal eyes so that the actual visual benefit could be assessed. Fortunately, adaptive optics provide just such a method. Figure 2-13 shows a simplified drawing of an adaptive optics system for the eye that is in use in our lab at the University of Rochester.[24] The complete system requires a wavefront sensor to measure the wave aberration of the eye and a wavefront corrector to compensate for the aberrations. The correcting element in our system is a deformable mirror with 37 actuators mounted behind it that can reshape the mirror in such a way as to correct most of the particular aberrations found in each patient's eye. In addition to the wavefront sensor and corrector, the adaptive optics system has an optical path that allows the subject to view visual stimuli, such as sine wave gratings or Snellen letters, through the deformable mirror. Subjects viewing the world through adaptive optics can have a sharper image

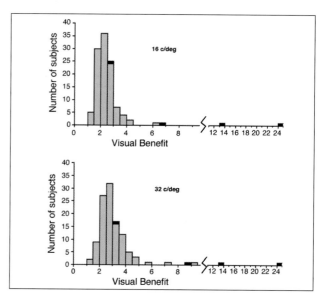

Figure 2-10. Histogram of the visual benefit, at 16 and 32 c/deg, of correcting higher-order aberrations in white light for a population of 109 normal subjects (gray) and a sample of four keratoconic patients (black). Pupil size is 5.7 mm.

than they have ever had before. Adaptive optics can also correct the aberrations for light leaving the eye, which makes it possible to obtain very high resolution images of the living retina[32] as well as to improve vision.

Contrast Sensitivity with and without Higher-Order Correction

To assess the benefit of correcting higher-order aberrations, we measured the contrast sensitivity of the eye following correction with adaptive optics compared with the contrast sensitivity following a conventional refraction to correct defocus and astigmatism only. Figure 2-14 shows the contrast sensitivity functions (lower) and visual benefit (upper) for two subjects with only defocus and astigmatism corrected (x symbols), after correcting the higher-order monochromatic aberrations as well as defocus and astigmatism (open circles), and after correcting both monochromatic aberrations and chromatic aberration (filled circles). In this case, visual benefit is calculated from the ratio of the CSFs instead of the ratio of MTFs, but its meaning is otherwise identical. Chromatic aberrations, both axial and transverse, were eliminated by using a narrow band interference filter between the eye and the stimulus.

The results are similar for both subjects. The contrast sensitivity when correcting most monochromat-

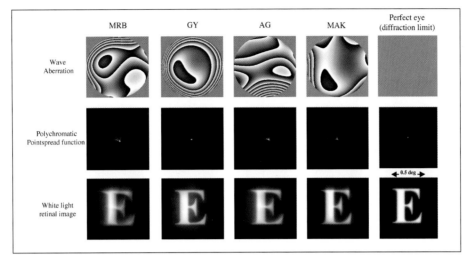

Figure 2-11. The wave aberration of four typical eyes and a perfect diffraction-limited eye for 5.7-mm pupils are shown at the top. Their corresponding PSFs, computed from the wave aberrations, are shown in the middle row. The bottom row shows the convolution of the PSF with a Snellen letter E, subtending 30 minutes of arc. This shows the retinal image of the letter given the wave aberration measured in each eye. Note the increased blurring in the real eyes compared with the diffraction-limited eye. The calculations were performed assuming white light, axial chromatic aberration in the eye, and that a wavelength of 555 nm was in best focus on the retina.

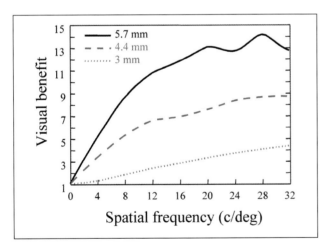

Figure 2-12. Average visual benefit in a sample of four keratoconic patients for three pupil diameters.

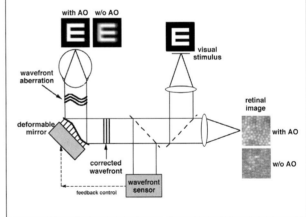

Figure 2-13. Schematic of the University of Rochester adaptive optics system for the human eye.

ic aberrations with a deformable mirror is higher than when defocus and astigmatism alone are corrected. This illustrates that higher-order aberrations in normal eyes reduce visual performance. Moreover, correcting both chromatic and monochromatic aberrations provides an even larger increase in contrast sensitivity.

Figure 2-14 also shows the visual benefit of correcting various aberrations, defined as the ratio of contrast sensitivity when correcting monochromatic and chromatic aberrations (filled circles) and when correcting monochromatic aberrations only (open circles) to that when correcting defocus and astigmatism only. Contrast sensitivity when correcting monochromatic aberrations is only improved by a factor of two on average at 16 and 24 c/deg. The maximum benefits for the two subjects are approximately a factor of 5.7 (YY) and 3.2 (GYY) at 16 c/deg

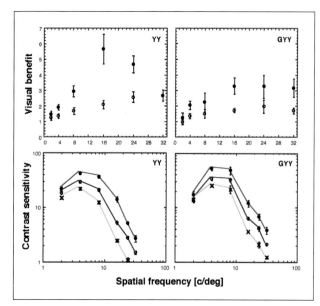

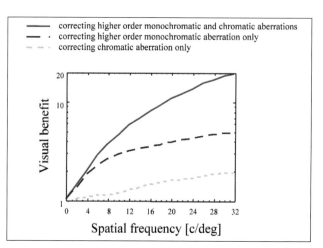

Figure 2-14. The measured contrast sensitivity (lower) and visual benefit (upper) for two subjects when correcting various aberrations in a 6-mm pupil: both monochromatic aberration and chromatic aberration (filled circles), monochromatic aberration only (open circles), and defocus and astigmatism only (x symbols).

Figure 2-15. The maximum visual benefit of correcting higher-order monochromatic aberrations and/or chromatic aberrations for a 6-mm pupil. A perfect correction method was assumed. The monochromatic MTFs were computed every 10 nm from 405 to 695 nm assuming an equally distributed energy spectrum. The reference wavelength assumed to generate no chromatic aberration was 555 nm where the photopic spectral sensitivity is maximal. The axial chromatic aberration data of Wald and Griffin[30] were used after rescaling them to the reference wavelength of 555 nm. Estimates of foveal TCA from Thibos, et al[53] were also considered in the calculation. For both monochromatic and white light, the amounts of defocus were chosen to maximize the MTF at 16 c/deg.

when both monochromatic and chromatic aberrations were corrected.

The Role of Chromatic Aberrations

The results in Figure 2-14 illustrate that the maximum increase in retinal image contrast that could be achieved requires correcting the chromatic aberrations as well as the monochromatic aberrations. Figure 2-15 shows the average maximum theoretical visual benefit computed from the wave aberrations of 17 normal eyes for a 6-mm pupil. For a 6-mm pupil, correcting monochromatic aberrations alone provides a large benefit of a factor of about five at middle and higher spatial frequencies. The theoretical benefit of correcting both chromatic and monochromatic aberrations is substantially larger than that when correcting higher-order monochromatic aberrations only. In theory, for these subjects, correcting both could increase contrast sensitivity by a factor of almost 20 at 32 c/deg. These theoretical benefits are larger than we measured empirically (see Figure 2-14), because the adaptive optics system is incapable of perfect correction.

Campbell and Gubisch[33] found that contrast sensitivity for monochromatic yellow light, which can-

not produce chromatic aberration, was only slightly greater than contrast sensitivity for white light. One of the reasons that axial chromatic aberration is not as deleterious under normal viewing conditions as one might expect is that it is overwhelmed by the numerous monochromatic aberrations.[34] This is shown in Figure 2-15. The visual benefit when only chromatic aberration is corrected is relatively small since the effect of higher-order aberrations on retinal image quality dilutes the benefit of correcting chromatic aberration. Similarly, chromatic aberration reduces the visual benefit when only monochromatic aberrations were corrected. But correcting both at the same time produces much larger benefits. The challenge is therefore to devise a method to correct the chromatic aberrations of the eye along with the monochromatic aberrations. This cannot be achieved with laser refractive surgery. Multilayer contact lenses that could correct chromatic aberration with conventional methods would be too bulky and decentration would obliterate any benefit. Reducing the bandwidth of illumination is simple to implement

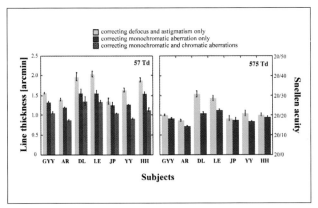

Figure 2-16. Measured visual acuity for seven subjects when correcting various aberrations in a 6-mm pupil. Two retinal illuminance levels, 57 (left) and 575 Td (right), were used. A color CRT was used to display the acuity target—a single letter E. The spectrum of the CRT was a reasonable example of the broadband spectrum considered in natural scenes. The letter E with one of four different orientations was displayed at 100% contrast. From trial to trial, the orientation of the letter was varied randomly among four orientations: the normal orientation and rotations of 90, 180, and 270 degrees. Subjects indicated the orientation of the letter by pressing one of four keys. The psychometric function based on 40 trials was derived using the QUEST procedure,[54] and acuity was taken as the line thickness of the letter for which 82% of responses were correct. Chromatic aberration was removed using a 10-nm bandwidth interference filter.

and is effective, but it also eliminates color vision and greatly reduces luminance. No practical solution to this problem currently exists.

Snellen Acuity with and without Higher-Order Correction

Due to the ubiquitous use of Snellen acuity in the clinic, we have also measured the increase in Snellen visual acuity provided by correcting higher-order aberrations as well as defocus and astigmatism. Figure 2-16 shows visual acuity at a low (57 Td, left) and a high (575 Td, right) retinal illuminance. Before the measurement, defocus and astigmatism were subjectively corrected with a trial lens if necessary. Correcting monochromatic aberrations provides an average increase for the seven subjects of a factor of 1.2 at 575 Td and 1.4 at 57 Td. Correcting both monochromatic and chromatic aberrations improves visual acuity by a factor of 1.6. Therefore, visual acuity reveals a small benefit of correcting higher-order monochromatic aberrations. All subjects reported an

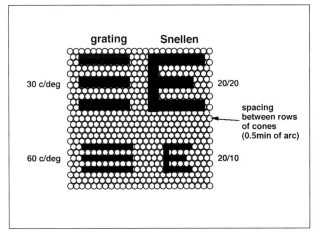

Figure 2-17. The grating and Snellen letter E sampled by the foveal cone mosaic with a triangular arrangement. 20/20 vision (5 minutes of visual angle) and 20/10 vision (2.5 minutes) correspond to 30 c/deg and 60 c/deg, respectively. The spacing between cones is about 0.5 minutes.

All subjects reported an obvious subjective increase in image sharpness when higher-order aberrations were corrected compared with the conventional refraction.

obvious subjective increase in image sharpness when higher-order aberrations were corrected compared with the conventional refraction.

Though reliable improvements in letter acuity can be measured when higher-order aberrations are corrected with adaptive optics, visual acuity is a far less sensitive measure of the benefits of correcting higher-order aberrations than contrast sensitivity. This is because the contrast sensitivity function is steep at the acuity limit and a large increase in contrast sensitivity slides the intersection of the function with the x axis only a short distance. Another reason why visual acuity may underestimate the benefit of correcting higher-order aberrations is that cone sampling considerations will ultimately limit acuity even when improvements in retinal image contrast can continue to provide improved contrast sensitivity at lower spatial frequencies. How does Snellen acuity compare with grating acuity? (see Chapter Seven.) Figure 2-17 shows a mosaic of foveal cones assuming triangular arrangement, the 20/20 and 20/10 letters E, and gratings of 30 and 60 c/deg. An approximate array of 10 x 10 cone samples the 20/20 letter. Clinical visual acuity is usually defined as letter acuity using a standard letter chart observed at a set distance. The size of the smallest letter that can be rec-

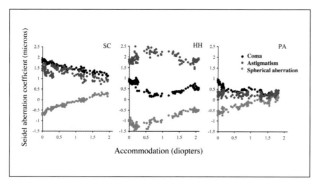

Figure 2-18. Changes in some of the eye's aberrations with accommodation. Pupil size is 4.7 mm. The Seidel aberrations were calculated from wave aberration measurements made with a realtime Hartmann-Shack wavefront sensor at a rate of 25 Hz, while the subjects smoothly changed accommodation from the far point to a vergence of about 2 D.

ognized is taken as the clinical visual acuity of the subject. The most widely used system of acuity notation is the Snellen fraction: V = d/D, where d is distance at which a given letter can just be discriminated and D is distance at which the same letter subtends 5 minutes of arc of visual angle. The reading distance is usually 6 meters (20 feet). At that distance, the letter size corresponding to 20/20 vision (6/6 in meters) is 5 minutes of arc in height. Acuity of 20/200 means that the subject can read at 20 feet a letter that subtends 5 minutes at 200 feet (ie, the smallest letter that this subject can read at 6 meters would subtend 50 minutes). A subject with 20/10 vision could read at 6 meters a letter that subtends 2.5 minutes of arc. The 20/20 letter E may be regarded as being composed of three black horizontal lines and two interdigitated white lines that have the same spacing as a grating with a spatial frequency of 0.5 c/min, or 30 c/deg. A 20/10 letter has the same stroke periodicity as a 60 c/deg grating. If human grating acuity approaches 60 c/deg, one may well wonder why the average Snellen acuity is not 20/10. For one thing, the detection of gratings is a very different task than the recognition of Snellen letters. In Snellen acuity, the subject can be influenced by literacy and past experience. Letters present low spatial frequency cues due to the symmetry or asymmetry in the form that can help recognize them. Grating targets usually extend over a larger visual angle than their equivalent Snellen letters, which increases their visibility. All these factors make the comparison between Snellen and grating acuity problematic. As mentioned above, increasing retinal image quality

with higher-order correction is generally expected to have a smaller effect on visual acuity, whether measured with gratings or letters. We suggest that visual benefit, as we have defined it based on retinal image contrast, is a more robust and useful measure of the outcome of correcting higher-order aberrations.

ADDITIONAL CONSIDERATIONS IN HIGHER-ORDER CORRECTION

We have already discussed the role that pupil diameter and chromatic aberration play in the visual benefit of higher-order correction. This section discusses additional factors that need to be considered to evaluate the ultimate benefits that customized correction will be able to produce.

Accommodation

Any attempt to improve the eye's optics with a customized correction will only be beneficial if the values of the eye's aberrations are relatively fixed. If, for any reason, the eye's optics are not stable, the ability to improve vision will be limited. The eye's higher-order aberrations change substantially with accommodation. What implications will this have for the visual benefit that could be obtained with a customized correction? Figure 2-18 shows how a few of the eye's aberrations (coma, astigmatism, and spherical aberration) varied for a 4.7-mm pupil in three subjects as they smoothly changed their accommodation from distant (far point) to near accommodation (a change of about 2 D or 0.5 meters).[35] Although the nature of the change in the eye's higher-order aberrations generally varies for different subjects, it is clear that for each subject there are substantial, systematic changes in the aberrations that depend on accommodative state. This means that a higher-order correction tailored for distance vision would not be appropriate for near viewing and vice versa.

For the same three subjects, the effect of accommodative state on the monochromatic visual benefit that could be attained with a higher-order correction is illustrated in Figure 2-19. The blue curve for each subject shows the visual benefit that would be obtained with the ideal corneal ablation profile designed to eliminate the eye's higher-order aberrations when the subject is accommodating at infinity. This is the maximum obtainable visual benefit for each subject. The pink curve shows the subjects' visual benefit obtained with this same ablation pro-

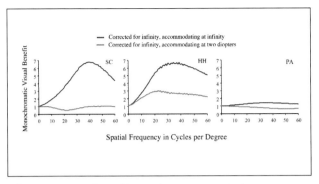

Figure 2-19. The effect of accommodative state on visual benefit. For the same three subjects as in Figure 2-3, the visual benefit in monochromatic light was computed for different accommodative states from wave aberrations measured with a Hartmann-Shack wavefront sensor. Pupil size is 4.7 mm.

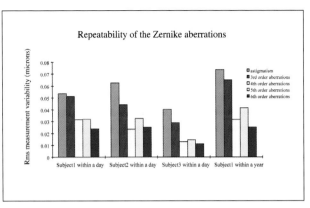

Figure 2-20. Repeatability of the Zernike aberration measurement for Zernike coefficients of different radial orders. This figure shows the average RMS variability of different orders of Zernike coefficients measured several times throughout a single day for three subjects. Pupil size was approximately 6 mm. The RMS measurement variability of the different Zernike orders over the course of 1 year is also shown for one of the subjects. The Zernike coefficients were measured with a Hartmann-Shack wavefront sensor. Since the measurement variability includes experimental errors specific to the particular Hartmann-Shack wavefont sensor, measurement noise, and errors due to pupil centration, it represents an upper bound to the actual instability in the wave aberration.

file, when the subject is actually accommodating at 2 D instead of infinity. It is important to keep in mind that defocus is not responsible for the drop in visual benefit. In fact it has been assumed that the subject has perfect accommodation. This was implemented by zeroing the residual Zernike defocus. (Note: although the focal plane for best image quality does not necessarily correspond to the plane where Zernike defocus is equal to zero, for relatively small pupil sizes and mild wave aberrations, zeroing the Zernike defocus is usually a good approximation to the best focal plane.) This shows that a customized corneal ablation profile tailored to perfectly correct all the higher-order aberrations at one accommodative state does little or no good when the accommodative state is substantially changed. In this situation the custom correction is little better, and maybe even somewhat worse, than a traditional spherocylindrical correction. Though the changes of the wave aberration with accommodation limits the conditions under which a customized static correction of the eye's aberrations would provide a benefit in young people who can still accommodate, it does not imply that such a correction would have no use. This limitation is not particularly severe because it does not apply to presbyopes. Even in younger people there would be value in designing the lens to correct for distance vision. The failure to focus correctly on the target, or accommodative lag, will also diminish the visual benefit of higher-order correction.

Slow Changes in the Wave Aberration Over Time

Another issue that is important to consider in

evaluating the feasibility of a customized corneal ablation procedure is whether, for a fixed accommodative state, the wave aberration is stable over long periods of time. If higher-order aberrations were not stable, there would be little point in performing a customized corneal ablation. This issue can be addressed by examining the repeatability with which the wave aberration can be measured within a single day and within an entire year. Figure 2-20 shows the root mean square (RMS) between-measurement variability in the wave aberration, expressed in microns, for the three subjects with 6 mm pupils. Each measurement was made with a long integration time to minimize the influence of short-term instability in the wave aberration, to be discussed later. Within-a-day variability depends on the Zernike order considered but generally ranges between 0.01 and 0.06 microns. This RMS within-a-day variability is about nine times smaller than the average magnitude of aberration for the second-order aberrations and about three times smaller than the average magnitude of aberration for the third- and fourth-order modes. It is likely that the actual variability in the wave aberration is smaller than this since much of the variability is probably due to changes in pupil position and other sources of measurement error rather than actual changes in the wave aberration that would affect vision.

Figure 2-20 also shows repeatability data for one eye over a much longer time scale. The wave aberration for this eye was measured on three occasions spanning more than an 8-month period and showed a RMS between-measurement variability of < 0.08 microns in every case, only slightly worse than the within-a-day variability. These results imply that for a fixed accommodative state, the wave aberration of the eye is stable both within a day and probably over a period of many months as well. Although similar data for more subjects would be required to make a definitive statement about longer periods, the evidence that is available indicates that a custom surgical procedure to correct higher-order aberrations would be of value to the patient for an extended period of time.

Although we believe the wave aberration to be fairly stable over relatively long time periods, it is known that spatial vision does deteriorate with age.[36] In addition to neural factors, a significant steady increment in ocular aberrations with age has been found,[37,38] which produces a degraded retinal image in the older eye. Both changes in the crystalline lens[39,40] and changes in the cornea[41,42] are responsible. However, the cause of the degradation of the eye's optical quality is the loss of the aberration balance between cornea and lens that seems to be present in the younger eye.[43] These factors ultimately limit the longevity of an effective customized correction.

Rapid Changes in the Wave Aberration Over Time

The experiments described above address the issue of the long-term stability of the wave aberration, but they do not consider the possibility that the short-term stability of the eye might be poor. Rapid temporal fluctuations in the wave aberration might also reduce the value of a static correcting procedure such as a customized corneal ablation. All the calculations described thus far have assumed that the eye's aberrations are perfectly static in time, and the contrast sensitivity measurements described earlier are usually conducted with paralyzed accommodation so that at least some of the dynamics would have been suppressed compared with normal viewing.

Microfluctuations in accommodation, even during attempted steady-state accommodation, have been

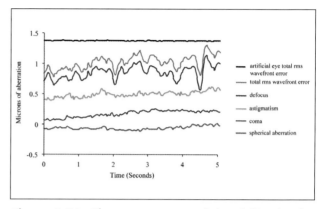

Figure 2-21. Short-term temporal instability in the eye's wave aberration. Aberrations were measured with a real-time Hartmann-Shack wavefront sensor while the subject attempted to fixate steadily on a high contrast target at 2 D. Pupil size is 4.7 mm.

documented and studied since 1951,[44,45] however measurement of the short-term instability of the eye's higher-order aberrations has not been possible until recently. Figure 2-21 shows the short-term temporal variability of the eye's total RMS wavefront error and some of the Zernike aberrations for one subject measured over 5 seconds. For comparison, the total RMS wavefront error measured for a static artificial eye is also shown.[46] It can be seen from this figure that the eye's higher-order aberrations do exhibit temporal instability, but by far the largest source of short-term instability in the eye's wave aberration is due to the microfluctuations in accommodation.

Figure 2-22 shows the theoretical effect of this short-term variability in the eye's aberrations on the maximum visual benefit that can be obtained in one subject with a perfect customized corneal ablation procedure for a 5.8-mm pupil. The calculations were performed assuming a perfect correction of the static component of the eye's wave aberration and also perfect correction of the eye's chromatic aberration, implying that a perfect corneal ablation procedure in the absence of temporal instability would result in diffraction-limited performance. The effect of temporal instability is similar to the effect of chromatic aberration in that it only fully reveals itself when higher-order aberrations are very small. The blue curve indicates the monochromatic visual benefit of a perfect correction, for this subject, if her aberrations were perfectly static. The pink curve shows how the visual benefit is decreased when the effect of the temporal instability in her wave aberration is taken into account. Temporal instability causes very little

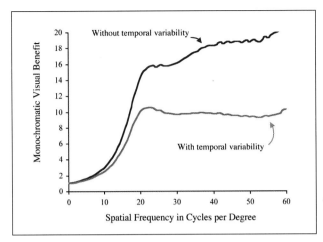

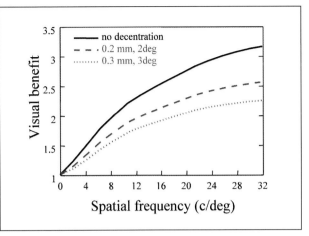

Figure 2-22. The effect of short-term temporal instability in the eye's wave aberration on the visual benefit of a perfect custom correction. The time-averaged monochromatic visual benefit for different conditions was calculated from wave aberration measurements made with a real-time Hartmann-Shack wavefront sensor. Pupil size is 5.8 mm. The blue curve is the benefit that could be obtained in the absence of temporal instability. This is the benefit that would be achieved with a perfect customized correction. The pink curve is the visual benefit obtained with a perfect customized correction of the static component of the eye's wave aberration when the effects of temporal instability are included. It is the best optical quality that can be achieved with any static correction method.

Figure 2-23. Mean visual benefit in white light across 10 eyes with 7-mm pupils, calculated when an ideal correcting method is perfectly centered and for decentrations within an interval of translation and rotation characterized with a standard deviation of 0.2 mm, 2 degrees and 0.3 mm, 3 degrees, respectively. The visual benefit was obtained as the ratio between the MTF in white light when the monochromatic aberrations are corrected and the MTF achieved with an optimum correction of defocus and astigmatism.

reduction in visual benefit for the low spatial frequencies and a reduction of almost a factor of two at higher spatial frequencies. Even so, the visual benefit for the perfect custom correction of the eye's static aberrations (pink curve) is still quite substantial, indicating that a perfect customized correction would still be of benefit to this subject.

Decentration Errors

The benefit from the correction of the higher-order aberrations will be reduced by decentration of the correcting method. A customized contact lens will translate and rotate to some extent with respect to the cornea. Also, the eye is not completely static during a laser refractive surgery procedure. Calculations suggest, contrary to what one might expect, that reasonable decentrations do not detract greatly from the potential benefit.[47,48] Even with fixed translations or rotations of up to 0.6 mm and 30 degrees, a correction of the higher-order aberrations would still yield an improvement over a typical spherocylindrical refraction.

> Even with fixed translations or rotations of up to 0.6 mm and 30 degrees, a correction of the higher-order aberrations would still yield an improvement over a typical spherocylindrical refraction.

Maximum translations and rotations reported for soft contact lenses[49] and measurements of the motion of the eye during the laser surgery treatment[50] allow us to estimate the typical decentration of an ideal correcting method. Figure 2-23 shows the impact of movements within a reasonable interval (characterized by a standard deviation of 0.2 to 0.3 mm for translation and 2 to 3 degrees for rotation) on the visual benefit in white light. The eye's chromatic aberration overwhelms the effect of residual aberrations caused by decentrations. The visual benefit is as high as 2.5 at 32 c/deg, only somewhat less than the ideal case with no decentration.

Correcting progressively higher orders of aberration will result in progressively lower tolerances to decentration. Figure 2-24 shows the impact of translation and rotation on a correction that includes different orders of aberration (up to second, third, fourth, fifth, and sixth order). The ordinate is a measure of the amount of residual aberrations remaining in the eye. While a perfectly centered correcting

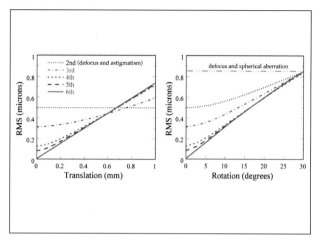

Figure 2-24. RMS of the residual wave aberration (mean value across 10 eyes, 7-mm pupils) as a function of fixed translations and rotations when the ideal correcting method corrects the higher-order aberrations up to second, third, fourth, fifth, and sixth order. For example, a method designed to compensate for the aberrations up to fourth order leaves the aberrations of order higher than fourth uncorrected and there is a residual RMS even with perfect centration due to the incomplete correction. The RMS is a measure of the total amount of aberration.

method continues to provide improvement in image quality when it is designed to correct more orders, the benefit of correcting additional orders decreases when decentration increases. This fact indicates that the higher-order corrections are more sensitive to translation and rotation. If the expected decentration of the correction is too large, then it is not worth correcting all the higher-order aberrations that one can measure. As a general statement, we can say that for translations of 0.3 to 0.4 mm and rotations of 8 to 10 degrees (expressed as standard deviations) there is still a reduction of about 50% of the higher-order aberrations.

THE RATIONALE FOR PURSUING HIGHER-ORDER CORRECTION

Even though we must consider the implications of the aforementioned hurdles in the path to effective customized correction, it is clear from the population statistics that substantial benefits can be had for some eyes in the normal population. As previously shown in Figure 2-12, there are some subjects who have a visual benefit of nearly one, indicating that they have excellent optics and would not benefit

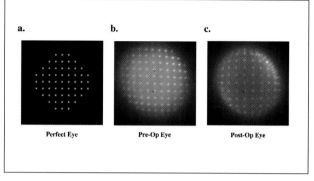

Figure 2-25. The Hartmann-Shack spot array pattern for a perfect eye (a), a normal aberrated eye (b), and the same eye following LASIK surgery (c).

Pathological patients, such as keratoconics, would experience the greatest gains in visual performance.

from a customized correction. However, there are also many normal subjects who possess inferior optical quality and would experience large visual benefits from a customized correction. Of course, pathological patients, such as keratoconics, would experience the greatest gains in visual performance.

In addition to correcting higher-order aberrations in these populations, it is important to examine and attempt to correct for the higher-order aberrations that are being introduced by current refractive surgical procedures. Figure 2-25 shows three images obtained from a Hartmann-Shack wavefront sensor. The details of its operation will be explained in Chapter Six. A perfect eye, shown in Figure 2-25a, produces a spot pattern that is regular and possesses uniform spots that are equally spaced. An aberrated eye produces a Hartmann-Shack array containing spots that are displaced from their ideal, perfect locations. The larger the displacements of these spots, the greater the amount of aberration that is present in an image. Adjacent to the perfect eye is the Hartmann-Shack array for a normal subject before LASIK surgery. The preoperative spherocylindrical refraction of this unoperated eye was -7.75 -2.00 x 57. The third picture in this sequence shows the Hartmann-Shack array for the same subject 4 months following the LASIK surgery. The postoperative refraction for this eye was +0.25 -0.50 x 172. As seen in the figure, the spots in the center of the pupil are fairly uniform and evenly spaced, while the spots in the periphery become distorted and elongated as the spacing between the spots becomes dramatically com-

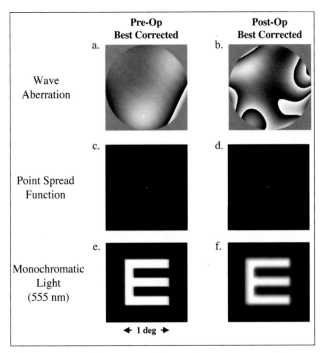

	Pre-Op Best Corrected	Post-Op Best Corrected

Figure 2-26. The wave aberrations across a 3-mm pupil for the LASIK patient's left eye before surgery with best correction (a), after surgery with best correction (b), and corresponding PSFs (c and d). For the wave aberrations shown in (a) and (b), the subject's best refraction was determined by adjusting the amount of defocus and astigmatism (or all three second-order Zernike modes) needed to maximize the Strehl ratio in the corresponding PSF. (e) and (f) show the result of convolving the letter E in monochromatic light (555 nm) with subject DE's best-corrected PSF before and after surgery. After surgery, higher-order aberrations become the dominant source of degradation in the quality of the E.

pressed. This indicates that the aberrations are becoming more severe as we move away from the center of the pupil.

We can more easily determine how the aberration structure of subject DE has changed following surgery by analyzing the pre- and postoperative Hartmann-Shack arrays to determine the corresponding wave aberrations. These results are shown in Figure 2-26 for a 3-mm pupil diameter and in Figure 2-27 for a 4.8-mm pupil diameter. The step size of an individual contour line in the wave aberration is 0.56 microns. Due to the large compression and overlapping of the spots in the periphery of the postoperative eye, we were unable to accurately determine the wave aberration for pupil diameters larger than 5 mm. The eye's PSF for any pupil size up to 5 mm

may then be determined from the wave aberration, yielding a complete description of the imaging properties of the entire eye. The PSF is an alternative representation of retinal image quality that captures exactly the same information as the combined MTF and phase transfer functions.

For the smaller pupil size of 3 mm, we see that there is not a dramatic difference between the wave aberration before and after surgery. This is to be expected since the eye's aberrations are mainly limited by diffraction for small pupil diameters. By convolving the letter E with the eye's PSF we can directly observe how the eye's wave aberration degrades the retinal image. Even for this small pupil size, the letter E shows a reduction in image quality after surgery when compared with the preoperative E, indicating that the surgery has produced higher-order aberrations.

The same trends occur to a larger degree in Figure 2-27 for the 4.8-mm pupil. The best-corrected postoperative LASIK eye produces a retinal image of the letter E whose quality is inferior to that formed by the best-corrected preoperative eye. As the pupil size increases from 3 to 4.8 mm, the postoperative LASIK patient has noticeably poorer retinal image quality than her typical, unoperated eye and would see even worse for larger pupil diameters. The wave aberration after surgery for the postoperative LASIK eye is fairly smooth in the center of the pupil, as evidenced by the low density of contour lines. However, the density of the contour lines increases at the edge of the pupil, indicating the presence of more severe aberrations in the periphery of the pupil. This increase in aberration structure at the pupil edge is primarily due to a steepening of the cornea near the transition zone of the ablation.[50]

The predominant higher-order aberration exhibited by this LASIK patient and several other LASIK patients[51,52] after surgery is spherical aberration (see Chapter Twenty for similar evidence obtained from corneal topographic measurements). Corneal topography correlates with wavefront variance.[53]

Figure 2-28 shows the increase in spherical aberration for this LASIK patient as a function of pupil diameter. Before surgery, the preoperative values of spherical aberration for subject DE are comparable to those expected from the normal population data. After surgery, the magnitude of spherical aberration in the post-LASIK eye becomes twice as large as the unoperated values. This postoperative value will become even larger as the pupil diameter increases from a moderate size of 4.8 mm to a fully dilated size

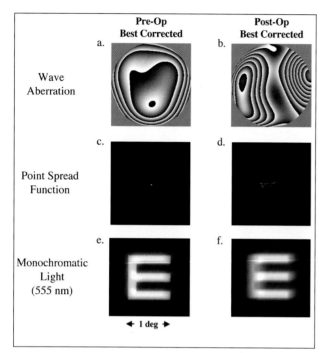

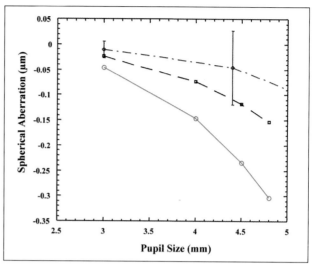

Figure 2-28. Spherical aberration (in microns) for the normal population of 109 subjects (dash-dotted), subject DE before LASIK surgery (dashed), and subject DE after LASIK surgery (straight line) as a function of pupil size. The error bars for the normal population represent plus and minus two standard deviations from the mean value, encompassing 95% of the normal population. The patient's preoperative values for spherical aberration fit in with the normal population. However, after LASIK surgery, the patient's spherical aberration doubles in magnitude as a result of the procedure.

Figure 2-27. The wave aberrations across a 4.8-mm pupil for the same LASIK patient's left eye before surgery with best correction (a), after surgery with best correction (b), and corresponding PSFs (c and d). The aberrations have become more severe for subject DE over this moderately larger pupil diameter. For the wave aberrations shown in (a) and (b), the subject's best refraction was again determined by adjusting the amount of defocus and astigmatism needed to maximize the Strehl ratio in their corresponding PSF. Subject DE's best-corrected PSFs before and after surgery were convolved with the letter E in monochromatic light (555 nm) to produce the retinal images shown in (e) and (f). After surgery, higher-order aberrations become the dominant source of degradation in the quality of the E.

of 6 or 7 mm, severely degrading nighttime vision.

The results from this LASIK patient and the population data suggest that there is a need to refine corrective techniques that can eliminate the eye's higher-order aberrations. Abnormal eyes, such as keratoconics, and eyes containing large amounts of higher-order aberrations, such as subject DE, will obviously benefit the most from a customized correction. Normal eyes, particularly in low illumination conditions with large pupil diameters, can also substantially benefit from a customized correction. Wavefront sensing is a key technology that will be instrumental in perfecting these techniques to maximize the potential benefit each individual patient will be able to receive from a customized correction.

REFERENCES

1. Willoughby Cashell GT. A short history of spectacles. *Proc Roy Soc Med.* 1971;64:1063-1064.
2. Rubin ML. Spectacles: past, present and future. *Surv Ophthalmol.* 1986;30:321-327.
3. Helmholtz H. *Helmholtz's Treatise on Physiological Optics.* New York, NY: Optical Society of America; 1924.
4. Liang J, Grimm B, Goelz S, Bille J. Objective measurement of the wave aberrations of the human eye using a Shack-Hartmann wavefront sensor. *J Opt Soc Am A.* 1994;A11:1949-1957.
5. Liang J, Williams DR, Miller DT. Supernormal vision and high-resolution retinal imaging through adaptive optics. *J Opt Soc Am A.* 1997;A14:2884-2892.
6. MacRae SM, Schwiegerling J, Snyder R. Customized corneal ablation and super vision. *J Refract Surg.* 2000;16:S230-S235.
7. Goodman JW. *Introduction to Fourier Optics.* 2nd ed. New York, NY: McGraw-Hill; 1996.
8. Williams DR. Topography of the foveal one mosaic in the living human eye. *Vision Res.* 1988;28:433-454.
9. Williams DR, Coletta NJ. Cone spacing and the visual resolution limit. *J Opt Soc Am A.* 1987;14:1514-1523.

10. Williams DR. Aliasing in human foveal vision. *Vision Res.* 1985;25:195-205.

11. Bergmann C. Anatomical and physiological findings on the retina. *Zeitschrift für rationelle Medicin II.* 1857;83-108.

12. Byram GM. The physical and photochemical basis of visual resolving power. Part II. Visual acuity and the photochemistry of the retina. *J Opt Soc Am A.* 1944;34:718-738.

13. Campbell FW, Green DG. Optical and retinal factors affecting visual resolution. *J Physiol.* 1965;81:576-593.

14. Williams DR, Sekiguchi N, Haake W, Brainard D, Packer O. The cost of trichromaticity for spatial vision. In: A Valberg, BB Lee, eds. *From Pigments to Perception: Advances in Understanding Visual Processes.* Series A. Vol 203. New York, NY: Plenum Press; 1991:11-22.

15. Helmholtz H. *Popular Scientific Lectures.* New York, NY: Dover Publications, Inc; 1962.

16. Smirnov MS. Measurement of the wave aberration of the human eye. *Biophysics.* 1962;7:766-795.

17. Van den Brink G. Measurements of the geometrical aberrations of the eye. *Vision Res.* 1962;2:233-244.

18. Berny F, Slansky S. Wavefront determination resulting from Foucault test as applied to the human eye and visual instruments. In: JH Dickenson, ed. *Optical Instruments and Techniques.* Newcastle, Scotland: Oriel Press; 1969:375-386.

19. Howland HC, Howland B. A subjective method for the measurement of monochromatic aberrations of the eye. *J Opt Soc Am A.* 1977;67:1508-1518.

20. Walsh G, Charman WN, Howland HC. Objective technique for the determination of monochromatic aberrations of the human eye. *J Opt Soc Am A.* 1984;A1:987-992.

21. Campbell MCW, Harrison EM, Simonet P. Psychophysical measurement of the blur on the retina due to optical aberrations of the eye. *Vision Res.* 1990;30:1587-1602.

22. Webb RH, Penney CM, Thompson KP. Measurement of ocular wavefront distortion with a spatially resolved refractometer. *Applied Optics.* 1992;31:3678-3686.

23. Platt B, Shack RV. Lenticular Hartmann-Screen. *Optical Science Center Newsletter.* Univerisity of Arizona. 1971;5:15-16.

24. Liang J, Williams DR. Aberrations and retinal image quality of the normal human eye. *J Opt Soc Am A.* 1997;A14:2873-2883.

25. Howland HC, Buettner J. Computing high order wave aberration coefficients from variations of best focus for small artificial pupils. *Vision Res.* 1989;29:979-983.

26. El Hage SG, Berny F. Contribution of crystalline lens to the spherical aberration of the eye. *J Opt Soc Am A.* 1973;63:205-211.

27. Artal P, Guirao A. Contribution of cornea and lens to the aberrations of the human eye. *Letters. Optics.* 1998;23:1713-1715.

28. Artal P, Guirao A, Williams DR. Aberrations of the internal ocular surfaces measured in vivo with a Hartmann-Shack sensor. *Invest Ophthalmol Vis Sci.* 1999;40(4):S39-S39.

29. Porter J, Guirao A, Cox IG, Williams DR. The human eye's monochromatic aberrations in a large population. *J Opt Soc Am A.* Submitted.

30. Wald G, Griffin DR. The change in refractive power of the human eye in dim and bright light. *J Opt Soc Am A.* 1947;37:321-336.

31. Artal P, Navarro R. Monochromatic modulation transfer function for different pupil diameters: an analytical expresion. *J Opt Soc Am A.* 1994;11:246-249.

32. Roorda A, Williams DR. The arrangement of the three cone classes in the living human eye. *Nature.* 1999;397:520-522.

33. Campbell FW, Gubisch RW. The effect of chromatic aberration on visual acuity. *J Physiol.* 1967;192:345-358.

34. Yoon GY, Cox I, Williams DR. The visual benefit of the static correction of the monochromatic wave aberration. *Invest Ophthalmol Vis Sci.* 1999;40(Suppl):40.

35. Artal P, Hofer H, Williams DR, Aragon JL. Dynamics of ocular aberrations during accommodation. Optical Society of America annual meeting; 1999.

36. Owsley C, Sekuler R, Siemsen D. Contrast sensitivity throughout adulthood. *Vision Res.* 1983;23:689-699.

37. Artal P, Ferro M, Miranda I, Navarro R. Effects of aging in retinal image quality. *J Opt Soc Am A.* 1993;10:1656-1662.

38. Guirao A, Gonzalez C, Redondo M, Geraghty E, Norrby S, Artal P. Average optical performance of the human eye as a function of age in a normal population. *Invest Ophthalmol Vis Sci.* 1999;40:203-213.

39. Cook CA, Koretz JF, Pfahnl A, Hyun J, Kaufman PL. Aging of the human crystalline lens and anterior segment. *Vision Res.* 1994;34:2945-2954.

40. Glasser A, Campbell MCW. Presbyopia and the optical changes in the human crystalline lens with age. *Vision Res.* 1998;38:209-229.

41. Oshika T, Klyce SD, Applegate RA, Howland HC. Changes in corneal wavefront aberrations with aging. *Invest Ophthalmol Vis Sci.* 1999;40:1351-1355.

42. Guirao A, Redondo M, Artal P. Optical aberrations of the human cornea as a function of age. *J Opt Soc Am A.* 2000;17:1697-1702.

43. Berrio ME, Guirao A, Redondo M, Piers P, Artal P. The contribution of the corneal and the internal ocular surfaces to the changes in the aberrations with age. *Invest Ophthalmol Vis Sci.* 2000;41(4):S105-S105.

44. Arnulf A, Dupuy O, Flamant F. Les microfluctuations d'accommodation de l'oiel et l'acuite visuelle pur les

diametres pupillaires naturels. *CR Hebd Seanc Acad Sci Paris.* 1951;232:349-350.

45. Arnulf A, Dupuy O, Flamant F. Les microfluctuations de l'oiel et leur influence sur l'image retinienne. *CR Hebd Seanc Acad Sci Paris.* 1951;232:438-450.

46. Hofer H, Artal P, Singer B, Aragon JL, Williams DR. Dynamics of the eye's wave aberration. *J Opt Soc Am A.* Submitted.

47. Guirao A, Williams DR, Cox IG. Effect of rotation and translation on the expected benefit of an ideal method to correct the eye's higher-order aberrations. *J Opt Soc Am A.* Submitted.

48. Guirao A, Williams DR, Cox IG. Effect of rotation and translation on the expected benefit of ideal contact lenses. In: *Vision Science and Its Applications. OSA Technical Digest.* Washington, DC: OSA; 2000.

49. Tomlinson A, Ridder III WH, Watanabe R. Blink-induced variations in visual performance with toric soft contact lenses. *Opt Vis Sci.* 1994;71:545-549.

50. Schwiegerling J, Snyder RW. Eye movement during laser in situ keratomileusis. *J Cataract Refract Surg.* 2000;26:345-351.

51. Oshika T, Klyce SD, Applegate RA, Howland HC, El Danasoury MA. Comparisons of corneal wavefront aberrations after photorefractive keratectomy and laser in situ keratomileusis. *Arch Ophhthtalmol.* 1999;127:1-7.

52. Thibos LN, Hong X. Clinical applications of the Shack-Hartmann aberrometer. *Opt Vis Sci.* 1999;76:817-825.

53. Williams DR, Yoon GY, Porter J, Guirao A, Hofer H, Cox I. Visual benefit of correcting higher order aberrations of the eye. *J Refract Surg.* 2000;16:5554-9.

54. Applegate RA, Hilmantel G, Howland HC, Tu EY, Starck T, Zayac EJ. Corneal first surface optical aberrations and visual performance. *J Refract Surg.* In press.

55. Thibos LN, Bradley A, Still DL, Zhang X, Howarth PA. Theory and measurement of ocular chromatic aberration. *Vision Research.* 1990;30:33-49.

56. Watson AB, Pelli DG. QUEST: A Bayesian adaptive psychometric method. *Perception & Psychophysics.* 1983;33:113-120.

57. Williams DR. Visibility of interference fringes near the resolution limit. *J Opt Soc Am A.* 1985;2:1087-1093.

BIBLIOGRAPHY FOR TABLE 2-1

Curcio CA, Sloan KR, Packer O, Hendrickson AE, Kalina RR. Distribution of cones in human and monkey retina: individual variability and radial asymmetry. *Science.* 1987;236:579-582.

Curcio CA, Sloan KR, Kalina RR, Hendrickson AE. Human photoreceptor topography. *J Comp Neurol.* 1990;292:497-523.

Miller WH. Ocular optical filtering. In: H Autrum, ed. *Handbook of Sensory Physiology.* Vol VII/6A. Berlin, Germany: Springer-Verlag; 1979: 70-143.

Østerberg GA. Topography of the layer of rods and ones in the human retina. *Acta Ophthalmol.* 1935;13:1-97.

Yuodelis C, Hendrickson A. A qualitative analysis of the human fovea during development. *Vision Res.* 1986;26:847-856.

Chapter Three

Ophthalmic Wavefront Sensing
History and Methods

Howard C. Howland, PhD

INTRODUCTION

Prior to the introduction of refractive surgery, the wave aberration of the eye played a very small role in anyone's thinking about the optics of the eye. This is because in normal eyes, even at relatively large apertures, the wave aberration generally does not degrade the image quality below 20/20 vision.

However, with the advent of refractive surgery, very large amounts of spherical aberration and coma were induced in eyes treated with radial keratotomy (RK), photorefractive keratectomy (PRK), or laser in situ keratomileusis (LASIK).[1,2] While generally not significant at small pupil sizes, these induced aberrations became important at low light levels and large pupil apertures. This spurred an increased interest both in the measurement of high-order monochromatic aberrations and techniques for eliminating them.

> With the advent of refractive surgery, very large amounts of spherical aberration and coma were induced in eyes

METHODS OF DETECTION OF WAVE ABERRATION

The primary methods of wave aberration detec-

tion and reconstruction have been based either on interferometry or ray tracing. The Twymann green interferometer (Figure 3-1), described in almost every book on physical optics, works by first dividing and then recombining a collimated beam of light after its divided beams have been reflected from test and reference surfaces. Only if the surfaces are identical and correctly aligned will no interference fringes be visible in the final, recombined beam. Otherwise, the resulting interference fringe pattern will provide a topographic map (in steps of one wavelength) of the wave aberration difference surface.

The interferometric method has not found much application in physiological optics primarily due to difficulties in stabilizing the eye and constructing appropriate reference surfaces with which to compare, for example, corneal shape.

All of the other methods have been based on ray tracing and reconstruction of the wave aberration surface by integrating the slopes of an array of beams intersecting the eye's entrance pupil. In physical optics, these methods were first realized by Hartmann[3] at the turn of the last century. About 5 years earlier, Tscherning[4] constructed and described an apparatus, which he named an "aberroscope"

> In physical optics, ray tracing methods were first realized by Hartmann (at the turn of the century and by Tscherning about 5 years earlier).

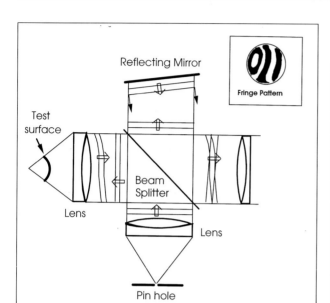

Figure 3-1. Twymann green interferometer. A collimated light source enters a beam splitter where light in one path is focused onto a curved surface (arrow; eg, a cornea) and reflected back through the beam splitter. This beam is then combined with (and interferes with) the second beam, which has passed through the beam splitter and is reflected from a reference reflecting mirror. If the test spherical surface is perfectly centered with its center at the focal point of the lens and the reference mirror is tilted, a set of perfectly parallel fringes would be seen by the observer.

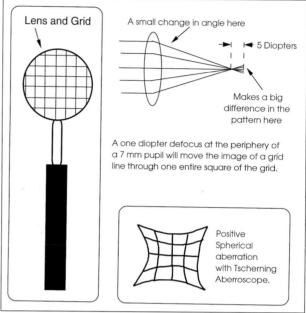

Figure 3-2. The Tscherning aberroscope. The aberroscope is shown at the left and consists of a +5 D lens with a grid consisting of about 1-mm squares. To use it, the subject views a distant point source of light that is focused in front of his or her retina by the aberroscope's lens. The grid is then shadowed on the subject's retina, and the distortions of the grid are noted and drawn by the subject. A grid corresponding to positive spherical aberration is depicted.

(Figure 3-2), from a grid superimposed on a 5 diopter (D) spherical lens. Viewing a distant point source of light through the aberroscope, a subject could see a shadow image of the grid on his or her retina. From the distortions of the grid, one could infer the aberrations of the eye.

Tscherning's aberroscope was attacked and dismissed by Gullstrand; and possibly due to this, its use was temporarily abandoned. Sixty years later, Bradford Howland invented the crossed cylinder aberroscope[5] (Figure 3-3) to investigate the aberrations of camera lenses. Instead of using a spherical lens to shadow the grid on the retina, he used a crossed cylinder lens of 5 D with the negative cylinder axis at 45 degrees. The advantages of this over the Tscherning aberroscope are:

- Diffraction blurs the grid lines along their axes, producing a sharper grid.
- The point of zero defocus of the eye is clearly indicated by the horizontal and vertical orientations of the central grid lines.

- The distorted grid lines represent the ray intercept plots of classical optics.

Another 20 years passed before a subjective aberroscope was used to investigate and characterize the monochromatic aberrations of 55 subjects.[6] The principal result of that study was that third-order coma-like aberrations dominate the aberration structure of the eye at all physiological pupil sizes. This was the first time that comatic aberrations had been meas-

> Third-order coma-like aberrations dominate the aberration structure of the eye.

ured, as opposed to estimated, in any eye. This study also introduced the use of Zernike polynomials to describe the wave aberration of the human eye.

The crossed cylinder aberroscope was improved by introducing an ophthalmoscopic track and photographing grid patterns on the retina,[7] making it an objective technique. More recently, an objective

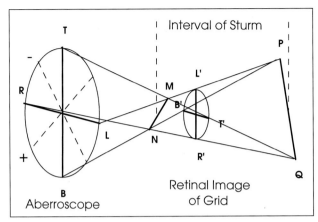

Figure 3-3. The optics of the crossed cylinder aberroscope. The construction and use are similar to that of the Tscherning aberroscope. However, in place of a +5 D spherical lens a ±5 D crossed cylinder lens is employed. This causes the grid to be shadowed in the interval of Sturm. In this arrangement, diffraction smears the images of the lines along their lengths, making the image sharper than that of the Tscherning aberroscope.

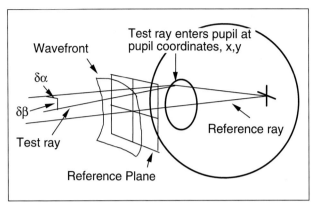

Figure 3-4. Optics of a spatially resolved refractometer. A reference beam enters the center of the pupil (or alternatively the entire pupil) and forms a reference mark at the fovea. A second beam, which can scan the pupil, enters a small portion of the pupil and its entrance angles are adjusted by the subject so that it intersects the reference mark at the fovea. From a knowledge of the entrance angles of the test ray at multiple positions on the pupil, the wavefront can be reconstructed.

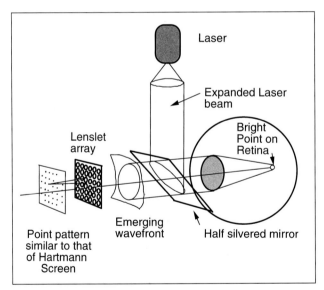

Figure 3-5. Optics of a Hartmann-Shack device. A laser beam is expanded, collimated, and focused to a point on the retina. The emerging beam from this point source is focused onto a lenslet array, which forms a point pattern that is captured by a video camera. The obtained pattern is compared with that of an aberration-free beam, and again the wavefront is computed from the displacements of the points from their unaberrated pattern.

Tscherning aberroscope method has been adapted for clinical use.[8]

Another subjective method to find the wave aberration of the human eye was that of Smirnov,[9] wherein a grid is viewed by the entire aperture of the eye minus a single central intersection, which is viewed through a small aperture and made to scan the entire pupil sequentially. Smirnov measured the topographies of seven eyes and commented on them.

More recently, Webb and colleagues[10] (Figure 3-4) made a modern implementation of Smirnov's method that computes the wave aberration and reduces it to Zernike polynomials in a matter of minutes. It shows remarkable repeatability.

Lastly, the Hartmann-Schack wavefront sensor (Figure 3-5), a method initiated in astronomy to analyze the aberrations of the atmosphere above a telescope in real time, was adapted by Bille and Liang in Heidelberg, Germany and developed by Liang, Williams, and colleagues in Rochester, NY to image the human fundus by removing the aberrations of the eye with a deformable mirror.[11] The measurement is made by focusing a bright spot of light on the retina and projecting the quasiplanar wave onto a matrix of lenslets that focus spots of light on a CCD video array. Just as in the Tscherning aberroscope, the displacement of the spots from their unaberrated positions yields the average slopes of the wavefront at each lenslet's position.

In conclusion, there exists today a variety of subjective and objective methods for assaying the wave aberration of human eyes, which span a wide range in cost, complexity, and accuracy. Due to the unique advantages of each method, we may expect to see their continued use in the future.

REFERENCES

1. Martinez CE, Applegate RA, Klyce SD, McDonald MB, Medina JP, Howland HC. Effect of pupillary dilation on corneal optical aberrations after photorefractive keratectomy. *Arch Ophthalmol.* 1998;116:1053-1062.

2. Oshika T, Klyce SD, Applegate RA, Howland HC, el Danasoury MA. Comparison of corneal wavefront aberrations after photorefractive keratectomy and laser in situ keratomileusis. *Am J Ophthalmol.* 1999;127(1):1-7.

3. Hartmann J. Bemerkungen ueber den Bau und die Justierung von Spektrographen. *Zeitschrift fuer Instrumentenkunde.* 1900;20:47.

4. Tscherning, M. Die monochromatischen Aberrationen des menschlichen Auges. *Z Psychol Physiol Sinn.* 1894;6:456-471.

5. Howland B. Use of crossed cylinder lens in photographic lens evaluation. *Applied Optics.* 1960;1587-1588.

6. Howland HC, Howland B. A subjective method for the measurement of monochromatic aberrations of the eye. *J Opt Soc Am A.* 1977;67:1508-1518.

7. Walsh G, Charman WN, Howland HC. Objective technique for the determination of monochromatic aberrations of the human eye. *J Opt Soc Am A.* 1984;1:987-992.

8. Mierdel P, Krinke HE, Wiegand W, Kaemmerer M, Seiler T. A measuring device for the assessment of monochromatic aberrations in human eyes. *Ophthalmologe.* 1997;94(6):441-445.

9. Smirnov HS. Measurement of the wave aberration in the human eye. *Biophys.* 1961;6:52-66.

10. He JC, Marcos S, Webb RH, Burns S. Measurement of the wavefront aberration of the eye by a fast psychophysical procedure. *J Opt Soc Am A.* 1998;15(9):2449-2456.

11. Miller DT, Williams DR, Morris G, Liang J. Images of cone photoreceptors in the living human eye. *Vision Res.* 1996;36(8):1067-1079.

Chapter Four

Retinal Imaging Using Adaptive Optics

Austin Roorda, PhD
David R. Williams, PhD

INTRODUCTION

The optical system of the human eye is fraught with aberrations. This fact was documented as early as 1801 by Thomas Young,[1] but perhaps Helmholtz stated it best when he wrote, "Now, it is not too much to say that if an optician wanted to sell me an instrument (the eye) which had all these defects, I should think myself quite justified in blaming his carelessness in the strongest terms and giving him back his instrument."[2] These ocular aberrations blur

> "Now, it is not too much to say that if an optician wanted to sell me an instrument (the eye) which had all these defects, I should think myself quite justified in blaming his carelessness in the strongest terms and giving him back his instrument."[2]

the retinal image and limit our ability to see, but they also impose a limit on one's ability to look into the eye since, for ophthalmoscopy, the optics of the eye serve as the objective lens. For years, these aberrations were considered to impose fundamental limits on what can be imaged[3] in the retina, but recent developments have demonstrated that these limits can be overcome. The most notable recent developments include the first application of the Hartmann-Shack wavefront sensing technique to accurately measure the aberrations of the human eye,[4,5] which was soon followed by the application of adaptive optics (AO) to compensate for these optical aberrations.[6]

HISTORY OF ADAPTIVE OPTICS

The original problem that AO was proposed to solve was that of image degradation arising in ground-based telescopes due to turbulence in the earth's atmosphere. Babcock, in 1953, wrote a paper, "The Possibilities of Compensating Astronomical Seeing" in which the basic concepts of an AO system were described.[7] Due to the technological difficulties associated with AO, it was not until 1977 that the first successful application was demonstrated.[8] The technological development was largely due to an infusion of funds from the military, who appreciated the potential benefits of AO largely for imaging (and targeting) foreign satellites from ground-based installations.[9] Much of the military's information was declassified in 1992, a move that accelerated progress for all applications, including astronomy and vision science. At the present time, AO technology is still maturing and developing, and there is much scope for improvement. Today, virtually every major telescope has or is planning to establish an AO program. By comparison, the history of AO for ophthalmic imaging is just over 10 years old. AO was first used in a scanning laser ophthalmoscope in 1989 by Dreher, et al.[10,11] Their wavefront corrector was a 13-element segmented mirror, and the correction was limited to the astigmatism of the eye. The information used to control the mirror was the patient's prescription since they had not yet developed to the wavefront sensing technology required to close the loop on the AO system. The images they obtained were only slightly better than without correction—not surprising given the low order of the correction. Nonetheless, they clearly appreciated the potential benefits of correcting the ocular aberrations with adaptive optics. It was not until 1997 that the first closed loop adaptive optics system for the eye was demonstrated to correct higher-order aberrations other than defocus and astigmatism.[6] This device provided the highest transverse resolution of images of the human retina to date, allowing single cells to be clearly resolved. It was also used to demonstrate that vision could be improved by correcting higher-order aberrations as well as the defocus and astigmatism corrected by ordinary spectacles.

METHODS

Mathematics of Imaging

In any optical system, the maximum frequency that can be transmitted is defined by

$$f_{cut\text{-}off} = \frac{d}{57.3\lambda}$$

where d is the diameter of the pupil and λ is the wavelength of the light. $f_{cut\text{-}off}$ is the maximum spatial frequency (in cycles per degree [c/deg]) that is transmitted through the optical system. For a diffraction-limited eye, spatial frequencies that are lower than the cut-off are imaged with increasing contrast to a maximum contrast of 100% at 0 c/deg. The curve that defines the transmitted contrast as a function of changing spatial frequency is called the *modulation transfer function*, or MTF. This formula sets a minimum on the pupil size that is required to image the smallest structures in the retina. For example, the foveal cones have a spatial frequency that peaks at about 120 c/deg. According to the formula, the minimum pupil size required to image these cones would have to be 4.3 mm (for 632 nm light). Practically, the size has to be greater because the transmitted contrast at the cut-off is, by definition, zero. The human eye is not diffraction-limited for pupil sizes greater than 1 mm² and even though information up to the cut-off frequency is still transmitted, it is transmitted with such low contrast that the effective cut-off frequency is much lower. Aberrations increase with pupil size to such an extent that the blur they cause more than offsets the gains in image quality that diffraction predicts. The

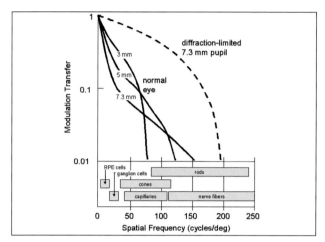

Figure 4-1. Modulation transfer functions and retinal features as a function of spatial frequency. The solid lines show the average MTFs for three pupil sizes: 3 mm (12 eyes), 6 mm (14 eyes), and 7.3 mm (14 eyes).[5] The diffraction-limited MTF for a 7.3-mm pupil is also shown (dashed line) to illustrate the improvements in contrast offered by correcting the aberrations of a 7.3-mm pupil. The lower part of the plot shows the typical sizes of photoreceptors,[33] ganglion cells,[34] RPE cells,[35] and capillaries[36] in the retina. Their spatial frequencies are based on their sizes. Because the sizes of the retinal cells change with location in the retina, they span a range of spatial frequencies. For example, cone photoreceptors are about 2.5 microns in the fovea but increase to about 10 microns in the far periphery.[24]

overall best pupil size for imaging over spatial frequencies from 0 to 30 c/deg is usually between 2 and 3 mm.[12] Figure 4-1 shows MTFs for the average human eye compared with the MTFs for the same eyes if they had diffraction-limited optics. So, in order to benefit from the larger pupils that the eye offers (up to ~8 mm), one must compensate for the aberrations.

The Adaptive Optics Ophthalmoscope

A schematic layout of the Rochester AO ophthalmoscope is shown in Figure 4-2. Like all AO systems, two main components—a wavefront sensor and a wavefront corrector—are required. The wavefront sensor is used to measure the aberrations of the optical system that are to be corrected. Different wavefront sensing techniques might be used, but the technique that is integrated into the Rochester AO ophthalmoscope is the Hartmann-Shack wavefront sensor.[6] The wavefront corrector in the Rochester ophthalmoscope is a deformable mirror, or DM (Xinetics,

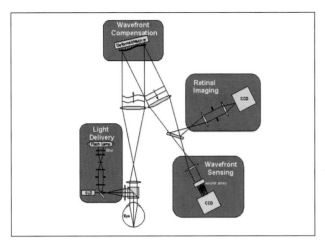

Figure 4-2. Optical system for wavefront sensing and correction. The eye focuses a collimated beam from a laser onto the retina. The light reflected from the retina forms an aberrated wavefront at the pupil, which is measured by the Hartmann-Shack wavefront sensor. A deformable mirror, conjugate with the pupil, is used to compensate for the eye's wave aberration. After compensation is achieved, the retina is imaged by sliding a mirror into place to open the retinal imaging arm. For imaging the retina, a krypton flash lamp delivers a 4-ms flash, illuminating a 1-degree diameter retinal patch.

> Piezoelectrics are electromechanical devices that can push or pull the mirror over a range spanning ±2 micrometers.

Inc, Deven, Mass). The DM is a 2-mm-thick aluminized reflecting mirror that is mounted onto a grid of 37 piezoelectric actuators. Piezoelectrics are electromechanical devices that can push or pull the mirror over a range spanning ±2 micrometers, allowing for compensation of wavefronts with peak-to-valley magnitudes of up to 8 micrometers. Alternative techniques to compensate the wavefront aberrations are being explored, but as yet, none have been demonstrated successfully. Nonetheless, an alternative choice is desirable given the high cost and large size of the deformable mirror system.

In the AO ophthalmoscope, the wavefront sensor and the DM are integrated into the same system. The patient sits in the instrument and his or her eye is brought into alignment with the instrument axis. The first aberration measurement of the eye is made with the DM in an initially flattened state. The wavefront sensor measures the slope of the wavefront at a discrete number of points, and the appropriate DM

actuator voltages that are required to compensate the aberrations are calculated and sent to the mirror. The mirror shape required to compensate the aberrations is simply one-half the magnitude of the actual wavefront aberration. Rather than attempting to correct the aberrations all in one step, an iterative procedure is used in which a small number of measurement and correction cycles converge smoothly on the best correction. The present system requires < 20 iterations and runs as fast as 30 Hz. Since there is a limited number of actuators in the DM and the eye has a small fraction of very high-order aberrations, a perfect correction is not possible. One usually continues the iterations until the wavefront aberration asymptotes to a minimum value. With a 37 actuator DM, the aberrations in the eye over a 6.8-mm pupil have been reduced to a root-mean-square wavefront error that is typically between 0.05 and 0.25 micrometers. Once the wavefront is flattened, a dichroic mirror that is placed in the path redirects light from the eye into the retinal camera, which looks at the retina through the compensating mirror. The human retina is not a source of light so, to take an image, the retina is flood-illuminated over a 1-degree circular patch with light from a krypton flash lamp. Narrow-bandwidth interference filters are placed in the illumination path to control the wavelength of the imaging light.

RESULTS

Photoreceptor Images

Human cone photoreceptors comprise the earliest stage in receiving the retinal image. Photoreceptor images are important for learning about the fundamental properties of vision as well as for diagnosing retinal disease. Most effort on the Rochester AO ophthalmoscope to date has been concentrated on imaging cone photoreceptors, and from that effort we have produced the best pictures ever of the cone mosaic in the living human eye. Examples of the types of images that can be obtained are shown in the three panels on Figure 4-3. The image on the left is a single snapshot taken after only defocus and astigmatism have been corrected in the eye.[6,13] Prior to the implementation of AO, this was the only correction

> We have produced the best pictures ever of the cone mosaic in the living human eye.

that was ever applied to improve image quality. In the case shown here, the subject's aberrations were sufficiently low so that some photoreceptor structure could be seen in the uncompensated images. This ability to resolve photoreceptors without using AO had already been documented by other groups who showed similar results.[14-17] Nonetheless, the improvements in image quality obtained after AO compensation (see the middle panel) are striking. In the compensated image, the fine structures are better resolved and have higher contrast than in the uncompensated image. The bright spots in the image are cone photoreceptors, which at this retinal location are about 5 micrometers in diameter. Nearly all photoreceptors are resolved in a single image. Registration of multiple images, as shown on the rightmost image, improves the signal:noise ratio in the image to an extent in which all photoreceptors are resolved.

Arrangement of S, M, and L Cones

Over 200 years ago, Thomas Young proposed that the human retina was comprised of three cone types,[1] but it was not possible to determine the spatial arrangement of those cones prior to the development of high-resolution imaging with AO. While retinal densitometry has been used for years to measure the pigment concentration in cone photoreceptors,[18] the advantage of using AO is that it allows one to perform the same measurements on individual photoreceptors. Full details of this experiment are described elsewhere,[13] but a brief description follows.

All photoreceptor images were taken with 550-nm light; a wavelength chosen to maximize the absorptance by L and M cone photopigment. Individual cones were classified by comparing images when the photopigment was fully bleached with those taken when it was either dark-adapted or exposed to a light that selectively bleached one photopigment. Images of a fully bleached retina were obtained following exposure to 550-nm light. Images of a dark-adapted retina were taken following 5 minutes of dark adaptation. To distinguish S from M and L cones, we compared fully bleached and dark-adapted images. Since the S cones absorb negligibly while the M and L cones absorb strongly at the imaging wavelength of 550 nm, the S cones reflect relatively more light than the M and L cones, which absorb the light and appear dimmer. Once the sparse population of S cones was identified, they were removed from analysis so that the M and L cones could be dis-

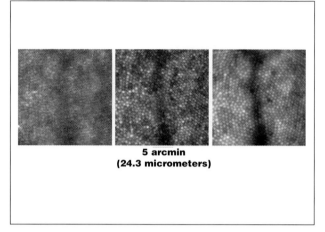

**5 arcmin
(24.3 micrometers)**

Figure 4-3. Images before and after adaptive compensation for the right eye of a living human subject. All three images are of the same retinal area located 1 degree from the central fovea. Images were taken with 550-nm light (25-nm bandwidth) through a 6-mm pupil. The dark vertical band down the center of each image is an out-of-focus shadow of a blood vessel. The leftmost image shows a single snapshot taken after defocus and astigmatism have been corrected. The middle image is a snapshot after additional aberrations have been corrected with adaptive optics. The rightmost image shows the benefits in image quality obtained by registering and averaging multiple frames, 61 in this example.

tinguished. To distinguish L from M cones, we took images immediately following either of two bleaching conditions. In the first bleaching condition, a dark-adapted retina was exposed to a 650-nm light that selectively bleached the L pigment. In the second, a 470-nm light selectively bleached the M pigment. The image following the 650-nm bleach revealed relatively brighter, low absorptance L cones that had been heavily bleached and darker, highly absorbing M cones spared from bleaching. The absorptance images for the 470-nm bleach showed the opposite. Densitometric measurements were repeated in this way until the signal:noise ratio in the data was sufficiently high to confidently identify the individual cones. A pseudocolor image of the arrangement of the cones for two humans and one macaque monkey retina is shown in Figure 4-4.

Angular Tuning

It is well known that human photoreceptors act as waveguides. High-resolution AO imaging can be brought to bear on some remaining questions about these waveguiding properties by looking at how

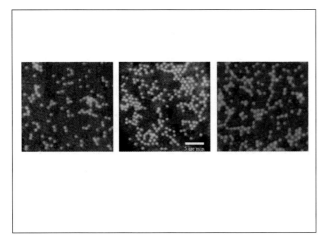

Figure 4-4. Pseudocolor images of the trichromatic cone mosaic in two human eyes and the eye of a macaque monkey. Blue, green, and red colors represent the short (S), middle (M), and long (L) wavelength-sensitive cones, respectively. The two human subjects have a more than three-fold difference in the number of L versus M cones.[13] In all cases, the arrangement of the M and L cones is essentially random.

each individual photoreceptor contributes to the overall directional properties. For example, it is suggested, based on psychophysics[19] and reflectometric measurements from an ensemble of cones[20] that all the cones are narrowly tuned. This question can be answered directly now that individual cones can be resolved in living eyes. In the AO ophthalmoscope, we can measure the directional properties of individual cones by determining how efficiently light is coupled into the cones as a function of illumination angle. If less light gets into a cone because it is illuminated away from the cone's optical axis, then the reflected light from that cone will also be less.[21,22] We took images of the same cone mosaic under identical conditions except that of the illumination angle. The illumination angle was controlled by translating a 2-mm entrance pupil beam to different locations in the pupil. In all cases we took images through a fixed 6-mm exit pupil, which was necessary to obtain sharp retinal images. The pair of images in Figure 4-5 shows striking changes in the amount of reflected light with a < 2-mm translation of the illumination beam location in the pupil.

Capillary Images

In Figure 4-2, the dark vertical band down the center of the image is the shadow of a capillary. A larger field view of the same retinal location is shown in

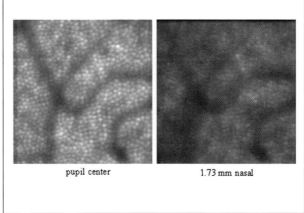

pupil center   1.73 mm nasal

Figure 4-5. Photoreceptor images taken with two different illumination angles. Both images were taken through a 6-mm pupil with the same energy of 550-nm light delivered through a 2-mm diameter entrance pupil. For the left image, the 2-mm pupil was located so that the photoreceptors were illuminated along the axis of the photoreceptors. In the right image, the same photoreceptors were illuminated with the entrance pupil displaced 1.73 mm in the nasal direction. Both intensity and contrast are reduced in the image taken with the offset illumination angle.

Figure 4-6. The pair of images in Figure 4-6 show that by adjusting the focus to a higher plane, the capillaries can be resolved. In this image the capillaries are resolved as distinct shadows that are back-illuminated by the underlying photoreceptor layer. This occurs at this retinal location. With a wavelength of 550 nm, the photoreceptors are the source of most of the scattered light from the retinal image. The capillaries in Figure 4-3 delineate the edge of the avascular zone and are the only images of capillaries from a living human retina from which the diameter can be measured. In this image, the capillary diameters were as small as 6 micrometers.[23]

THE FUTURE OF ADAPTIVE OPTICS FOR OPHTHALMOSCOPY

Clinical Applications

Early diagnosis and treatment of retinal disorders have been hampered by the inability to resolve microscopic structures in the living human eye. In many cases, the retinal disease is detected only after significant and irreversible retinal damage has

It is important that we develop instruments that are sensitive to the specific changes, like photoreceptor loss, that are known to occur with these disorders.

occurred. Since early detection and appropriate treatment is the best way to maintain good vision, it is important that we develop instruments that are sensitive to the specific changes, like photoreceptor loss, that are known to occur with these disorders. The increased contrast and resolving power offered with AO will provide this sensitivity. Moreover, this increased sensitivity will open the possibility of testing the effectiveness of treatment interventions and also learning more about the mechanisms of the retinal disease.

To date, little AO imaging effort has been spent on the study of features other than the cone photoreceptors, but to develop the instrument for clinical applications, it is desirable to expand the range of features that can be imaged (eg, rods, nerve fibers and retinal pigment epithelium cells). Rods outnumber the cones by 20:1 in the human eye.[24] They are not important for central vision, but they have important roles in peripheral and night vision, and rods are also the first photoreceptors to drop off in common retinal diseases like retinitis pigmentosa. Rods have never been resolved with the AO ophthalmoscope, but it remains a real possibility and a future challenge. Nerve fibers have diameters of about 3 microns and the striated patterns they produce are readily seen in conventional fundus images. With AO, we should be able to resolve individual nerves fibers and even measure their diameters. Problems with the retinal pigment epithelium (RPE) are implicated in several important retinal diseases, and the ability to image the mosaic of RPE cells may help us better diagnose and learn about the disease process. The difficulty with imaging RPE cells is not that they are too small but because they have such low contrast. The low contrast is mainly due to the fact that to see the RPE, one must look through the strong reflection from the photoreceptor layer. Imaging modalities that can potentially combine AO imaging with optical sectioning, such as the scanning laser ophthalmoscope, might be the best method to image these structures.

Flood Illumination Ophthalmoscopy or Scanning Laser Ophthalmoscopy

A scanning laser ophthalmoscope (SLO) differs

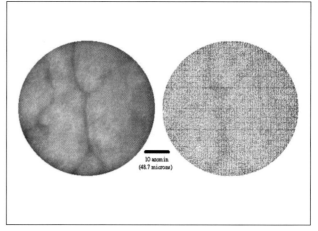

Figure 4-6. One-degree images of the same retinal location at two different focal planes in the right eye of a living human subject. In the left image, capillaries as small as 6 microns are resolved. By focusing deeper into the retina, the underlying photoreceptors are resolved and the capillaries appear as faint shadows. These images are from a location 1 degree from the central fovea, which is located to the right in the direction of decreasing photoreceptor diameter.

from conventional imaging in that the SLO captures an image over time by detecting the scattered light from a focused point as it scans across the retina in a raster pattern.[25] This different imaging modality offers several noted advantages over conventional ophthalmoscopes. First, one can use more sensitive detectors, such as a photomultiplier tube or an avalanche photodiode, to detect the light rather than using an inherently noisier and less sensitive CCD camera. More importantly, SLOs are relatively insensitive to image degradation due to scatter in the optics and they have the ability to perform optical sectioning in the retina. The latter two advantages are facilitated by passing the detection light through a small aperture conjugate to the retina, called the confocal aperture, prior to detection.

SLOs are similar to conventional ophthalmoscopes in that they suffer from the same image quality losses from aberrations since they also use the optical system of the eye as the objective lens for imaging. Hence, it follows that the AO technique can offer the same benefits of this imaging technique. The Rochester ophthalmoscope incorporates AO into a conventional imaging system that uses flood illumination and a CCD camera. With this device, a nearly three-fold benefit in lateral resolution has been realized. By incorporating AO into a SLO, the same lateral improvement is possible but the more significant improvement will be up to a ten-fold increase in optical slicing capability. This improvement in optical sectioning is important because current instruments report a maximum resolution (FWHM of the axial point spread function) of > 300 micrometers, which is about the thickness of the neural retina. Improved axial sectioning should allow imaging of and increase the contrast of specific layers in the retina such as nerve fibers, photoreceptors, or the RPE.

Alternate Technologies

Developing and expanding the scope of the use of AO for basic and clinical investigations will require that AO technology become simpler to use, more compact, and less expensive. The DM is the most effective technology for AO, but these devices are large and expensive, and a cheaper, smaller version of DM technology is not likely. However, alternate technologies are on the horizon. For more details on these alternate technologies the reader is referred to some recent publications.[26-28] For vision science, the best choice for an alternate wavefront corrector may depend on the particular imaging application. For example, the requirement of using polarized light for liquid crystal wavefront correcting devices might be a drawback for some applications but an advantage for others. Economical wavefront correctors such as custom contact lenses, membrane mirrors, or bimorph mirrors (which correct fewer aberrations) might be sufficient for many applications. On the other hand, for the best imaging possible, high temporal bandwidth to compensate for small eye movements, tear film changes, and accommodative fluctuations will be necessary. Significant improvements in image quality are accomplished with a static correction of the aberrations in the eye, but continued research on the dynamics of the eye's wavefront aberration has identified that further improvements in image quality are possible by compensating with a closed-loop bandwidth of 20 Hz.[29]

Beyond Imaging

Since AO can be used to image the retina with high spatial resolution, it follows that AO can be used to deliver light to the retina with the same precision. This opens a number of possibilities that range from studying the perception of aberration-free retinal images to realizing the potential for pinpoint laser treatment of the retina.

Prior to the development of AO for vision appli-

Using AO, any complex aberration-free image can be projected on the retina.

cations, studies of the perception of high spatial frequency retinal images could only be done by producing interference fringes on the retina.[30,31] This was and remains a very useful and productive technique, but the complexity of the retinal image is limited to sinusoidal gratings. Using AO, any complex aberration-free image can be projected on the retina. Projection of such images is already being used to test the potential benefits of aberration-correcting refractive surgical techniques.[32] While there are some obvious benefits to vision, such as an improvement in contrast sensitivity, it remains to be seen whether or not hyperacuity tasks might be compromised. Delivering small spots of color to the single photoreceptor cells might also be used to learn about the early stages of color processing in the human retina.

For clinical applications, laser systems can be equipped with AO to potentially pinpoint the treatment of features as small as individual capillaries or single cells. Using this technology, laser treatments like photocoagulation or photodynamic therapy can be restricted to a localized region, thereby preserving neighboring functional tissue in the retina. Finally, a real-time high-resolution image offers the opportunity to do eye tracking measurements with unprecedented resolution.

Laser systems can be equipped with AO to potentially pinpoint the treatment of features as small as individual capillaries or single cells.

CONCLUSION

AO in ophthalmoscopy is still a young field. Both the technology and the ideas of how to apply it are still developing. With new technologies on the horizon and a host of new scientists and companies developing their own AO programs, the future promises to be exciting and productive for years to come.

REFERENCES

1. Young T. On the mechanism of the eye. *Philosophical Transactions of the Royal Society of London.* 1801;91:23-88.

2. Helmholtz H. *Helmholtz's Treatise on Physiological Optics*. Rochester, NY: Optical Society of America; 1924.

3. Snyder AW, Miller WH. Photoreceptor diameter and spacing for highest resolving power. *J Opt Soc Am A*. 1977;67:696-698.

4. Liang J, Grimm B, Goelz S, Bille JF. Objective measurement of wave aberrations of the human eye with use of a Hartmann-Shack wavefront sensor. *J Opt Soc Am A*. 1994;11:1949-1957.

5. Liang J, Williams DR. Aberrations and retinal image quality of the normal human eye. *J Opt Soc Am A*. 1997;14(11):2873-2883.

6. Liang J, Williams DR, Miller D. Supernormal vision and high-resolution retinal imaging through adaptive optics. *J Opt Soc Am A*. 1997;14(11):2884-2892.

7. Babcock HW. The possibilities of compensating astronomical seeing. *Pub Astr Soc Pac*. 1953;65:229-236.

8. Hardy JW, Lefebvre JE, Koliopoulis CL. Real-time atmospheric compensation. *J Opt Soc Am A*. 1977;67:360-369.

9. Benedict R, Breckinridge JB, Fried DL. Atmospheric-compensation technology: introduction. *J Opt Soc Am A*. 1994;11(1):257-262.

10. Dreher AW, Bille JF, Weinreb RN. Active optical depth resolution improvement of the laser tomographic scanner. *Applied Optics*. 1989;28:804-808.

11. Bille JF, Dreher AW, Zinser G. Scanning laser tomography of the living human eye. In: BR Masters, ed. *Noninvasive Diagnostic Techniques in Ophthalmology*. New York, NY: Springer-Verlag; 1990:528-547.

12. Campbell FW, Gubisch RW. Optical quality of the human eye. *J Physiol*. 1966;186:558-578.

13. Roorda A, Williams DR. The arrangement of the three cone classes in the living human eye. *Nature*. 1999;397:520-522.

14. Miller D, Williams DR, Morris GM, Liang J. Images of cone photoreceptors in the living human eye. *Vision Res*. 1996;36(8):1067-1079.

15. Roorda A, Campbell MCW. Confocal scanning laser ophthalmoscope for real-time photoreceptor imaging in the human eye. Vision science and its applications. *Technical Digest, OSA*. Washington, DC: Optical Society of America; 1997:1,90-93.

16. Wade AR, Fitzke FW. In vivo imaging of the human cone-photoreceptor mosaic using a confocal laser scanning ophthalmoscope. *Lasers Light Ophthalmol*. 1998;3:129-136.

17. Marcos S, Navarro R, Artal P. Coherent imaging of the cone mosaic in the living human eye. *J Opt Soc Am A*. 1996;13(5):897-905.

18. Rushton WAH, Baker HD. Red/green sensitivity in normal vision. *Vision Res*. 1964;4:75-85.

19. MacLeod DIA. Directionally selective light adaptation: a visual consequence of receptor disarray? *Vision Res*. 1974;14:369-378.

20. Marcos S, Burns SA. Cone spacing and waveguide properties from cone directionality measurements. *J Opt Soc Am A*. 1999;16:995-1004.

21. van Blokland GJ. Directionality and alignment of the foveal receptors, assessed with light scattered from the human fundus in vivo. *Vision Res*. 1986;26:495-500.

22. Burns SA, Wu S, Chang He J, Elsner AE. Variations in photoreceptor directionality across the central retina. *J Opt Soc Am A*. 1996;14:2033-2040.

23. Williams DR, Liang J, Miller D, Roorda A. Wavefront sensing and compensation for the human eye. In: RK Tyson, ed. *Adaptive Optics Engineering Handbook*. New York, NY: Marcel Dekker; 1999:287-310.

24. Curcio CA, Sloan KR, Kalina RE, Hendrickson AE. Human photoreceptor topography. *Journal of Comparative Neurology*. 1990;292:497-523.

25. Webb RH, Hughes GW, Pomerantzeff O. Flying spot TV ophthalmoscope. *Applied Optics*. 1980;19:2991-2997.

26. Tyson RK. *Principles of Adaptive Optics*. 2nd ed. San Diego, Calif: Academic Press; 1998.

27. Tyson RK, ed. *Adaptive Optics Engineering Handbook*. New York, NY: Marcel Dekker; 2000.

28. Séchaud M. Wavefront compensation devices. In: F Roddier, ed. *Adaptive Optics in Astronomy*. Cambridge, England: Cambridge University Press; 1999:57-91.

29. Hofer H, Artal P, Aragon JL, Williams DR. Dynamics of the eye's wave aberration. *J Opt Soc Am A*. Submitted.

30. Westheimer G. Modulation thresholds for sinusoidal light distributions on the retina. *J Physiol*. 1960;152:67-74.

31. Arnulf MA, Dupuy MO. La transmission des contrastes par le système optique de l'oeil et les seuils de contrastes retinines. *CR Acad Sci Paris*. 1960;250:2757-2759.

32. Yoon G, Cox I, Williams DR. The visual benefit of static correction of the monochromatic wave aberration. *Invest Ophthalmol Vis Sci*. 1999;40(4Suppl):40.

33. Curcio CA, Hendrickson A. Organization and development of the primate photoreceptor mosaic. In: NN Osborne, GJ Chader, eds. *Progress in Retinal Research*. Oxford, England: Pergamon; 1991:89-120.

34. Kolb H, Linberg KA, Fisher SK. Neurons of the human retina: a Golgi study. *Journal of Comparative Neurology*. 1992;318:147-187.

35. Zinn KM, Benjamin-Henkind JV. Anatomy of the human retinal pigment epithelium. In: KM Zinn, MF Marmor, eds. *The Retinal Pigment Epithelium*. Cambridge, England: Harvard University Press; 1979: 3-31.

36. Snodderly DM, Weinhaus RS, Choi JC. Neural-vascular relationships in central retina of macaque monkeys (Macaca fascicularis). *Journal of Neuroscience*. 1992;12(4):1169-1193.

Chapter Five

Physics of Customized Corneal Ablation

David Huang, MD, PhD

INTRODUCTION

In a broad sense, refractive surgeons are performing customized corneal ablation today. After all, we do not apply the same laser ablation to every eye. Each ablation in laser-assisted in situ keratomileusis (LASIK) and photorefractive keratectomy (PRK) is tailored to the eye's subjective spherocylindrical refraction. Our current usage of the term "custom cornea," however, refers specifically to laser ablation of the cornea customized to each eye's higher-order as well as spherocylindrical aberrations. Eliminating higher-order aberrations may allow us to achieve a supranormal vision ("20/10 perfect vision"). Reduction of higher-order aberrations is also useful in restoring vision to a normal level in pathologic conditions such as corneal scar, ectasia, and complicated keratorefractive surgery. In either case, customized corneal ablation requires more precision in all aspects of the surgery. More precise control of laser ablation is required. Novel wavefront sensors are needed to precisely map the aberrations of the eye. Accurate alignment of laser ablation with either a wavefront or corneal topographic map is also necessary.

In order to use, evaluate, and improve the "custom cornea," the ophthalmic surgeon needs to understand the physical principles behind the technology. This introductory chapter will cover these principles in broad terms.

WHY, WHAT, AND HOW OF WAVEFRONT OPTICS

Why Wavefront?

In order to achieve super normal vision, it is essential to correct the wavefront aberration of the entire optical system of the eye. If one only corrects corneal topographic aberration, vision would still be limited by aberrations in the posterior corneal surface, the crystalline lens, and the remaining refractive elements in the eye.

> If one only corrects corneal topographic aberration, vision would still be limited by aberrations in the posterior corneal surface, the crystalline lens, and the remaining refractive elements in the eye.

What is a Wavefront?

Wavefront optics is not a familiar subject to most people outside of the field of optical engineering and physics. In this introductory chapter, we start with a graphic explanation of wavefront. A more comprehensive treatment of the subject can be found in Chapter Six.

Light is a traveling electromagnetic wave. A wavefront is a continuous isophase surface. To simplify our mental picture from three to two dimensions,

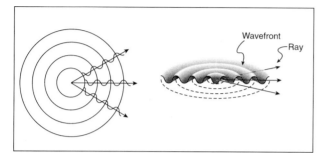

Figure 5-1. The relationship between wavefront and rays in a surface wave example.

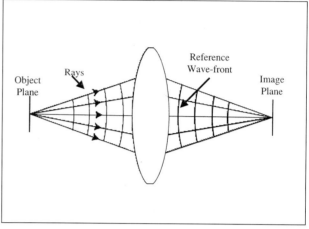

Figure 5-2. An ideal optical system. Light from the object plane is focused by the lens and converges at the image plane. Deviation from the ideal wavefront defines aberration.

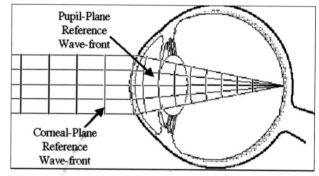

Figure 5-3. An ideal eye. Deviation from the ideal wavefront defines aberration.

let's first consider waves on the surface of water. Imagine throwing a stone into still water and observing the expanding circles of waves. If we take a snapshot of this wave at one point in time (Figure 5-1), we can draw circular wavefronts across the crests (phase 0) of the waves. We can also draw the wavefronts at any arbitrary reference phase, such as the troughs (phase π), or the midpoint of descent (phase $\pi/2$). Note that the wavefronts are perpendicular to the direction of travel, which can be represented by rays (see Figure 5-1). For optical waves, there is one more dimension, and a wavefront is a surface instead of a line.

Both wavefronts and rays can be used to describe wave propagation. For example (Figure 5-2), an optical wavefront from a point source propagates through a lens. As the wave travels through the lens, the speed of propagation is slowed because the lens

> As the wave travels through the lens, the speed of propagation is slowed because the lens material has a higher index.

material has a higher index of refraction than the optical media surrounding it (generally air). The center of the lens is thicker and therefore retards the center of the wavefront relative to the periphery. The differential slowing imparted by the shape of the convex lens in air converts the incoming diverging (convex) wavefront into a converging (concave) wavefront on exit (see Figure 5-2). In the absence of aberration, wavefront converges to a diffraction-limited spot at the focus. Wavefront aberration is defined by the deviation of the actual wavefront from an ideal reference wavefront that is centered on the focus (see Figures 5-2 and 5-3)

The propagation can also be described by ray optics. Recall that rays are at all points perpendicular to the wavefront. At the lens surfaces, the incoming diverging rays are refracted according to Snell's law at each lens location and, again, converge toward the focus. The deviation of the rays from the perfect focus ray path can be used to derive the wavefront aberration.

How is Wavefront Aberration Used to Guide Corneal Ablation?

Wavefront aberration can be corrected at a number of locations in the eye. If one were to implement the correction by inserting an intraocular lens (IOL) implant, then the correction should be guided by the wavefront aberration at the plane of the lens implant (see Figure 5-3). For customized corneal ablation, the ablation pattern is derived from the wavefront aberration at the corneal plane. Defining ocular aberration by the wavefront just outside the eye follows the

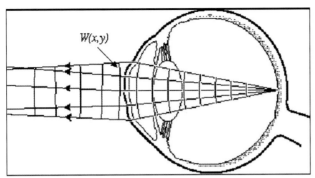

Figure 5-4. Wavefront aberration exiting the eye from a foveal point source.

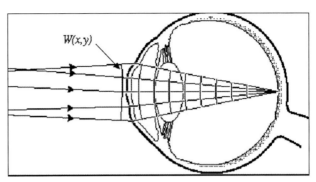

Figure 5-5. Entrance wavefront needed to nullify ocular aberrations.

convention of Smirnov.[1] Most references follow the Howland convention,[2-4] which defines ocular aberration by the wavefront at the pupil plane (see Figure 5-3). Because the corneal plane is not far from the pupil plane, measurements of $W(x,y)$ at the two planes produce similar results. They can be interconverted by calculations that assume a standard optical model of the eye.

Wavefront aberration of the eye is defined as the deviation of the actual wavefront from an ideal reference wavefront emanating from a foveal point source. For an eye focused at infinity, the ideal wavefront exiting the aberration-free eye is a flat plane (see Figure 5-3). In a real eye, there are optical aberrations, and the exit wavefront deviates from that of the plane wave (Figure 5-4). This wavefront aberration is $W(x,y)$, where x and y are the horizontal and vertical axes. $W(x,y)$ is conventionally measured in microns.

Now we reverse the direction of propagation and watch $W(x,y)$ enter the eye (Figure 5-5). By symmetry, we can see that $W(x,y)$ will perfectly cancel out

> Diffraction of light limits the size of the focussed spot even in the absence of optical aberration. The diffraction limit depends on the wavelength and numerical aperture.

ocular aberrations and focus to a point (strictly speaking, a diffraction-limited spot) at the fovea. Diffraction of light limits the size of the focussed spot even in the absence of optical aberration. The diffraction limit depends on the wavelength and numerical aperture. In order for a point source from infinity to achieve perfect focus in this aberrated eye, we need a lens at the corneal surface that converts the flat

wavefront to $W(x,y)$. This lens can be etched onto the corneal surface by customized ablation. Removal of 1 micron of corneal tissue reduces wavefront retardation by ncornea - nair microns. Therefore, the equation for the customized corneal ablation depth $A(x,y)$ needed to correct ocular wavefront aberration $W(x,y)$ is (equation 1):

$$A(x,y) \times (n_{cornea} - n_{air}) = C - W(x,y)$$

where n_{cornea} = corneal index of refraction, n_{air} = refractive index of air, and C is the smallest constant depth needed to keep $A(x,y)$ from becoming negative anywhere. Ablation depth $A(x,y)$ cannot take on a negative value because ablation cannot add tissue to the cornea. C = the maximum value of $W(x,y)$ over the optical zone.

Equation 1 is a basic starting point for designing wavefront-guided ablation. A more comprehensive treatment of the subject is found in Chapter Eight. As with the Munnerlyn formula for spherocylindrical ablation, equation 1 ignores the eye's response to laser ablation. In the context of PRK, Munnerlyn describes this simplifying assumption very well in his classic paper[5]: "The following analysis assumes that if an area of the epithelium is removed and a portion of the stroma is ablated, the epithelium will regrow with a uniform thickness and produce a new corneal curvature determined by the new curvature of the stroma."

Reality differs from this assumption and modification of the corneal surface does occur after both PRK and LASIK.[6,7] To realize the full potential of custom cornea, we will eventually need to understand and deal with the corneal biological response. Biomechanical changes are part of the corneal response and are discussed in Chapter Nine.

The introduction of mapping devices for ocular aberrations has accelerated recently due to commercial interest. The rapid proliferation of new devices leaves many of us struggling to understand the physical principles behind each of them. I hope the following classification schemes will help readers quickly catch up with this growing field. These devices are described in detail in Chapters Twelve through Seventeen. We will adopt the name "wavefront sensor" to describe all these devices because the wavefront aberration map is their final output.

Wavefront sensors can be divided into subjective and objective types. Subjective methods require response from the subject and usually take more time. Subject motion and cooperation are limitations. Objective methods use imaging systems to analyze reflections from the ocular fundus. Since fundus reflection can arise from multiple chorioretinal layers, the reference focal plane is not as well defined as that for subjective methods, which are based on light perception at photoreceptor layer. Chorioretinal structures that backscatter into objective wavefront sensors are generally within 200 microns of the photoreceptor plane. The axial length of the eye is approximately 23 mm. Therefore, the uncertainty is roughly 1% (200 microns/23 mm). The eye's focusing power is about 60 D. Therefore, objective wavefront sensors can be wrong by up to 0.6 D in defocus. For astigmatism and even higher-order terms, 1% error should be insignificant. This focal plane uncertainty is relatively small and should be important only for the defocus (spherical equivalent) term. Wavefront sensors can also be classified by the kind of optical information that is directly measured.

EXIT WAVEFRONT FROM AN ILLUMINATED FOVEAL SPOT

In this class of instruments, the fovea is illuminated and the backscattered wavefront is measured (see Figure 5-4). In the Hartmann-Shack wavefront sensor (Chapters Twelve and Thirteen), the slope of the exit wavefront W(x,y) is mapped with a Shack lenslet array. The wavefront can also be mapped with an interferogram.[8] This class of instruments can provide rapid single-shot wavefront measurement. These devices work best when backscattering from the fovea closely approximates a point source. Challenges to this ideal include multiple scattering

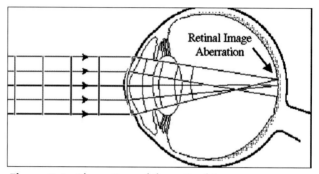

Figure 5-6. Aberration of the retinal image.

from choroidal structures, interference speckle from coherent light sources (eg, lasers), and limits to the brightness and quality of foveal illumination.

ENTRANCE WAVEFRONT NEEDED TO CANCEL OCULAR ABERRATION

In this class of instruments, patches of the corneal surface are probed with incoming light beams to determine the ray directions needed to overcome aberrations and focus at the fovea (see Figure 5-5). The map of ray directions is used to derive the entrance wavefront W(x,y) needed to cancel ocular aberration (Figure 5-6). In the spatially resolved refractometer (Chapter Sixteen), the subject provides feedback by manually steering the probe beam. The Nidek slit skioloscope (Chapter Seventeen) is an objective variant in which the direction of a slit beam entering the eye is rapidly scanned and the fundus reflection is measured by a detector array. The slit axis is then successively rotated to map the wavefront aberration over the entire cornea. These instruments are intrinsically sequential and may take more time to acquire data. However, objective measurements can be acquired in a rapid sequence.

ABERRATION OF RETINAL IMAGE

In these instruments, an image is projected on the retina. The image can be a grid or a point. The deviation of the retinal image from the ideal is used to compute the ocular aberration by a ray-tracing algorithm. The Howland cross cylinder aberroscope (both subjective and objective) projects a grid line pattern.[2] The Tscherning-type aberroscope (see Chapter Ten) projects a grid pattern of points simultaneously. The Tracey system (see Chapter Fifteen) projects a point grid pattern sequentially. The double-pass ophthalmoscope projects a single point and uses the retinal point spread function to compute ocular aberration.[9] These instruments must assume an idealized eye model in order to perform the ray-tracing computation that derives the wavefront aberration at the corneal or pupil plane.

TOPOGRAPHY-GUIDED ABLATION

Corneal topography can only measure the aberration of the corneal surface. Therefore, on its own, it cannot measure or guide the elimination of all ocular aberrations. However, there may be situations in which corneal topography may be superior to wavefront sensors. Placido ring-based corneal topography is a mature technology. It maps the surface of the cornea based on several thousand sampled points on the reflected ring pattern. By comparison, wavefront sensors typically sample only a few hundred points.[10,11] In cases in which corneal aberration is predominant and contains small-scale irregularities (scar, dystrophy, ectasia, and surgical complications such as steep central islands), corneal topography may be able to map ocular aberration with higher resolution than current wavefront sensors. These patients are highly motivated to receive custom ablation to relieve their visual disability from poor acuity, ghosting, glare, and halos. Therefore, topography guidance will likely be an important part of customized corneal ablation.

The basic formula for topography-guided ablation is simple in form (equation 2):

$$A(x,y) = C - (T[x,y] - T_{target}[x,y])$$

where $A(x,y)$ is the ablation pattern, $T(x,y)$ is the actual corneal elevation topography, $T_{target}(x,y)$ is the target corneal topography one wishes to achieve, and C is the smallest constant depth needed to keep $A(x,y)$ from becoming negative anywhere. Ablation depth $A(x,y)$ cannot take negative value because ablation cannot add tissue to the cornea. C = the maximum value of $(T[x,y] - T_{target}[x,y])$ over the optical zone.

There are several limitations to the accuracy and completeness of corneal topography in practice. Placido ring-based devices measure the local radial slope of the cornea at discrete sampling points. Slope data are converted to height topography by an integration operation starting from the center outward.

This integration introduces error in a cumulative fashion; therefore, height estimate becomes less reliable further from the center. The coverage of the ring projections on the cornea can be obscured by the nose and brow. The tear film is variable over time and often there are poorly wet areas on the cornea where measurement cannot be made. These patches of missing slope data can introduce large errors into height calculations. With all these limitations, Placido ring-based topography is still the most successful technology so far.

A tricky step in topography-guided ablation is the determination of the target topography $T_{target}(x,y)$. Theoretically, $T_{target}(x,y)$ should be a parabolic surface with the right refractive power to achieve emmetropia or other postoperative refractive targets. In practice, the spherical equivalent power of the preoperative cornea and the spherical equivalent refraction of the preoperative eye may be difficult to determine in cases with severe aberration and poor best-corrected visual acuity. One may need to use rigid contact lens over-refraction to estimate these quantities. The surgeon's judgment may also enter into this art. More detailed descriptions of topography-guided ablation (Chapters Eighteen through Twenty-Four) and surgeon-guided ablation (Chapters Twenty-Five through Twenty-Nine) are found in the last two sections of the book.

LASER PHYSICS

Photons: Particles of Light

While the propagation of light is described very well by electromagnetic wave theory, many aspects of the interaction between light and matter can only be understood through quantum mechanics. A basic tenet of quantum mechanics is that physical systems such as atoms and molecules can be found, upon measurement, in discrete energy states. Light interacts with these physical systems by the absorption or emission of photons. When an atom transitions from a higher energy state E_2 to a lower energy state E_1, a photon of energy $E = E_2 - E_1$ is emitted. When an atom transitions from the lower to higher state, a photon is absorbed. The energy of the photon is related to its frequency v by $E = hv$, where h is Plank's constant.[12] The wavelength λ of the photon is related to its frequency by the relation $\lambda = c/v$, where c is the speed of light in vacuum.

LASER: LIGHT AMPLIFICATION BY STIMULATED EMISSION

When a photon of energy E travels through a medium, it can induce atomic transitions by either absorption or emission. When there are more atoms or molecules in a higher energy state E_2 than in the lower energy state E_1 ("population inversion"), the probability of a stimulated emission is higher than absorption. Thus, light is amplified by gaining more photons as it passes through the gain medium. This action defines LASE (light amplification by stimulated emission).[12]

A laser is most often constructed as an oscillator (Figure 5-7), where light bounces back and forth between two end mirrors. The two mirrors form the laser cavity. Each time light completes a roundtrip between the mirrors, energy is gained by passage through the gain medium and lost by transmission through the output end mirror. Oscillation is maintained by population inversion in the gain medium. To obtain population inversion, energy is replenished by a pump source, which can be electrical, optical, or chemical. The laser output is shaped by the gain medium, the resonant modes of the laser cavity, and other cavity elements. Since light circulates through a typical laser cavity about a billion times per second, extremely powerful control of the laser output can be obtained. The laser can be made to output a very narrow wavelength range ("monochromicity") or a broad wavelength range. The laser output can be very constant or concentrated in extremely short pulses. The spatial coherence imposed by the cavity resonance means that lasers can often be focused to near diffraction-limited spots.

A method of producing a powerful short pulse from a laser is Q-switching.[12] The quality factor Q is proportional to the ratio of the optical energy in the laser cavity over the power dissipated by the cavity. Thus, a high Q cavity leaks energy very slowly while a low Q cavity loses energy quickly. In Q-switching, the "Q" of the laser cavity is lowered by some means during the pumping phase (see Figure 5-7). Low Q in the cavity prevents amplification of cavity oscillation, so the gain in the laser medium can be built up to a very high level. Once the population inversion in the medium reaches its peak, the Q is suddenly switched to a high value. This causes a very rapid buildup of the oscillation that quickly drains energy in the laser medium by the output of a giant laser pulse. The duration of the pulse is a few nanosec-

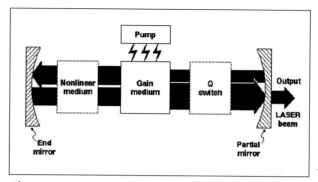

Figure 5-7. Laser oscillator.

onds to hundreds of nanoseconds (a few to a few hundred roundtrips in the cavity).

A nonlinear medium can be placed inside the laser cavity to modify the laser output (see Figure 5-7). The nonlinear medium can be used to generate an extremely short pulse in the picosecond or femtosecond scale, to convert the laser output to a different wavelength by second harmonic generation, or optical parametric oscillation.[12]

Laser Ablation Rate

Removal or ablation of tissue requires that the amount of laser energy absorbed per tissue volume is sufficient to break up the tissue through chemical decomposition, mechanical stress, and/or heating. As laser light travels deeper into tissue, absorption decreases the fluence (energy per area) until it falls below the threshold for ablation. Below threshold, tissue remains in place, but thermal coagulation may still occur. Ablation is a dynamic and complex event[13] that is only described approximately by the following equation, which assumes fluence decreases with depth in an exponential fashion described by the Lambert-Beer's law. Empirically, the depth of ablation is approximately related to the incident fluence by (equation 3)[14]:

$$d = m \times \ln(F/F_{th}) \text{ for } F > F_{th} > 0$$

where d is the ablation depth per pulse, m is the slope efficiency of ablation, F is the incident fluence of the laser pulse, and F_{th} is the threshold fluence for ablation.

The ablation efficiency m is usually close to but not identical to the absorption length measured under nonablative conditions. The ablation efficiency m is measured in units of microns and corresponds to the ablation depth per pulse at a pulse fluence 2.7 times that of threshold (e = 2.7 is the basis of the natural logarithm). For efficient tissue ablation, one should operate at a fluence level that removes approximately *m* microns per pulse. Thus, *m* is of an important measure of the precision of ablation when comparing the various lasers available for laser vision correction. Smaller *m* corresponds to less ablation depth per pulse and finer precision.

The ablation parameters are determined primarily by the wavelength and pulse duration. For precise ablation, it is desirable to have the laser radiation absorbed over a superficial depth of a few microns or less. This is possible in the far ultraviolet (UV) (150 to 200 nm) where there is strong absorption by peptide bonds,[15] and at the water absorption peak in the mid-infrared (IR) (3 microns). It is also desirable to have a short pulse duration that does not permit heat to diffuse into deeper layers. On a micron scale, a laser pulse duration of less than 1 microsecond is needed to avoid thermal diffusion.

Ultraviolet Lasers and Photodecomposition

In order to directly breakup an organic molecule, the photon energy must surpass that of the intramolecular bonding energy. Photons in the far UV range are capable of ablating tissue through this "photodecomposition" mechanism.[16] The photochemical interaction also powers the expansion and ejection of tissue material. This differs from photothermal ablation, where tissue heating and phase changes provide the energy for expansion and ejection. When photodecomposition is the predominant mechanism, tissue ablation occurs at a lower fluence and tissue heating is greatly reduced. This is why the UV excimer lasers are often touted as being "cool" lasers. At the 193-nm ArF (argon flouride) excimer wavelength, thermal effect is small and thermal coagulation of adjacent tissue becomes negligible. This clean ablation characteristic is one reason why the 193-nm laser dominates vision correction.

The dynamic event of tissue ejection during excimer laser ablation has been studied using high-speed photography.[17,18] Immediately after the ablation, hot gaseous products leave the ablation site and expand rapidly outward. The expansion and cooling forms a low pressure zone that draws in surrounding air, which constricts the base of the ejection plume and forms a mushroom cloud appearance. Subsequent recirculation of ablation products toward the low pressure zone forms ring vortices. Eventually, most of the ejected material dissipates with air flow while part of it falls back unto the tis-

sue surface. With a larger ablation diameter, the plume evolves more slowly and more ablated material redeposits on the center of the ablation zone. Both the airborne and redeposited material can block subsequent laser pulses. This has been implicated as a mechanism that contributes to the formation of steep central islands with broadbeam laser ablation.[18]

The practical methods of generating far UV pulses at this time include the excimer lasers and harmonic generation from lasers of longer wavelengths.

The active gain medium of the excimer lasers is a transient rare gas-halogen molecular state that emits

> The ArF excimer laser at 193 nm has been found to be optimal for tissue ablation in the context of vision correction.[16]

a photon on dissociation. Different molecular combinations emit different wavelengths ranging from 157 to 10,600 nm. The ArF excimer laser at 193 nm has been found to be optimal for tissue ablation in the context of vision correction.[16] At shorter wavelengths, beam delivery systems are very difficult to build because of lack of optical material that can transmit and withstand the radiation. At longer wavelengths, thermal effects become increasingly dominant over the photodecomposition mechanism, and thermal coagulation of adjacent tissue becomes significant.[19] At 193 nm, the ablation efficiency *m* is approximately 0.3 microns and collateral thermal damage to adjacent tissue is negligible.[20,21] This is the most precise laser currently being used for corneal ablation.

Harmonic generation using output from the Nd:YAG laser is an alternative method for generating UV radiation. The Q-switched Nd:YAG laser is a very efficient basis for generating nanosecond laser pulses at 1064-nm wavelength. Passage of the 1064-nm radiation through a nonlinear medium allows the up conversion of two 1064-nm photons into a more energetic 532-nm photon. A cascade of this up conversion process can be used to generate 213-nm laser pulses (Figure 5-8). The 213-nm laser has absorption length[15] twice that of the ArF excimer laser. However, the ablation efficiency appears to be only slightly deeper (0.4 microns),[22] and collateral thermal damage is less than 1 micron deep.[23] A potential disadvantage of the fifth harmonic generation is that pulse-to-pulse energy fluctuation is increased roughly five-fold by the harmonic generation process, which can reduce the accuracy of laser ablation.

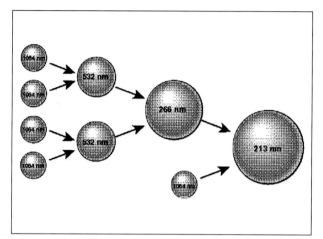

Figure 5-8. Fifth harmonic generation from 1064-nm Nd:YAG laser. Five 1064-nm hpotons are combined in a cascade up conversion to obtain a more energetic 213-nm photon.

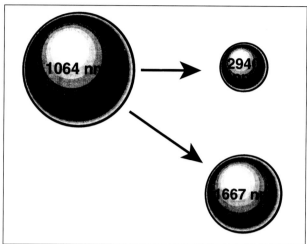

Figure 5-9. Down conversion in an optical parametric oscillator divides the energy in a 1064-nm photon between two photons of longer wavelengths.

Infrared Lasers

Laser output at a mid-IR wavelength of around 3 microns is strongly absorbed by tissue water. Several mid-IR sources have been tested for corneal ablation. In general, because there is no photochemical decomposition, mid-IR lasers have larger ablation depth per pulse and produce more thermal coagulation of adjacent tissue. The Q-switched Er:YAG laser at 2.94 microns and 100 nanoseconds has an ablation efficiency of 4 microns.[14] Down conversion of the Q-switched Nd:YAG laser with the optical parametric oscillator (OPO, Figure 5-9)[24] or the Raman shift (Figure 5-10)[25] can produce mid-IR pulses of less than 10 nanoseconds. One report[24] showed that the OPO can produce ablation depths per pulse under 1 micron and a thermal coagulation zone of 0.1 to 0.2 microns, which are comparable to the 193-nm excimer laser. The lack of thermal damage is explained by an ablation mechanism called "photospallation," where tissue is removed by a fast expanding bipolar pressure wave that induces a strong mechanical tension at the surface of the tissue. Further studies are needed to determine whether photospallation by nanosecond or subnanosecond mid-IR pulses will eventually rival the clinical results of the 193-nm excimer.

ACCURACY OF ABERRATION CORRECTION

The goal of eliminating higher-order aberrations from the eye demands more accuracy in both measurement and ablation. The required resolution

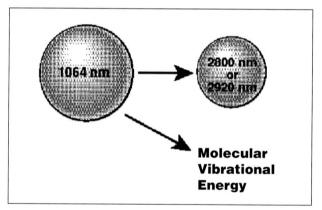

Figure 5-10. Down conversion by Raman shift. A 1064-nm photon is absorbed and a less energetic photon at a longer wavelength is emitted. The balance of energy is left behind as vibration energy in the Raman medium.

increases with increasing Zernike-order aberration. To understand these issues, we will review the representation of optical aberrations (Zernike polynomials), establish the relevant criteria for optimal optical and visual performance, and compare these criteria to the performance of current lasers and wavefront sensors.

Zernike Polynomials

Wavefront aberrations can be represented by a series of terms called Zernike circle polynomials.[26] Zernike polynomials can also be used to represent an optical surface such as corneal elevation topography.[27] Zernike polynomials are ideal for describing the optics of the eye because they are defined based on a circular geometry (the cornea and pupil have circular geometry), can be interpreted in terms of common optical elements, and are mathematically well-behaved.

The Zernike term Z_n^m is defined by a radial order n and an azimuthal frequency m. m is never larger than n and $m-n$ must be an even integer (see Appendix One for standards for expressing the Zernike polynomial for ocular optics). They are defined inside a unit circle. For our application, we would normalize the radial dimension against the radius of the optical zone (radius = 3 mm for a 6-mm diameter circular optical zone). The lowest-order Zernike polynomials are familiar quantities. Z_0^0 is a flat piston, such as a flat circular phototherapeutic keratectomy (PTK) ablation. Z_1^1 and Z_1^{-1} represent tilts along the vertical and horizontal meridians. Z_2^0 represents defocus or spherical equivalent refractive error. Z_2^2 and Z_2^{-2} are cardinal (against- and with-the-rule) and oblique (45/135 degrees) astigmatisms. Zernike polynomials provide us with a tool to separate these spherocylindrical aberrations from higher-order aberrations. A more detailed treatment of Zernike polynomials is found in Chapter Six.

Zernike polynomials have nice mathematical properties, such as orthogonality, normality, and completeness. Completeness means that any aberration over a circular aperture can be completely represented by a series of Zernike polynomial terms. Orthogonality means that each Zernike term can be arithmatically manipulated and recombined separately. For example, lenticular and corneal components of Z_2^2 (cardinal astigmatism) can be simply added arithmatically to give the Z_2^2 for the eye. Orthogonality is lacking in our traditional definitions of positive and negative cylinders. For example, 1 D of positive corneal cylinder at axis 180 degrees plus 1 D of positive lenticular cylinder at axis 30 degrees do not add up to 2 D of positive cylinder along any axis. In order to add them by simple arithmetic, they need to be broken down into orthogonal terms. One diopter of positive cylinder at axis 180 degrees is broken down into 0.5 D of Z_2^0 (defocus or spherical equivalent) and 1 D of Z_2^2 (cardinal astigmatism). Normality means that the unit measures of Zernike terms are adjusted so that they contribute equally to the root mean square (RMS) wavefront aberration. For example, 1 micron RMS of Z_2^0 plus 1 micron RMS of Z_2^2 equals $\sqrt{2}$ microns of combined RMS aberration. The RMS wavefront aberration of an optical system is directly related to its

An aberration-free optical system has a Strehl ratio of 1. Strehl ratio decreases with increasing aberration.[30]

Strehl ratio, a measure of optical performance.[30] The Strehl ratio is the ratio between the actual and ideal values of maximum light intensity at the focus. An aberration-free optical system has a Strehl ratio of 1. Strehl ratio decreases with increasing aberration.[30]

Wavefront Elevation

Criteria for Optical and Visual Performance

There are two approximate criteria on how much wavefront aberration can be present in a near diffraction-limited optical system. Both are based on a cutoff Strehl ratio of 0.8.

The Marechal criteria[26] states that an optical system can be regarded as well-corrected when the normalized intensity at the diffraction focus is ≥ 0.8 and that this condition is equivalent to the requirement that the RMS departure of the wavefront from a reference sphere that is centered on the diffraction focus shall not exceed the value $\lambda/14$, where λ is the wavelength of light.

Rayleigh's quarter wavelength rule[26] is based on the amplitude of maximum wavefront departure rather than the RMS departure. Rayleigh showed that when a system suffers from primary spherical aberration of such an amount that the wavefront in the exit pupil departs from the Gaussian reference sphere by less than a quarter wavelength, the intensity at the Gaussian focus is diminished by < 20%. Other types of aberration also roughly follow this $\lambda/4$ rule.

In the human eye, how many orders of Zernike terms must we eliminate in order to achieve a diffraction limit? By applying the Marechal criterion, Liang and Williams showed that correction of up to fourth-order (up to $Z_4^{\pm 4}$) Zernike terms is sufficient for a 3.4 mm pupil, and correction of up to eighth-order terms is needed for a 7.3 mm pupil.[10]

Besides monochromatic optical aberration, human vision is also limited by chromatic aberration and photoreceptor spacing; thus the more relevant criteria relates to visual performance as a whole rather than optical performance in isolation. However, it is also harder to establish visual performance criteria with our current state of knowledge. Experience with adaptive optics correction of the eye's monochromatic aberrations suggest that correction of up to fourth-order Zernike terms is sufficient for reaching the photoreceptor resolution limit in some subjects. Chapter Two provides a detailed account of how visual performance is related to optical aberrations.

Precision of Laser Ablation

In order to bring the eye to near diffraction-limited performance, the laser system must be able to sculpt the cornea with sufficient precision to meet the Rayleigh and Marechal criteria we just discussed.

Where the ablation depth is small, the precision of laser ablation is limited by the ablation depth per pulse. Current ArF excimer lasers used in vision correction operate at an ablation depth per pulse of roughly 0.25 microns. This corresponds to a change in wavefront retardation of 0.09 microns (equation 1). When applied to the average visible wavelengths (green light at 0.51 microns), the Rayleigh quarter wavelength rule requires that the wavefront departure be < 0.13 microns. Therefore, the 193-nm excimer laser satisfies the Rayleigh rule. The 213-nm fifth harmonic of the Nd:YAG laser has also demonstrated this level of precision.

The RMS accuracy of laser ablation is influenced by many factors. Pulse-to-pulse energy fluctuation affects all lasers. For broadbeam lasers, beam profile inhomogeneity, plume dynamics,[18] and aperture steps can all introduce errors. Small spot scanning lasers are limited by eye-tracking accuracy. Whether these lasers satisfy the Marechal criterion can only be determined empirically. I doubt that broadbeam lasers can satisfy the $\lambda/14$ criterion based on clinical experience with steep central islands and other types of ablation irregularity. Small spot scanning lasers with accurate eye tracking are likely to be essential to customized corneal ablation.

Precision and Accuracy of Wavefront Sensors

According to the Marechal criterion, wavefront sensors for a custom cornea need to measure wavefront elevation with a RMS precision and accuracy of better than $\lambda/14$. For green light, $\lambda/14$ is 0.04 microns.

The precision of a wavefront sensor can be easily gauged by the variability of repeat measurements. This performance figure should be routinely reported for any study using a wavefront sensor. The repeatability of ocular wavefront mapping appears to be limited at about $\lambda/14$ by the variability of the eye.[10] A Hartmann-Shack wavefront sensor can have an intrinsic repeatability of $\lambda/487$.[10]

The accuracy of wavefront sensors needs to be measured against a reference optical system with well-characterized optical aberrations. A trefoil phase plate has been proposed as a reliable standard that is relatively insensitive to displacement and tilt in a test setup.[4]

Transverse Resolution

Resolution of Wavefront Measurement

The transverse (x-y) resolution requirement for wavefront sensors proves to be relatively easy to satisfy. Wang, et al showed that a uniform sampling of 80 points is sufficient for the computation of eighth-order Zernicke coefficients.[30] Radial sampling (such as the Nidek slit skioloscope) requires more elements to achieve similar performance, depending on the specific sampling pattern.[30]

Spot Size for a Scanning Laser

The transverse resolution requirement for aberration correction with a scanning laser depends on the order of aberration one wishes to correct. An approximate guide to the spot size requirement is illustrated in Figure 5-11. The highest order monomial in a Zernike polynomial of order n is $(r/R)^n$, where r is the radial distance and R is the radius of the optical zone. This monomial varies most rapidly near the edge of the optical zone. In order to at least approximately reproduce this rapid spatial variation, the full-width-half-maximum (FWHM) laser spot size should be less than twice the distance between the half-maximum point of $(r/R)^n$ and the edge of the optical zone. Therefore, the FWHM spot size needs to be less than $2 R (1 - 0.5^{1/n})$. For an optical zone radius of 3 mm, the maximum FWHM spot size for fourth-order correction is 1.0 mm (see Figure 5-11). For eighth-order correction, it is 0.5 mm. These conclusions are confirmed in more detailed numerical simulations of ablation outcome with beam diameters between 0.5 and 2.0 mm (full results to be published). Thus, scanning lasers with 2-mm spot diameters are inadequate for correction of higher-order aberrations. Current scanning lasers with 1-mm spot diameter may be adequate for the correction of aberrations up to fourth-order Zernike terms.

Are Current Systems Accurate Enough for Customized Corneal Ablation?

The above review indicates that at least some of the current wavefront sensors and small-beam scanning laser systems are precise and accurate enough to correct a significant fraction of the eye's higher-order aberrations. This is what makes the custom

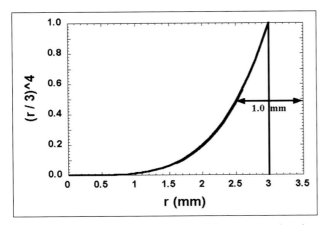

Figure 5-11. Graphic estimation of the FWHM that fits the fourth-order monomial, assuming a 3 mm radius optical zone.

cornea challenge so exciting. There is no fundamental physical reason why we should not succeed. The main stumbling blocks to success are likely to come from the variability of the eye itself. During surgery, the variability of corneal hydration may limit the accuracy of tissue removal even with a perfectly accurate laser. The cornea responds to the surgery with epithelial thickness modulation, hydration shifts, structural changes, and stromal remodeling. These changes may be difficult to predict. The cornea and lens undergo aging changes that may degrade the aberration correction over time. Only long-term clinical experience will tell us how much real-life benefit we will derive from a custom cornea.

REFERENCES

1. Smirnov MS. Measurement of wave aberration in the human eye. *Biophysics.* 1961;6:52-64.

2. Howland HC, Howland B. A subjective method for the measurement of monochromatic aberrations of the eye. *J Opt Soc Am A.* 1977;67(11):1508-1518.

3. Charman WN. Wavefront aberration of the eye: a review. *Optom Vis Sci.* 1991;68(8):574-583.

4. Thibos LN, Applegate RA, Schwiegerling JT, et al. Standards for reporting the optical aberrations of eyes. In: V Lakshminarayanan, ed. *Vision Science and its Applications.* Washington, DC: Optical Society of America; 2000.

5. Munnerlyn CR, Koons SJ, Marshall J. Photorefractive keratectomy: a technique for laser refractive surgery. *J Cataract Refract Surg.* 1988;14(1):46-52.

6. Gauthier CA, Fagerholm D, Epstein D, et al. Failure of mechanical epithelial removal to reverse persistent hyperopia after photorefractive keratectomy. Comments. *J Refract Surg.* 1996;12(5):601-6.

7. Gauthier CA, Holden BA, Epstein D, et al. Factors affecting epithelial hyperplasia after photorefractive keratectomy. Comments. *J Cataract Refract Surg.* 1997;23(7):1042-50.

8. Malacara D, DeVore SL. Interferogram evaluation and wavefront fitting. In: D Malacara, ed. *Optical Shop Testing.* John Wiley & Sons, Inc; 1992:455-499.

9. Artal P, Santamaria J, Bescos J. Retrieval of wave aberration of human eyes from actual point spread function data. *J Opt Soc Am A.* 1988;A5:1201-6.

10. Liang J, Williams DR. Aberrations and retinal image quality of the normal human eye. *J Opt Soc Am A.* 1997;14(11):2873-2883.

11. Liang J, Grimm B, Goelz S, et al. Objective measurement of wave aberrations of the human eye with the use of a Hartmann-Shack wave-front sensor. *J Opt Soc Am A.* 1994;11(7):1949-1957.

12. Yariv A. *Optical Electronics.* 3rd ed. New York, NY: Holt, Rinehart and Winston, Inc; 1985.

13. Sauerbrey R, Pettit GH. Theory for the etching of organic materials by ultraviolet laser pulses. *Applied Physics Letters.* 1989;55(5):421-3.

14. Mrochen M, Semshichen V, Funk RH, et al. Limitations of erbium:YAG laser photorefractive keratectomy. *J Refract Surg.* 2000;16(1):51-9.

15. Pettit GH, Ediger MN. Corneal-tissue absorption coefficients for 193- and 213-nm ultraviolet radiation. *Applied Optics.* 1996;35(19):3386-3391.

16. Trokel SL, Srinivasan R, Braren B. Excimer laser surgery of the cornea. *Am J Ophthalmol.* 1983;96(6):710-5.

17. Puliafito CA, Stern D, Krueger RR, et al. High-speed photography of excimer laser ablation of the cornea. *Arch Ophthalmol.* 1987;105(9):1255-9.

18. Noack J, Tonnies R, Hohla K, et al. Influence of ablation plume dynamics on the formation of central islands in excimer laser photorefractive keratectomy. *Ophthalmology.* 1997;104(5):823-30.

19. Krueger RR, Trokel SL, Schubert HD. Interaction of ultraviolet laser light with the cornea. *Invest Ophthalmol Vis Sci.* 1985;26(11):1455-64.

20. Kitai MS, Popkov VL, Semchishen VA, et al. The physics of UV laser cornea ablation. *IEEE J Quant Electron.* 1991; 27:302-307.

21. Krueger RR, Trokel SL. Quantitation of corneal ablation by ultraviolet laser light. *Arch Ophthalmol.* 1985;103(11):1741-2.

22. Dair GT, Pelouch WS, van Saarloos PP, et al. Investigation of corneal ablation efficiency using ultraviolet 213-nm solid state laser pulses. *Invest Ophthalmol Vis Sci.* 1999;40(11):2752-6.

23. Gailitis RP, Ren QS, Thompson KP, et al. Solid state ultraviolet laser (213 nm) ablation of the cornea and synthetic collagen lenticules. *Lasers Surg Med.* 1991;11(6):556-62.

24. Telfair WB, Puliafito CA, Dobi ET, et al. Histological

comparison of corneal ablation with Er:YAG laser, Nd:YAG optical parametric oscillator, and excimer laser. *J Refract Surg.* 2000;16(1):40-50.

25. Stern D, Puliafito CA, Dobi ET, et al. Infrared laser surgery of the cornea. Studies with a Raman-shifted neodymium:YAG laser at 2.80 and 2.92 micron. *Ophthalmology.* 1988;95(10):1434-41.

26. Born M, Wolf E. *Principles of Optics.* 7th ed. Cambridge, England: Cambridge University Press; 1999.

27. Schwiegerling J, Greivenkamp JE, Miller JE. Representation of videokeratoscopic height data with Zernike polynomials. *J Opt Soc Am A.* 1995;12(10):2105-2113.

28. Thibos LN, Wheeler W, Horner D. Power vectors: an application of Fourier analysis to the description and statistical analysis of refractive error. Comments. *Optom Vis Sci.* 1997;74(6):367-75.

29. Huang D, Stulting RD, Carr JD, et al. Multiple regression and vector analyses of laser in situ keratomileusis for myopia and astigmatism. *J Refract Surg.* 1999;15(5):538-49.

30. Wang JY, Silva DE. Wavefront interpretation with Zernike polynomials. *Applied Optics.* 1980;19(9):1510-1518.

Wavefront-Guided Custom Ablation

BASIC SCIENCE SECTION

Chapter Six

Assessment of Optical Quality

Larry N. Thibos, PhD
Raymond A. Applegate, OD, PhD

Contemporary visual optics research is changing our mindset, our way of thinking about the optical system of the eye, and in the process is redefining the field of visual optics. In the past, optical imperfections of the eye were conceived as simple refractive errors—defocus, astigmatism, and perhaps a bit of prism. Although clinical students learned about other kinds of optical imperfections, such as spherical aberration, coma, oblique astigmatism, and the other Seidel aberrations, those concepts were confined to courses in optical theory, not to clinical practice. This is for good reason: these higher-order aberrations of the eye could not be measured routinely in the clinic, and even if they could, we did not have the means to correct them optically at a reasonable cost to patients. Furthermore, since the effects of such aberrations on visual function were largely unknown, there was little reason to suppose that correcting them would do any good for the patient's vision. However, the introduction of laser refractive surgery, with its potential for removing as well as introducing unwanted optical aberrations into the eye, demands changes in established ways of thinking and answers to these unresolved issues.

Today, optical imperfections of the eye are being re-examined within a comprehensive theoretical framework that expresses the combined effect of all the eye's aberrations in a two-dimensional aberration map of the pupil plane. An aberration map is similar in concept to corneal topographic maps used

> An aberration map is similar in concept to corneal topographic maps used to describe the corneal surface.

to describe the corneal surface. The major difference is that a corneal map describes the curvature of a physical surface, whereas an aberration map describes the difference between a wavefront of light and a reference wavefront. By concentrating our attention on light instead of the refracting surface, we gain an ability to compute image quality on the retina for simple points of light, for clinical test targets, or for any complex object in the real world. For example, Figure 6-1 shows a wavefront aberration map for a defocused eye from which the retinal image of an acuity chart may be computed. Such computations are poised to become routine clinical tools of the future for predicting the visual benefit of aberration correction to the patient, and for explaining the risks and visual consequences of unintended increases in optical aberrations following refractive surgery or other forms of treatment.

Customized corneal ablation is a surgical procedure designed to improve the optical quality of the eye, thereby improving vision. To assess the outcome of this procedure requires measures of the direct effect on retinal image quality and secondary effects on visual performance and the quality of visual experience. A variety of methods for specifying optical quality are well established in the field of optics and may be readily applied to the optical image on the retina. Similarly, a variety of visual performance measures are sensitive to the optical quality of the retinal image and therefore may be used to assess the effect of refractive surgery on vision. However, optical limits normally imposed by the eye's optical aberrations may recede in the near future if refractive surgery, contact lenses, or intraocular lenses (IOLs) improve retinal image quality beyond limits imposed by the neural component of the visual system. If this occurs, then common measures of visual performance such as letter acuity, which are traditionally regarded as good measures of optical quality of the retinal image, may no longer be optically limited. When this happens, visual performance will be limited instead by the neural architecture and physiology of the retina and visual brain, thereby generating a demand for new measures of vision that are sensitive to even the smallest departures from perfect retinal image quality.

MEASURES OF OPTICAL QUALITY

The quality of an optical system may be specified in three different, but related, ways. The first method is to describe the detailed shape of the image for a simple geometrical object such as a point of light, or a line. The distribution of light in the image plane is called a *point spread function* (PSF) for a point object or a *line spread function* (LSF) for a line object. Simple measurements derived from these functions, such as the width (blur circle diameter) or height (Strehl ratio) of the intensity distribution, are taken as figures of merit that capture the blurring effects of optical imperfections.

The second method is a description of the loss of contrast suffered when an image of a sinusoidal grating object is cast. The sinusoidal grating is a very special object in optics because it has the unique property of producing images of the same form. In other words, a sinusoidal grating object forms sinusoidal images with the same spatial frequency (expressed in cycles/degree) and the same orientation. Thus, gratings make it easy to specify the optical effect of the

This property of sinusoidal grating objects, known as "preservation of form," is strictly true only if the aberrations of the imaging system remain the same over the full extent of the object.

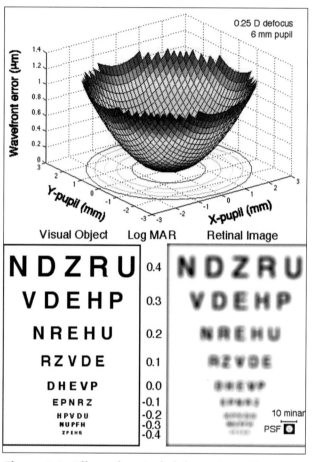

Figure 6-1. Effect of optical defocus (0.25 D, 6-mm pupil diameter) on the aberration map (top) and simulated retinal image of an eye chart (bottom). Method of calculation is to first determine the PSF, which is then convolved with the eye chart to yield the retinal image.

In visual science, a grating is usually described in *polar* form in terms of its spatial frequency and orientation. An alternative—*rectangular* form in terms of spatial frequency in two orthogonal x- and y-directions—is usually preferred in mathematical treatments

imaging system in terms of just two parameters: spatial contrast and spatial phase. The ratio of image contrast to object contrast captures the blurring effects of optical imperfections, and the variation of this ratio with spatial frequency and orientation of the grating object is called the modulation transfer function (MTF). The difference between the spatial phase of the image and the phase of the object captures the prismatic displacements induced by optical imperfections. The variation of this phase difference with spatial frequency and orientation of the grating object is called the phase transfer function (PTF). Taken together, the MTF and PTF define the optical transfer function (OTF) of an imaging system. One of the most important results of optical theory in the 20th century is the linking of the PSF, LSF, MTF, PTF, and OTF by means of a mathematical operation known as the Fourier transform.[1,2] Furthermore, given these characterizations of an imaging system, one may use optical theory to compute the expected retinal image for any visual object, thus overcoming the great handicap imposed on clinicians and visual scientists by the natural inaccessibility of the retinal image.

This chapter examines a third method for specifying optical quality in terms of underlying optical aberrations rather than the secondary effect of those aberrations on image quality. Such a description may be couched in terms of the deviation of light rays from perfect reference rays (ray aberrations) or in terms of the deviation of optical wavefronts from the ideal reference wavefront (wavefront aberrations). This aberration method is a more fundamental approach to the description of optical imperfections of eyes, from which all of the secondary measures of optical quality described above (PSF, LSF, MTF, PTF and OTF) may be derived. It is also the most useful approach for customized corneal ablation since the aberration function of an eye is a prescription for optical perfection.

DEFINITION AND INTERPRETATION OF ABERRATION MAPS

From a clinical perspective, perhaps the most useful interpretation of optical aberration maps is in terms of errors of optical path length (OPL). The OPL concept specifies the number of times a light wave must oscillate in traveling from one point to another. Since the propagation velocity of light is slower in the watery refractive media of the eye than in air, more oscillations will occur in the eye compared to the same physical distance in air. Thus, by defining OPL as the product of physical path length with refractive index, OPL becomes a measure of the number of oscillations executed by a propagating ray of light. This is an important concept because light rays emitted by a point source will propagate in many directions, but if all the rays have the same OPL, then every ray represents the same number of oscillations. Consequently, light at the end of each ray will have

the same temporal phase and this locus of points with a common phase represents a *wavefront* of light. A propagating wavefront of light is defined by the locus of points in space lying at the same OPL from a common point source of light. To define the aberrations of an optical system, we compare the OPL for a ray passing through any point (x,y) in the plane of the exit pupil, with the chief ray passing through the pupil center (0,0). The result is called the optical path difference (OPD). The aberration structure of the eye's optical system is summarized by a two-dimensional map showing how OPD varies across the eye's pupil.

For a perfect imaging system, the OPL is the same for all light rays traveling from the object point to the image point; therefore, OPD = 0 for all (x,y) locations in the pupil. In the case of an eye, this means that rays of light from a single point object that pass through different points in the pupil will arrive at the retinal image point having oscillated the same number of times. Such rays will have the same temporal phase and will therefore add constructively to produce a perfect image. If, on the other hand, light passing through different points in the pupil arrive with different phases because they traveled along paths of different OPLs, then the system is aberrated and the quality of the image will suffer. Thus, by conceiving of optical aberrations as differences in optical path length it is easy to see how aberrations might arise due to:

1. Thickness anomalies of the tear film, cornea, lens, anterior chamber, posterior chamber, etc.
2. Because of refractive index anomalies of the ocular media that might accompany inflammation, disease, aging, etc.
3. Because of decentering or tilting of the various optical components of the eye with respect to each other.

A concrete example of the OPL concept is illustrated in Figure 6-2. For a myopic eye with no other aberrations, the optical path is shorter for rays passing near the pupil margin compared to rays passing through the pupil center. Consequently, the best retinal image of a point object will be formed if we compensate for this variation in optical path length by placing the point source at the eye's far point. Now the wavefront of light enters the eye as a concave wavefront such that the central rays arrive at the eye before the marginal rays, giving them a head start so that when they follow a longer optical path through the eye, they arrive in-phase with the marginal rays.

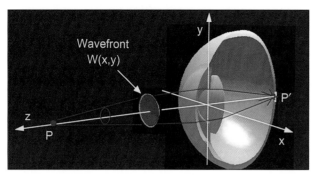

Figure 6-2. Example of a diverging wavefront from source P being focused to retinal point P′ by a myopic eye. Reversing the direction of light propagation, light reflected from retinal point P′ emerges from the eye as a wavefront converging on point P. When referenced to the x-y plane of the pupil, the wavefront shape W(x,y) is also an aberration map of the eye.

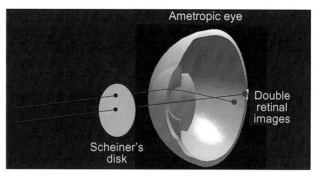

Figure 6-3. Scheiner's disk isolates rays, allowing their aberrated direction of propagation to be traced. An ametropic eye will form two retinal images for each object point when viewing through a Scheiner disk with two apertures.

In short, to obtain the optimum retinal image requires the optical distance from each object point to its image be the same for every path through the pupil. The wavefront aberration map indicates the extent to which this ideal condition is violated.

By reversing the direction of light propagation in Figure 6-2, we achieve a more practical definition of an aberration map for the eye. It follows from the preceding discussion that if the retinal point P′ is a source of light reflected out of the eye, then the shape of the emerging wavefront is determined by the variation of OPL across the eye's pupil. If the eye is optically perfect and emmetropic, this reflected wavefront would be a plane wave propagating in the positive z-direction. Thus, for distance vision, any departure of the emerging wavefront from the x-y plane is an optical aberration. On the other hand, for near vision the reflected wavefront emerging from the eye must be compared with a spherical wavefront centered on the fixation point. In practice, the distance W(x,y) between the reflected wavefront emerging from the eye and the corresponding reference sphere is taken as a measure of the wavefront aberration function of the eye for the given viewing distance. By convention, positive aberrations occur when the marginal ray travels a shorter OPL than does the central (chief) ray, as in the case of a myopic eye shown in Figure 6-2. Therefore, by this sign convention, W(x,y) = -OPD(x,y).

In summary, the shape of a wavefront of light reflected out of the eye from a point source on the retina is determined by the OPD for rays passing through each point in the eye's pupil. Therefore, a map of OPD across the pupil plane is equivalent to a mathematical description, W(x,y), of the shape of the aberrated wavefront that emerges from the eye. Either may be used as an aberration map of the eye. Such maps are fundamental characterizations of the optical quality of the eye that may be used to compute other common metrics of image quality (eg, the PSF or OTF) from which we may compute the expected retinal image of any visual target.

METHODS FOR MEASURING ABERRATION MAPS OF EYES

The current explosion of interest in optical aberrations of eyes has been spawned by new technology resting on an ancient principle. Nearly 400 years ago, the celebrated Jesuit philosopher and astronomer Christopher Scheiner, professor at the University of Ingolstadt and a contemporary of Kepler and Galileo, published his 1619 treatise *Optical Foundations of the Eye* some 75 years prior to the invention of the wave theory of light by Huygens. This pioneering book[3] described a simple device (illustrated in Figure 6-3) that is widely known in ophthalmology as *Scheiner's disk*. Scheiner reasoned that if an optically imperfect eye views through an

Scheiner reasoned that if an optically imperfect eye views through an opaque disk containing two pinholes, a single distant point of light such as a star will form two retinal images.

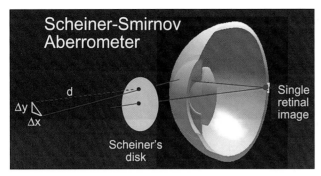

Figure 6-4. Smirnov's aberrometer used the principle of Scheiner's disk to measure the eye's optical imperfections separately at every location in the eye's entrance pupil.

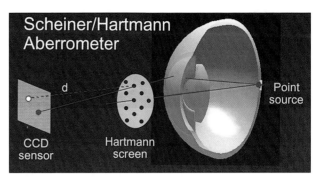

Figure 6-5. The Hartmann screen used to measure aberrations objectively is a Scheiner disk with numerous apertures.

opaque disk containing two pinholes, a single distant point of light such as a star will form two retinal images. If the eye's imperfection is a simple case of defocus, then the double retinal images can be brought into register by viewing through a spectacle lens of the appropriate power. This design idea for an optometer for measuring refractive errors of eyes was first proposed by Porterfield in 1747 and was afterward improved by Thomas Young in 1845.

A simple lens will not always bring the two retinal images into coincidence, however, so a more general method is needed for quantifying the refractive imperfection of the eye at each pupil location. Smirnov[4] was first to extend Scheiner's method by using a fixed light source for the central reference pinhole and a moveable light source for the outer pinhole, as illustrated in Figure 6-4. By adjusting the moveable source horizontally and vertically, the isolated ray of light is redirected until it intersects the fixed ray at the retina and the patient now reports seeing a single point of light. Having made this adjustment, the displacement distances Δx and Δy are measures of the ray aberration of the eye at the given pupil point.

Independent of these developments in ophthalmology, Scheiner's simple idea was re-invented by Hartmann for measuring the ray aberrations of mirrors and lenses.[5] Hartmann's method was to perforate an opaque screen with numerous holes, as shown in Figure 6-5. Each hole acts as an aperture to isolate a narrow bundle of light rays so they could be traced to determine any errors in their direction of propagation. Since rays are perpendicular to the propagating wavefront, any error in ray direction is also an error in wavefront slope. Thus, Hartmann's method is commonly referred to a *wavefront sensor*.

> Shack and Platt invented a better Hartmann screen using an array of tiny lenses that focus the light into an array of small spots, one spot for each lenslet.[5]

Seventy years later, Shack and Platt invented a better Hartmann screen using an array of tiny lenses that focus the light into an array of small spots, one spot for each lenslet.[5] Their technique came to be known as Shack's modified Hartmann screen, or Shack-Hartmann for short. To see how the array of spot images can be used to determine the shape of the wavefront, we need to look at the wavefront in cross-section, as shown in Figure 6-6. For a perfect eye, the reflected plane wave will be focused into a perfect lattice of point images, each image falling on the optical axis of the corresponding lenslet. By contrast, the aberrated eye reflects a distorted wavefront (Figure 6-7). The local slope of the wavefront is now different for each lenslet; therefore, the wavefront will be focused into a disordered collection of spot images. By measuring the displacement of each spot from its corresponding lenslet axis, we can deduce the slope of the aberrated wavefront as it entered the corresponding lenslet. Mathematical integration of slope yields the shape of the aberrated wavefront, which can then be displayed as an aberration map.

The first use of a Shack-Hartmann wavefront sensor to measure aberrations of human eyes was in 1994 by Liang and colleagues,[6] thus completing this historically meandering path to discover a fast, objective, reliable method for assessing the aberration structure of human eyes. Liang's concept of a Scheiner-Hartmann-Shack aberrometer is shown schematically in Figure 6-8. Because the shape of an aberrated wavefront changes as the light propagates,

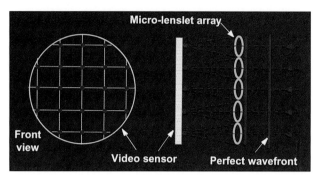

Figure 6-6. The Shack-Hartmann wavefront sensor forms a regular lattice of image points for a perfect plane wave of light.

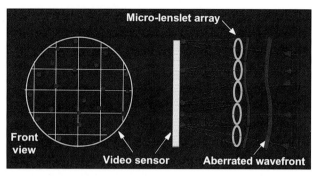

Figure 6-7. The Shack-Hartmann wavefront sensor forms an irregular lattice of image points for an aberrated wavefront of light.

it is important to analyze the reflected wavefront as soon as it passes through the eye's pupil. To do this, a pair of relay lenses focuses the lenslet array onto the entrance pupil of the eye. Optically, then, the lenslet array appears to reside in the plane of the eye's entrance pupil where it can subdivide the reflected wavefront immediately as it emerges from the eye. The array of spot images formed by the lenslet array is captured by a video sensor and then analyzed by computer to estimate the eye's aberration map.

Normal and Clinical Examples

Four examples of aberration maps for normal healthy eyes are shown in Figure 6-9. By using a grayscale to encode wavefront height, we capitalize on the human visual system's natural ability to infer depth and structure from shading. The maximum difference between the highest and lowest points on each of these maps is about 1 µm, which is a bit more than one wavelength of the light used to measure the eyes' aberrations (0.633 µm). Perhaps the most distinctive feature of these maps is the irregular shape of their smoothly varying shapes. Another important feature of aberration maps from normal eyes is the tendency to be relatively flat in the center of the pupil with aberrations growing stronger near the pupil margin. This is consistent with the literature showing that image quality is relatively good for medium-sized pupils but deteriorates as pupil diameter increases.[7,8]

For comparison, Figure 6-10 shows four examples of clinically abnormal eyes. Qualitatively, these maps have the same irregular, smoothly varying shapes as in normal eyes. The main difference is that the magnitude of the aberrations is about ten-fold larger; therefore, image quality is about ten-fold worse than

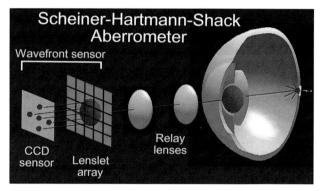

Figure 6-8. The modern aberrometer built on the Scheiner-Hartmann-Shack principle uses relay lenses to image the lenslet array into the eye's pupil plane. A video sensor (CCD) captures an image of the array of spots for computer analysis.

normal. Another important abnormality of the keratoconic patient (B) in this figure and, to a lesser extent, the dry-eye patient (A) is the tendency to have large aberrations in the middle of the pupil. The implication of this result is that image quality will be subnormal for small pupils as well as for large pupils.

Limitations

Classical analysis of data from a Shack-Hartmann wavefront sensor takes no account of the quality of individual spots formed by the lenslet array. Only the displacement of spots is needed for computing local slope of the wavefront over each lenslet aperture. However, experience has shown that the quality of dot images can vary dramatically over the pupil of a human eye as illustrated in Figure 6-11. The presence of blurred spots indicates a violation of the underlying assumption that the wavefront is locally

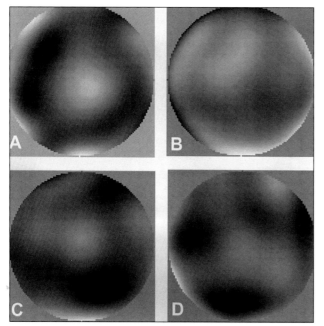

Figure 6-9. Examples of higher-order aberration maps for four normal, healthy individuals reconstructed from measurements taken with an Scheiner-Hartmann-Shack aberrometer, similar to that shown in Figure 6-8. Light areas in the map indicate the reflected wavefront is phase-advanced; dark areas indicate phase-retardance. The maximum difference between high and low points on each map is about 1 micrometer (Zernike orders 0-2 omitted for clarity).

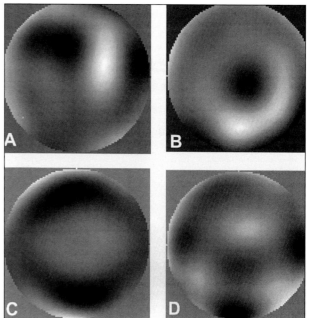

Figure 6-10. Examples of higher-order aberration maps from eyes with four different clinical conditions. A: dry eye; B: keratoconus; C: LASIK surgery; D: cataract. The maximum difference between high and low points on each map is about 10 micrometers except (D), which is closer to 1 micrometer (Zernike orders 0-2 omitted for clarity).

flat over the face of the lenslet. Two possible reasons are illustrated in Figure 6-12.

The first possibility is that the gross aberrations of the eye are so large that the wavefront is significantly curved over the area of the lenslet. The result is a blurry spot that is difficult to localize. If the aberrations are large enough, neighboring spots can even overlap, which considerably complicates the analysis. The second possible limitation involves irregular aberrations on a very fine spatial scale. Perturbations of the wavefront within the lenslet aperture are too fine to be resolved by the wavefront sensor using classical methods. Rather than displacing the spots laterally, these "micro-aberrations" scatter light and blur the spots formed by the aberrometer. Although these blurry spots are problematic, they nevertheless contain useful information about the degree and location of scattering sources inside the eye, which may prove useful in clinical applications.[9]

Taxonomy of Optical Aberrations

One systematic method for classifying the shapes of aberration maps is to conceive of each map as the weighted sum of fundamental shapes or basis functions. One popular set of *basis functions* are the Zernike polynomials. This set of mathematical functions are formed as the product of two other functions, one of which depends only on the radius r of a point in the pupil plane, and the other depends only on the meridian Θ of a point in the pupil plane. The former is a simple polynomial of the nth degree and the latter function is a harmonic of a sinusoid or cosinusoid. A pictorial dictionary of the first 28 Zernike polynomials is arranged in the form of a pyramid of basis functions in Figures 6-13a and b. Every aberration map can be represented uniquely by a weighted sum of these functions. The process of determining the weighting coefficient required to describe a given

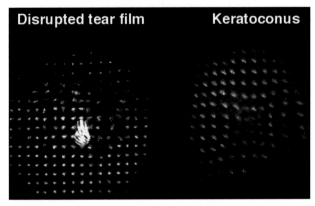

Figure 6-11. Examples of selective loss of image quality in individual spots for eyes with two different clinical conditions.

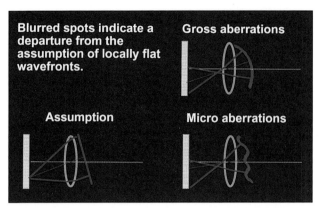

Figure 6-12. Blurring of individual spots detected by a Shack-Hartmann wavefront sensor may indicate the presence of gross aberrations of large magnitude or micro-aberrations. In either case, the blur is due to violation of the underlying assumption that the wavefront is locally flat over the lenslet aperture.

aberration map is a least-squares curve-fitting process called Zernike decomposition, which results in a vector of Zernike coefficients. Mathematical details may be found in several standard reference works.[10,11]

Recently, the Optical Society of America sponsored a taskforce of visual optics researchers to develop standards for reporting optical aberrations of eyes. Recommendations of this taskforce were presented at the 2000 Topical Meeting on Vision Science and Its Applications and will be published in full in a future issue of *Trends in Optics and Photonics*, published by the Optical Society of America.[12]

DERIVATIVES OF THE ABERRATION MAP

Klein and colleagues have suggested[13] using the slopes (first partial derivatives in x and y directions) and curvature (average of second partial derivatives in x and y) of the aberration map to supplement the interpretation of the wavefront aberration function W(x,y). As illustrated in Figure 6-14, the slope of the wavefront aberration map may be interpreted as the *transverse ray aberration*, which is defined by angle τ between the aberrated ray and the nonaberrated reference ray. The associated focusing error is called the *longitudinal ray aberration* and is equal to $1/z$ diopters (D), which may be computed as the ratio of transverse aberration to ray height in the pupil plane.

To illustrate the derivatives of the aberration map, we evaluated the wavefront error for the Indiana eye model, a simple, reduced eye model with an aspheric refracting surface that has proved useful on previous occasions for studying the aberrations of the human eye.[14] In the specific example illustrated in

Figure 6-15, the pupil diameter was 6 mm and the conic constant of the surface was set to 0.6, a value that generates a degree of spherical aberration that is typical of human eyes.[15] The wavefront aberration map W(x,y) for this model at the wavelength 589 nm (Figure 6-15A) is nearly flat in the middle of the pupil but becomes increasingly curved near the pupil margin.

Slope (Transverse Aberration)

In a symmetrical optical system, the transverse aberration τ may be measured in any meridian, but for nonsymmetrical systems it is typically computed as the partial derivative of the aberration function in the vertical as well as horizontal directions. One way to simultaneously visualize the variation of the vertical and horizontal components of transverse aberration is with a vector field (Figure 6-15B). Each arrow represents the transverse ray aberration for the pupil location marked by the tail of the arrow. The lengths of the horizontal and vertical components of each arrow give the horizontal and vertical components of angle τ, respectively. The calibration arrow in the lower left corner is 1 milliradian in length. The arrows all point toward the center of the pupil for this model eye, indicating that the light reflected out of the eye forms a converging wavefront. The arrows are longer near the pupil margin, indicating the steeper slope expected of spherical aberration.

In a perfect optical system, every ray from a point object will intersect the retina at the same location, but in an aberrated system the intersection will be

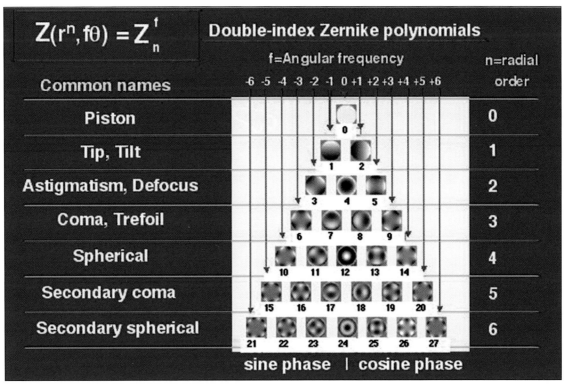

Figure 6-13a. Pictorial directory of Zernike modes used to systematically represent the aberration structure of the eye.

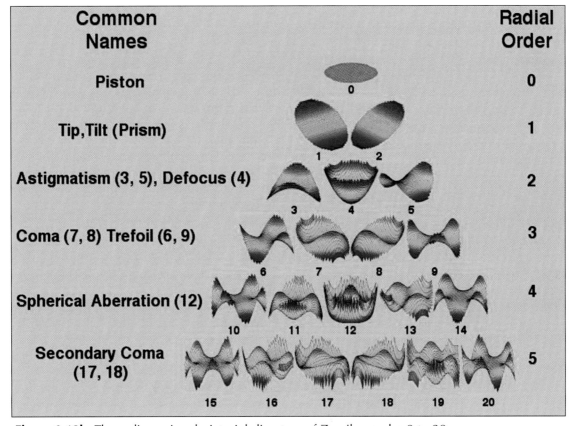

Figure 6-13b. Three-dimensional pictorial directory of Zernike modes 0 to 20.

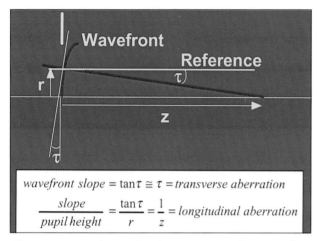

wavefront slope $= \tan\tau \cong \tau =$ *transverse aberration*

$$\frac{slope}{pupil\ height} = \frac{\tan\tau}{r} = \frac{1}{z} = longitudinal\ aberration$$

Figure 6-14. Relationship between wavefront, its first and second derivatives, and measures of transverse aberration (t) and longitudinal aberration (1/z).

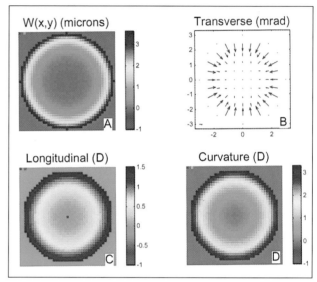

Figure 6-15. Four methods for displaying an aberration map. A: Height of reflected wavefront from the (x,y) plane perpendicular to the path of the chief ray (line-of-sight for foveal vision). B: Vector field map showing the displacement of each spot image from the optical axis of the corresponding lenslet. C: Axial power map obtained by dividing average wavefront slope at each pupil location by the radial distance of the point from the pupil center. D: Local curvature in the wavefront obtained by applying the Laplacian operator to the wavefront. Maps in C and D are calibrated in diopters.

displaced by an amount and direction indicated by the arrows in Figure 6-15B. We can then visualize where each ray strikes the retina by collapsing all of the arrows so that their tails coincide (the ideal image point) with the head of each arrow, showing where the ray from the corresponding pupil location intersects the retina. In optical engineering, such visualization would be called a "spot diagram" and would be taken as a discrete approximation to the continuous PSF.

Slope Per Unit of Pupil Radius (Longitudinal Aberration)

From the geometry of Figure 6-14 we noted that the ratio of wavefront slope to r, the distance from the pupil center to the given point on the wavefront, is the inverse of the distance between pupil center and the point where the aberrated ray crosses the optical axis. This latter quantity is the traditional definition of longitudinal ray aberration (also known as axial power). In general, the longitudinal aberration has horizontal and vertical components just like the transverse aberration, which reflects the fact that the refracted ray may be skew to the optical axis. In practice we simplify the situation by resolving the transverse ray arrow into radial and tangential components and then use the radial component to compute the longitudinal aberration. This allows us to reduce a vector plot, as in Figure 6-15B, into a scalar plot (Figure 6-15C).

If the eye suffers only from defocus, then the longitudinal aberration is constant and equal to the spherical refractive error of the eye. For other aberra-

tions, such as coma or spherical aberration, the longitudinal aberration varies with pupil location and may be depicted with a longitudinal aberration map like that shown in Figure 6-15C. The scale of this map is calibrated in diopters to enhance its clinical interpretation. For this particular example, the increased power near the margin represents 1.7 D of spherical aberration, which is the same result obtained by finite ray tracing.[15]

Curvature (Local Power)

The second derivative of the aberration function measures the rate of change of slope of the wavefront (ie, local curvature). The average curvature in the horizontal and vertical directions is called the Laplacian of the aberration map. An example of the Laplacian curvature map for the Indiana eye model is shown in Figure 6-15D. The scale of this map is also calibrated in diopters to enhance its clinical interpretation. Notice that the longitudinal aberration underestimates local curvature, which means that local segments of the wavefront come to focus

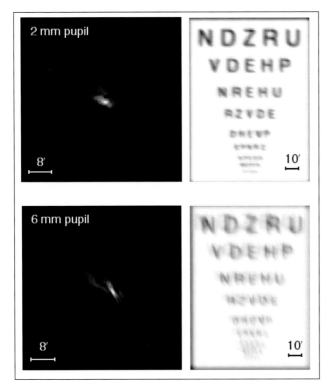

Figure 6-16. PSFs (left panels) and simulated retinal images of an eye chart (right panels) for the eye in Figure 6-10C analyzed for two pupil diameters (2 mm, 6 mm).

before the rays intersect the optical axis. Some difference is to be expected because the traditional measure of longitudinal aberration is proportional to wavefront slope, whereas curvature is a measure of the rate of change of slope.

RELATED MEASURES OF OPTICAL QUALITY

PSF and Strehl's Ratio

The PSF is computed as the squared magnitude of the Fourier transform of a complex-valued pupil function built from the aberration map. Since the PSF represents the intensity distribution of light in the image of a point source, it should be a highly localized, bright spot. Diffraction sets a lower limit to the diameter of the spot and an upper limit to the intensity in the center of the spot. A common metric of image quality, called *Strehl's ratio*, is computed as the ratio of the actual intensity in the center of the spot to the maximum intensity of a diffraction-limited spot.

As pupil diameter increases, the intensity of a diffraction-limited spot increases faster than the intensity of an aberrated spot, which tends to reduce Strehl's ratio. It is not uncommon for the PSF of human eyes to have multiple peaks, which complicates the simple notion of Strehl's ratio. More importantly, it signals the formation of two or more point images for a single point object. This condition of di- or polyplopia has great clinical significance because of its implications for visual performance and the quality of visual experience.[16,17]

Examples of PSFs computed from the wavefront aberration function displayed in Figure 6-10C are shown for small and large pupils in Figure 6-16. In the dark, this patient's natural pupil diameter was 6 mm, which was large enough to expose significant amounts of aberration introduced by refractive surgery. The effect of these aberrations was to blur the central spot while simultaneously spreading some of the light into a long, secondary, wispy tail. Since each point of light in an object will produce this same type of pattern, the retinal image of an eye chart will be blurred and contain a second, lower-contrast ghost image that hampers legibility. This situation may be contrasted with the much improved image quality for daylight viewing through a 2-mm pupil, which is small enough to exclude most of the aberrations of this patient's eye. Under these conditions the PSF is more compact, which results in a clearer, more focused retinal image.

> The reader should be aware that to meet publication standards, PSFs are usually scaled arbitrarily to use the full range of gray levels available for reproduction. The results are potentially misleading. In reality, the total amount of light in the PSF is determined by the intensity of the point source, the eye's pupil diameter, and absorption losses in the ocular media.

MTF, PTF, and OTF

The OTF, comprised of the MTF and PTF, is computed as the inverse Fourier transform of the PSF. The MTF component represents the contrast of the retinal image for a sinusoidal grating target of 100% contrast. Diffraction sets an upper limit to the contrast of the retinal image and therefore the ratio of MTFs for a real eye to a diffraction-limited optical system is a measure of the losses of contrast due to aberrations. One implication of the Fourier transform relationship between the OTF and the PSF is that Strehl's ratio, defined as the ratio of intensities at the center of the test PSF and a diffraction-limited PSF, is equal to the volume under the OTF of an aberrated system divided by the volume under the OTF for the same system without aberrations. In general, the OTF, PSF, and MTF are two-dimensional functions of spatial frequency and orientation, or equivalently, of spatial frequency in the x and y directions. Such functions may be reduced to one-dimensional graphs by averaging across orientation, a process called radial averaging.

Radially averaged MTFs for the LASIK patient in Figure 6-16 are shown in Figure 6-17 for small and large pupils. The transfer of contrast from object to image is from three to five times lower for the 6-mm pupil condition compared to the 2-mm condition over most of the visible range of spatial frequencies. It is to be expected that these optical losses would be reflected directly in visual performance measurements of contrast sensitivity for grating targets.

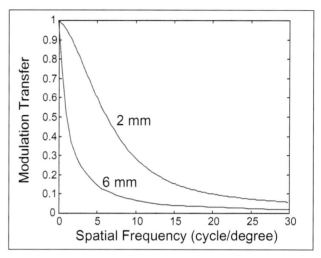

Figure 6-17. Radially averaged MTFs for the eye in Figure 6-10C analyzed for two pupil diameters (2 mm, 6 mm).

ACKNOWLEDGMENTS

Preparation of this chapter was supported by National Institutes of Health (National Eye Institute) grants R01-EY-05109 to Dr. Thibos and R01-EY-08520 to Dr. Applegate and an unrestricted grant to the Department of Ophthalmology from Research to Prevent Blindness, New York, NY.

REFERENCES

1. Gaskill JD. *Linear Systems, Fourier Transforms, and Optics.* New York, NY: John Wiley & Sons; 1978.

2. Goodman JW. *Introduction to Fourier Optics.* New York, NY: McGraw-Hill; 1968.

3. Scheiner C. Oculus, sive fundamentum opticum. *Innspruk.* 1619.

4. Smirnov MS. Measurement of the wave aberration of the human eye. *Biofizika.* 1961;6:687-703.

5. Shack RV, Platt BC. Production and use of a lenticular Hartmann screen. *J Opt Soc Am A.* 1971;61:656.

6. Liang J, Grimm B, Goelz S, Bille J. Objective measurement of the wave aberrations of the human eye using a Hartmann-Shack wavefront sensor. *J Opt Soc Am A.* 1994;11:1949-1957.

7. Campbell FW, Gubisch RW. Optical quality of the human eye. *J Physiol.* 1966;186:558-578.

8. Liang J, Williams DR. Aberrations and retinal image quality of the normal human eye. *J Opt Soc Am A.* 1997;14:28:73-2883.

9. Thibos LN, Hong X. Clinical applications of the Shack-Hartmann aberrometer. *Optom Vis Sci.* 1999;76:817-825.

10. Born M, Wolf E. *Principles of Optics.* 7th ed. Cambridge, England: Cambridge University Press; 1999.

11. Malacara D. *Optical Shop Testing.* 2nd ed. New York, NY: John Wiley & Sons, Inc; 1992.

12. Thibos LN, Applegate RA, Schwiegerling JT, Webb R. Standards for reporting the optical aberrations of eyes. *Trends in Optics and Photonics.* In press.

13. Klein SA, Garcia DD. Alternative representations of aberrations of the eye. *Vision Science and Its Applications.* Washington, DC: Optical Society of America; 2000:115-118.

14. Thibos LN, Ye M, Zhang X, Bradley A. The chromatic eye: a new reduced-eye model of ocular chromatic aberration in humans. *Applied Optics.* 1992;31:3594-3600.

15. Thibos LN, Ye M, Zhang X, Bradley A. Spherical aberration of the reduced schematic eye with elliptical refracting surface. *Optom Vis Sci.* 1997;74:548-556.

16. Woods RL, Bradley A, Atchison DA. Consequences of monocular diplopia for the contrast sensitivity function. *Vision Res.* 1996;36:3587-3596.

17. Woods RL, Bradley A, Atchison DA. Monocular diplopia caused by ocular aberrations and hyperopic defocus. *Vision Res.* 1996;36:3597-3606.

Chapter Seven

Visual Performance Assessment

Raymond A. Applegate, OD, PhD
Gene Hilmantel, OD, MS
Larry N. Thibos, PhD

INTRODUCTION

For the first time in history, it is possible to clinically measure the optical defects of the eye beyond sphere and cylinder, quickly and efficiently in the clinical environment. By all indications, this technology will soon work its way into clinical practice. There are several companies that are currently employing or planning to employ such technology to design refractive corrections intended to improve the optical quality of the retinal image beyond what is achievable with traditional spherocylindrical corrections. These "ideal" corrections may come in the form of customized corneal ablative corrections, contact lenses, intraocular lenses (IOLs), or in combination.[1]

At the time of writing, it is not clear that ideal corrections can be implemented routinely or that such corrections will routinely result in *supervision*. Supervision is vision that is significantly improved over that provided by more traditional forms of correction. In fact, surgeries to date (as of May 2000) generally increase corneal[2-5] and total eye aberrations.[6] Nonetheless, preliminary results with wavefront-guided surgery are encouraging (a decrease in the surgically induced aberrations) and pose several questions with respect to the measurement of visual performance. What will the world look like with supervision? Do we have tests of visual performance

> Supervision is vision that is significantly improved over that provided by more traditional forms of correction.

capable of quantifying the visual improvement in a clinically significant manner? When therapy induces new aberrations, do we have the tests necessary to quantify the visual complaints of our patients that have 20/20 vision but do not see as well as they used to, or whose vision changes with pupil size, or with time of day? To answer these questions, this chapter will:

1. Review the fundamental limits to visual performance imposed by optical imaging and photoreceptor sampling to determine the potential gains offered by ideal corrections.

2. Examine the losses in vision induced by less than ideal refractive corrections and their implications for visual testing.

3. Examine the nature of traditional and new clinical tests of visual performance in the context of fundamental limitations and the visual impact of less than ideal refractive corrections.

4. Identify the characteristics of the ideal clinical test to measure subtle gains and losses in visual function.

FUNDAMENTAL LIMITS TO VISUAL PERFORMANCE

What gains in visual performance are expected with "ideal" refractive corrections? Improving the optical transfer function (OTF) by removing optical aberrations increases the contrast and spatial detail of the retinal image. In a healthy visual system, these retinal image gains obtained from improving the OTF are reflected in percepts having higher contrast (increased modulation transfer) and sharper edges (decreased phase errors). These two components (modulation transfer and phase transfer) of the OTF are pupil size dependent and key to understanding the optical quality of the retinal image.

Diffraction-Limited Modulation Transfer Function

As discussed in greater detail in Chapter Two and elsewhere,[1,7-10] the importance of pupil size to modulation transfer can be easily seen by viewing plots of the diffraction-limited modulation transfer function (MTF) of the eye for a variety of pupil sizes (Figure 7-1). The diffraction-limited MTF displays the ratio of image modulation (contrast) to object contrast for perfect ocular optics as a function of the spatial frequency of a sinusoidal grating. The advantage of using sinusoidal gratings is two-fold. Sinusoidal objects are transferred to the image plane as demodulated (decreased contrast) sinusoidal images of the same frequency. (Phase changes are reflected as a shift in the location of the grating image with respect to object location and do not alter the nature of the sinusoidal luminance pattern or its image modulation. Nonetheless, phase changes are very important and will be discussed later in this chapter.) Second, through Fourier analysis, more complex patterns can be constructed as a summation of sinusoidal gratings of various frequencies, orientations, modulations, and phases. Conversely, objects can be decomposed into a series of sinusoidal gratings of various frequencies, orientations, modulations, and phases. Such decomposition allows the modulation of each frequency component to be reduced to reflect the impact of the visual system on object contrast. In turn, these demodulated spatial frequencies permit the reconstruction of an image as the eye would see it. For these reasons, the MTF and the phase transfer function (PTF) are standard measures of optical quality in the optical industry.

Notice in Figure 7-1 that the eye's diffraction-limited MTF reveals several interesting facts:

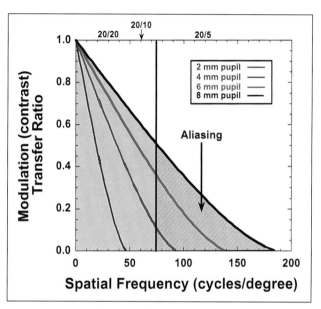

Figure 7-1. Diffraction-limited MTFs for four pupil sizes. If the object has 100% contrast, the stippled area identifies the spatial frequencies and contrast levels over which detection and recognition ("clear vision") are theoretically possible in the normal eye. The crossed-hatched area identifies the spatial frequencies and contrast levels over which detection of aliased images is possible. The area above the uppermost curve represents contrast that cannot be achieved in the retinal image. Calculations of the MTFs were made using 555-nm light and methods detailed by Smith's equation 11.38.[30]

1. Only for a uniform field (0 spatial frequency) is the object modulation (contrast) transferred to the image plane with 100% efficiency (a modulation factor of 1). This efficiency is independent of pupil size.

2. For all other frequencies, the modulation (contrast) transfer ratio is less than 1 and is pupil size dependent.

3. For higher spatial frequencies, the modulation (contrast) transfer ratio increases as pupil size increases.

4. The cut-off frequency (the spatial frequency at which the modulation goes to 0) increases as pupil size increases.

Diffraction-Limited Phase Transfer Function

The OTF is made up of two principle components: the MTF discussed above and the PTF. The PTF describes the phase shift of the image with respect to the object (Figure 7-2) as a function of spatial frequency. In a diffraction-limited optical system, object

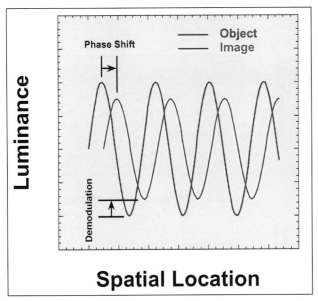

Figure 7-2. Luminance as a function of location for a sinusoidal object and image showing a 25% demodulation from object to image with a 100-degree phase shift, causing a change in image location.

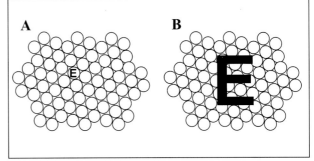

Figure 7-3. A: if a letter E is imaged such that it falls within the borders of a single photoreceptor, then the letter E cannot be differentiated from a period. B: to be seen as a letter, the E must be sampled by enough photoreceptors to differentiate the letter's component parts (reprinted with permission from Applegate RA. Limits to vision: can we do better than nature? *J Refract Surg*. In press).

location and image location are identical and there are no phase shifts. In an aberrated optical system, phase shifts can become very important and can lead to what is commonly called spurious resolution and decreased visual performance. These effects are discussed later in the chapter.

Retinal Limitations

So far we have limited our discussion to optical considerations. There is also a fundamental retinal limitation to visual performance: the ability of the photoreceptors to sample the retinal image (see Chapter Two). Photoreceptors in the foveola are on the order of 2 micrometers in diameter. The response of the photoreceptor to an input signal is graded based on photon capture within the photoreceptor. That is, within a single photoreceptor, spatial (shape) information is lost. Consequently, to differentiate a letter E from a period, the components of the letter E must be distributed over an adequate number of receptors to allow the components of the letter to be detected (Figure 7-3). Thus, the coarseness of the foveola photoreceptor mosaic limits letter acuity independent of the quality of the optics to somewhere between 20/8 and 20/10 (depending on the biological variation in foveolar receptor diameters for the particular eye of interest). At spatial frequencies beyond 75 cycles/degree (c/deg) (20/8) visual

percept will be distorted (aliased), limiting the ability of the nervous system to interpret a high-quality retinal image (see Figure 7-1). Therefore, in an optically aberrated eye capable of neural-limited acuity (20/8 to 20/10), improving the optics cannot improve acuity but will improve contrast for larger pupils.

Receptor sampling limits should not be interpreted to mean that the visual system is incapable of seeing targets having finer detail. This simply is not true. The visual system can see targets having finer detail; however, they will not appear in their true form. Because of receptor undersampling, the appearance of the image is distorted, forming what is commonly called an alias percept of the actual object (Figure 7-4). That is, the percept of the actual object takes on an appearance that can be quite different from the actual object. Consequently, photoreceptor sampling fundamentally limits acuity for larger pupils in the diffraction-limited eye.

LOSSES IN VISION INDUCED BY LESS THAN IDEAL REFRACTIVE CORRECTIONS AND THEIR IMPLICATIONS FOR VISUAL TESTING

In reality, we can only approach the diffraction limit as we correct higher and higher orders of ocular aberrations. The fact that we can only approach the ideal raises an interesting question: Do the same

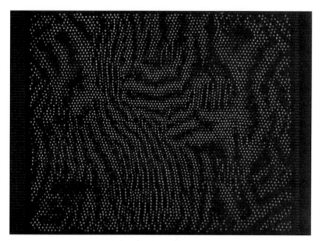

Figure 7-4. A simulated retinal view of an 80 c/deg grating (notice the edges of the pattern show the grating) being sampled by a primate foveolar retinal receptor mosaic. Undersampling creates an alias percept of the grating that appears as zebra stripes (photo courtesy of David Williams. Reprinted with permission from Applegate RA. Limits to vision: can we do better than nature? *J Refract Surg.* 2000;16:5547-5551).

gains in contrast and cut-off frequency exist when aberrations remain in the system (the system is not diffraction limited)?

MTF and Aberrations

Counter to the diffraction-limited case, in an optically aberrated system large pupils can be a disadvantage. First, the modulation transfer ratio can go negative, indicating a phase shift (light bars are now dark and dark bars are light). Second, in the diffraction-limited case (see Figure 7-1), the modulation transfer ratio first goes to zero at the cut-off frequency and remains at zero. In the aberrated case, the function can cross zero several times before reaching the cut-off frequency. The extent of these effects is dependent on the magnitude and type of the residual optical aberration. To illustrate this point, in Figure 7-5 we plot MTFs for four pupil diameters in the presence (thinner lines) and absence (thicker lines) of 0.50 diopters (D) defocus.

These effects are better illustrated by looking at the change in the modulation transfer ratio and the first zero crossover of the MTF caused by moderate aberrations (Figure 7-6). Both of these figures show that with moderate defocus, increasing pupil diameter decreases optical performance. Consequently, to maximize the benefit of increasing the pupil diameter (decreased f#) the system needs to be essentially aberration free.

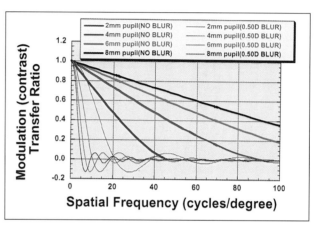

Figure 7-5. Diffraction-limited (no blur) MTFs (thick color-coded lines) and 0.50 D of defocus MTFs (color-coded thin lines) for four different pupil sizes. Calculations of the diffraction-limited MTFs were made using 555-nm light and methods detailed by Smith's equation 11.36. Calculations of the defocus MTFs were made using a geometric approximation detailed by Smith's equation 11.40.[30] Negative values reflect a phase shift and are discussed in the next section. (Note: A small error in the geometric approximation can be appreciated most clearly by the crossover of the 2-mm defocus MTF and the 2-mm diffraction MTF at low spatial frequencies. For larger pupil sizes in which the wavefront error is greater than 1 wavelength, the error in the geometric approximation of the defocus case is, for all practical purposes, inconsequential.)

Notice in Figures 7-5 and 7-6 that:
1. Counter to the diffraction-limited case, the larger the pupil the larger the loss in image contrast and cut-off frequency.
2. The defocus-induced losses in image contrast and cut-off frequency for the 2-mm pupil are less than for larger pupils, demonstrating why pinhole testing is effective clinically.

Phase and Aberrations

So far, we have emphasized the effects of optical aberrations on retinal image contrast and the resulting visual perception. Equally important are shifts in spatial phase induced by optical aberrations. It is well known, for example, that defocus can introduce phase reversals into images so that dark bars become light and light bars become dark, an effect sometimes called spurious resolution (Figure 7-7). Similar effects occur for other aberrations besides defocus, which can lead to subtle notches and other anomalies in the contrast sensitivity function (CSF).[11,12]

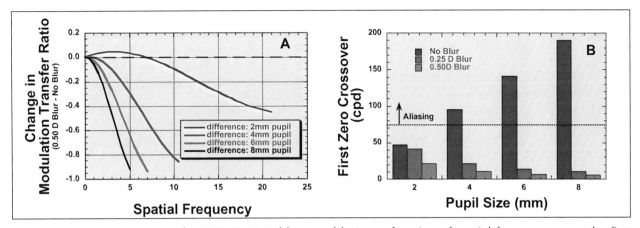

Figure 7-6. A: the change in the MTF (0.50 D blur—no blur) as a function of spatial frequency up to the first zero crossover. Notice that the loss in MTF increases as pupil size increases. (The small gain in the MTF for the 2 mm pupil between 0 and approximately 7 c/deg is an error in the calculation due to ignoring the effects of diffraction in the calculation of the blur MTF.) For larger pupils, this error is essentially zero. B: the MTF first zero crossover frequency as a function of pupil size for three levels of defocus.

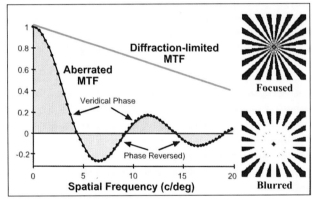

Figure 7-7. Schematic of a defocused MTF showing phase reversal. On the right is a focused image and blurred image of the same pattern showing phase reversal for higher frequencies (ie, notice how the higher frequency white part of the pattern just off center aligns with the dark part of the pattern in the periphery) (courtesy of Arthur Bradley).[31]

Therefore, one of the potential benefits of correcting ocular aberrations is that errors in spatial phase are corrected. This benefit is likely to be substantial for many aspects of visual function.

For example, the visual task of letter discrimination is strongly affected when optical defocus introduces phase reversals into some spatial frequency components of the target but not others (Figure 7-8). The upper row of images in Figure 7-8 demonstrates the devastating effect of phase reversals on letter legibility caused by optical blur. However, when these phase reversals are corrected, as shown in the bottom

> Phase reversals caused by optical aberrations can be more important than loss of contrast.

row of images, we see that the decrease in contrast induced by blur has relatively little impact. This simple demonstration shows that the phase shifts and phase reversals caused by optical aberrations can be more important than loss of contrast.

Chromatic Aberration, Spherical Aberration, and the Neural Transfer Function

So far we have limited our discussion to monochromatic light, simple defocus, and phase. We have ignored the effects of chromatic aberration and have not shown the relationship between the neural threshold function and the optical MTF. In Figure 7-9, we model these interactions for a 6-mm pupil using the Indiana model eye. Introducing chromatic defocus (green line) into the model reduces the MTF significantly from the diffraction-limited case (black line). The MTF suffers more when spherical aberration is introduced, and performance is even worse when chromatic and spherical aberration are combined in the model.

The vertical separation between these curves tells us that by correcting the eye's chromatic aberration we could expect about five-fold improvement in image contrast at 30 c/deg. The improvement in image contrast would be approximately twelve-fold if we corrected the eye's spherical aberration, and we

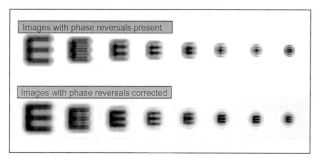

Figure 7-8. A blurred letter E with phase reversals at higher frequencies (top) and without phase reversal (bottom). Notice how phase reversal degrades the percept of the letter to the point in which the smaller letters (higher frequencies) are no longer legible (figure courtesy of Arthur Bradley).[31]

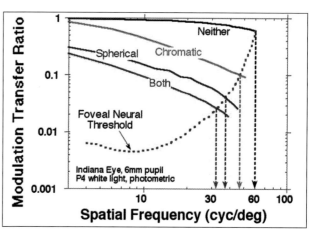

Figure 7-9. MTFs for a diffraction-limited case (black line), the chromatic aberration (green line), typical spherical aberration (blue line), both spherical and chromatic aberrations (red line), and the foveal neural threshold function. The foveal neural thresholds are measured by using gratings formed on the retina through interference, bypassing the optics of the eye. The points where each MTF crosses the foveal neural threshold function defines the limiting spatial frequency that the model can "see" (dashed arrows).

get approximately twenty-five-fold improvement in contrast at 30 c/deg by correcting both chromatic and spherical aberration.

Anticipated improvements in spatial resolution are not as dramatic as the improvements in contrast. The spatial frequency limit of detection without aliasing for the visual system is indicated graphically by the intersection of the optical MTF with the neural threshold function. This intersection occurs at approximately 30 c/deg (20/20) when both aberrations are included in the model. The intersection increases to 60 c/deg (20/10), a two-fold increase when both aberrations are removed. We may conclude from this analysis that the benefits of aberration correction are proportionally greater when measured in the contrast domain than when measured in the spatial domain.

Do clinical tests capitalize on these theoretical considerations to optimize sensitivity? In the next section we will examine current methods to measure visual performance in the context of these theoretical considerations and the demands of the clinical environment.

TRADITIONAL MEASURES OF VISUAL PERFORMANCE

Clinically defining the quality of the visual percept is much more complex than defining the quality of the retinal image using objective measurement techniques (see Chapter Six) or theoretical considerations discussed above and in Chapter Two. The retinal image defines the input to the visual system. The visual percept forms the basis for the final behavioral output after considerable cognitive processing. A

proper treatment of the conversion of the retinal image to a visual percept is well beyond the scope of this chapter. Here we will try to give the reader a feel for the complexity and the issues involved in assessing visual performance, followed by a discussion of commonly used clinical measures of visual performance.

Visual performance is multidimensional, with each dimension having its own set of tests. There are tests of color vision, temporal resolution (flicker fusion), variations in peripheral contrast sensitivity (perimetry), peripheral acuity, texture processing, motion processing, dynamic visual acuity (acuity while observing a moving target), visual attention (simultaneously identifying objects at two locations), localization (vernier) acuity, stereopsis, and many others. Although some of these may seem esoteric, some measure important aspects of visual function and are likely to work their way to prominence, particularly given the aging population. For example, a test of "useful field of vision" has been developed, which measures a subject's ability to identify the location of a car silhouette, eccentrically placed, while simultaneously performing a visual task at the point of fixation. Results from this test show a good correlation with incidence of automobile crashes in older drivers.[13]

Further, many aspects of human performance,

though strongly dependent upon vision, do not require exceptional visual acuity and are not harmed by mildly reduced acuity. For example, driving a car[14] or shooting basketballs[15] is essentially unimpaired by having 20/40 rather than 20/20 or better acuity. On the other hand, some tasks are exquisitely sensitive to high levels of visual performance. In the Air Force it is common wisdom that in a visual dogfight between two jet fighters, it is usually the pilot who first sees the enemy plane on the horizon who triumphs. For tasks such as these, improvements in the optics of the eye achieved through wavefront-guided laser surgery may mean the difference between success and failure. Superior vision does not necessarily mean exceptional performance; however, those who perform exceptionally generally have superior vision.

> Superior vision does not necessarily mean exceptional performance; however, those who perform exceptionally generally have superior vision.

Measuring visual performance in a meaningful manner is not a simple matter and principles of proper testing are often ignored in the clinical environment. The inherent variability of biological systems and the interpretive process dictate that reliable and sensitive tests must employ:

1. Small increments in task difficulty
2. Multiple trials at each level
3. A "forced-choice" methodology[16-18]
4. Scoring to the finest practical scale (eg, scoring by the number of letters read rather than by the number of lines read)

Acuity charts that have inconsistencies in letter size progression and number of letters per line (like the Snellen chart) make consistent scoring by the letter difficult. Further, and perhaps most importantly, clinicians and technicians are often satisfied if the patient can read the 20/20 line even though he or she may be able to read the 20/10 line. As a consequence, a patient who formerly had 20/10 vision can come in complaining of a vision loss that goes undetected. Such an experience leaves the patient thinking that he or she must be imagining things; or for the more confident patient, he or she may feel (more correctly) that you and your staff do not know what you are doing.

As a consequence of these and other factors (eg, quality of life measures), there is no one "silver bul-

> Acuity charts that have inconsistencies in letter size progression and number of letters per line (like the Snellen chart) make consistent scoring by the letter difficult.

let" test for measuring the quality of the visual percept and/or its impact on the quality of life. Despite this fact, every patient and clinician appropriately wants to know if refractive therapy improves vision. So what clinical tests best meet this need and why? Here we will focus on tests that are of particular relevance to refractive surgery and evaluating good but not perfect ocular optics. These tests center on tests of spatial processing (eg, acuity and contrast sensitivity).

CONTRAST SENSITIVITY

Although we would like to measure the MTF of the entire visual system (optics and neural pathways combined), such a MTF cannot be directly measured. To similarly characterize the visual system, one can measure the ability of the observer to detect sinusoidal gratings at threshold contrast as a function of spatial frequency. The resulting function is called the *contrast sensitivity function* (CSF). To carefully and accurately measure the CSF is too time consuming for routine clinical use (generally 15 to 20 minutes per eye), particularly given current insurance reimbursement for such testing. Further, testing with sinusoidally varying luminance patterns is insensitive to changes in phase. Nonetheless, understanding how the visual system responds to contrast as a function of spatial frequency provides excellent insight into currently used clinical tests of spatial vision and those likely to meet clinical needs in refractive surgery.

In Figure 7-10, notice that with increasing spatial frequency, contrast sensitivity increases to a peak and then decreases. The decrease in contrast sensitivity at low spatial frequencies is attributable to neural processing.[19] The decrease in contrast sensitivity after the peak at moderate spatial frequencies is principally due to ocular optics.[19] In eyes that have excellent optics, the highest spatial frequency detected without aliasing will be neural limited. Functional human spatial vision is defined by space under the curve.

The CSF provides information about the visual system that is not given by high-contrast acuity. For example, contrast sensitivity is more strongly related

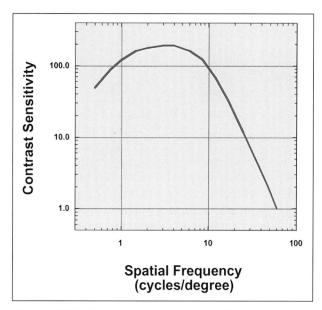

Figure 7-10. Typical log contrast sensitivity as a function of log spatial frequency for a normal eye.

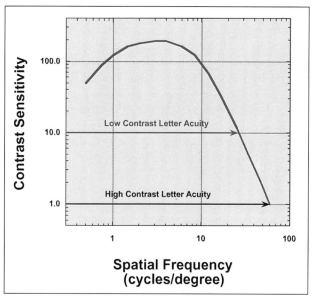

Figure 7-11. CSF showing that testing high or low contrast acuity samples spatial vision at a fixed contrast level and finds one point on the CSF curve. Acuity testing determines the highest spatial frequency (smallest letter) that can be seen at the fixed contrast level. Contrast is not varied in these tests.

to certain visual tasks, such as face recognition, than is visual acuity.[20] Further, it is possible for high-contrast acuity to remain normal or near normal, while contrast sensitivity in the midspatial frequencies is decreased. Such a mid-frequency loss results in objects having a "washed out" appearance. Likewise, it is also possible for contrast sensitivity to be improved by custom ablation, while acuity remains constant. Consider a patient who has 20/15 or better acuity best-corrected before surgery. After refractive surgery that successfully eliminated the spherical and cylindrical error and reduced the higher-order optical aberration, photoreceptor spacing will quickly limit improvement in acuity. Nevertheless, such a surgical outcome will result in higher contrast images with crisper borders,[1,21] making it easier for the individual to drive or perform other tasks under foggy conditions or dim illumination. Such benefits are more likely to be reflected in measures of contrast sensitivity than they are in more traditional clinical measures like high-contrast acuity.

High-Contrast Visual Acuity

As the name implies, high-contrast visual acuity employs high-contrast letters of varying size to measure the smallest letters a patient can correctly identify. Letters are complex targets made up of a large number of frequencies having numerous orientations and modulations. Despite their complex

nature, as letters get smaller and smaller the spatial frequency content shifts to higher spatial frequencies. Consequently, in CSF space, high-contrast acuity is a psychophysical measure that marches horizontally across the spatial frequency axis (toward smaller letters) near 100% contrast (CS of 1) until it hits the CSF curve (Figure 7-11). As a result, high-contrast acuity is a surrogate measure of the highest spatial frequency that the visual system can process accurately (ie, the smallest high-contrast letter that can be read).

An advantage of high-contrast acuity tests is that they are relatively insensitive in the normal or near normal eye to minor changes in pupil size and minor variations in the higher-order aberrations. Consequently, high-contrast visual acuity is not particularly sensitive to more subtle visual complaints commonly offered by refractive surgery patients (eg, the patient who reports, "I may see 20/20, but I do not see as well as I did, particularly at night").

Low-Contrast Acuity

Using letters of constant low contrast shifts the acuity measurement line vertically in CSF space (see Figure 7-11). Notice that spatial frequencies requiring high contrasts will be below the detection threshold.

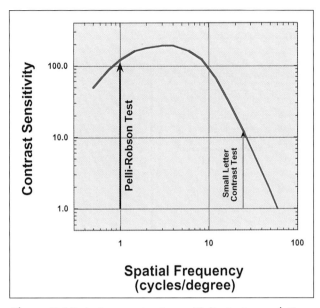

Figure 7-12. Letter contrast sensitivity tests use letters of a constant size (spatial frequency) and gradually decrease contrast of the letters.

A consequence of high spatial frequencies being below the threshold of detection and lower overall contrast for all frequencies is that the borders of visible letters are less distinct (letters are harder to read). Lowering letter contrast increases the test sensitivity, and more subtle changes in optical quality can be detected. Two prominent versions of the low-contrast acuity test are the Regan charts and the Bailey/Lovie low-contrast chart. The Regan charts[22] consist of four charts, each having a different contrast ranging from 4% to 96% (Weber contrast, $\Delta I/I$). The Bailey/Lovie low contrast (18% Weber contrast) chart appears on the back of their high-contrast charts. Both capitalize on state-of-the-art chart design by having a fixed number of letters in each line, a fixed scalar between lines, and separation between letters dependent on letter size.[20,22-24] At least three studies have found low-contrast acuity to be a more sensitive measure of changes in visual function after refractive surgery than high-contrast acuity.[6,25,26] Despite these findings, the correlation between high- and low-contrast acuity remains high ($r^2 = 0.87$), suggesting that the gains in test sensitivity are not as large as might be hoped.[27]

Pelli-Robson Large Letter Contrast Sensitivity

The Pelli-Robson test uses letters of equal legibili-

ty and a constant large size (20/640 or approximately 1 c/deg) and, unlike high- or low-contrast acuity, varies the contrast between letter presentations (Figure 7-12). Three letters are presented at each of 16 contrast levels. The letter contrast changes 0.15 log units for each level, starting at about 100% and decreasing to about 0.9%. The test has been shown to have good reliability[17] in measuring low frequency contrast sensitivity and has gained a fair amount of popularity among clinicians testing for neural problems. The choice of the large letter places the fundamental spatial frequency of the letter into the low frequency roll-off in the CSF due principally to neural processing. Using such a low spatial frequency makes the test more sensitive to neurologically induced changes in contrast sensitivity than optically induced changes. The reason is simple. Minor changes in optical properties have a greater effect on the higher spatial frequencies than they do on the low spatial frequencies, as seen in Figures 7-5 through 7-7 and 7-9. Although it is wise to switch to the contrast domain to test for optical changes likely to be induced by refractive surgery, test sensitivity to improvements or degradations in the eye's optics will be increased by using smaller letters where the fundamental frequency is securely in the steep portion of the CSF and more sensitive to changes in the eye's optical properties.

Small Letter Contrast Test

A fairly new test, Rabin's small letter contrast test,[28] capitalizes on the steep slope of the CSF in the moderate to high spatial frequencies, which are more sensitive to changes in optical quality than lower frequencies (see Figure 7-12). As a consequence of the steep slope, small amounts of blur cause relatively large changes in contrast sensitivity and only small changes in spatial frequencies (Figure 7-13). The small letter contrast test is similar to the Pelli-Robson chart in that all letters are the same size, and successive rows have lower contrast. However, instead of using large letters, the letter size is approximately 20/25 (24 c/deg). There are 14 lines in the test with 10 letters in each line. Contrast decreases by 0.1 log unit on each successive line.[28] Unlike tests of contrast using sinusoidal gratings, this test should be sensitive to phase shifts as well as gains or losses in the MTF. Despite its excellent design, the Rabin small letter contrast test has seen little clinical use to date.

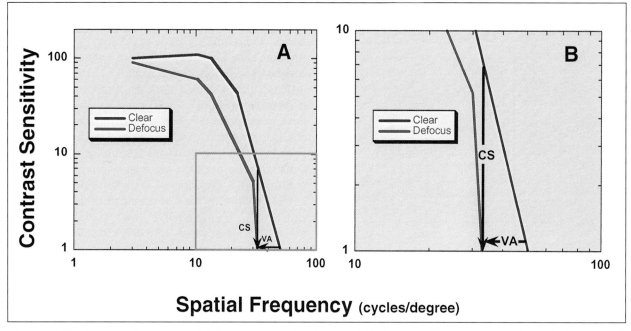

Figure 7-13. A: a small amount of defocus causes the CSF to shift down, which causes a minor shift in cut-off frequency and a large change in contrast at high frequencies. B: an enlargement of the light green square in panel A (adapted from Rabin J, Wicks J. Measuring resolution in the contrast domain: the small letter contrast test. *Optom Vis Sci.* 1996;73:398-403).

THE IDEAL CLINICAL TEST OF VISUAL FUNCTION

In the normal visual system we would like to believe that visual performance tests are a good surrogate measure for the optical quality of the retinal image. That is, as the retinal image improves, test performance improves and as the retinal image degrades, test performance degrades. Such an ideal test is fantasy. Visual systems vary in their capacity to interpret the retinal image and form a percept. It is unrealistic for such tests to perfectly mimic retinal image quality.

Fortunately, the reliance on visual performance tests to serve as a surrogate measure of retinal image quality will likely disappear over the next several years as sensitive new objective tests of retinal image quality make their way to the market. These new aberrometers will be able to quantify the aberration structure of the eye well beyond simple sphere and cylinder. In this new setting, visual performance tests will be used to define the relationship between retinal image quality and visual performance with the better tests correlating closely with the quality of the retinal image. Differences between retinal image quality and new tests of visual performance will be used to explore the nature of refractive amblyopia and new causes of refractive amblyopia. For example, it may be the case that "ideal" refractive corrections improve the retinal image quality but that visual performance does not improve to the neural limit accordingly.[1]

Only one study has been published (as of April 2000) correlating the change in total eye aberrations induced by refractive surgery to measures of visual performance. Using a Tscherning aberroscope, Seiler, et al[6] measured 15 eyes before and 3 months after myopic photorefractive keratectomy (PRK). Visual performance was measured using high-contrast acuity, low-contrast acuity, and glare acuity testing. The increase in the total wavefront error was correlated most strongly with the loss in low-contrast acuity (r = -0.89), followed by glare visual acuity (r = -0.52), and then high-contrast acuity (r = -0.50).

WHAT DESIGN CHARACTERISTICS SHOULD IDEAL VISUAL PERFORMANCE TESTS HAVE?

Key design characteristics include:

1. Ease of use for clinicians and technical support staff.
2. Easy for the patient to understand.
3. Fast—the test should be able to be administered and scored in less than 1 minute per eye.
4. Variable contrast and spatial frequency.
5. Small increments in task difficulty.
6. Multiple trials at each test level.
7. Use a "forced-choice" methodology.
8. Computer generated, scored, and random generation of test targets.
9. Allow the pupil to physiologically dilate.
10. Infrared pupil size monitoring.

The Rabin small letter contrast test meets many of these test requirements. However, it cannot be overemphasized that visual function following refractive surgery is highly dependent upon pupil size. Much of the interest in visual performance after refractive surgery is concerned with large pupil conditions. The reason is two-fold. First, aberrations induced by refractive surgery (as performed prior to the year 2000) increased dramatically under large

> Much of the interest in visual performance after refractive surgery is concerned with large pupil conditions.

pupil conditions (see Chapter Twenty). Consequently, visual performance decreased with increasing pupil size.[2,25,26] Second, the effects of diffraction increase with decreasing pupil size. Thus, the visual benefit (more contrast and sharper borders)[8,21] of correcting the eye's higher-order aberrations is increasingly masked by diffraction as pupil size decreases. Consequently, until ideal corrections are perfected it is important for clinicians and scientists to report pupil sizes or lighting conditions when reporting results of visual performance tests.

Tests Allowing Large Physiological Pupil Diameters

Current visual performance tests (eg, high- or low-contrast acuity) are generally performed under conditions of high illumination and consequently small pupil conditions. In order to measure visual acuity under large pupil conditions, it has been necessary to either artificially dilate the pupil with mydriatics or use low levels of lighting for the white chart background and for the surrounding environment.

As an alternative, Stanley Klein has suggested a new type of chart using single bright letters presented against a dark background (on a monitor) in a dark room and decreasing letter size to threshold.[29] Under these conditions the pupil would be physiologically dilated. This innovative concept may be considered a new twist on what may be one of the oldest methods of testing visual acuity. One can imagine shepherds in ancient Greece sitting in a field at night comparing their abilities to resolve two closely positioned stars. Klein's suggestion lends itself to modern methods of computer display with all its advantages. However, as currently suggested, Klein's test does not capitalize on the sensitivity of the contrast domain to subtle changes in optical quality. The test could be easily altered to test in the contrast domain similar to the Rabin small letter contrast test.

SUMMARY

New refractive therapy, whether it increases or reduces ocular higher-order aberrations (beyond sphere and cylinder), is changing how we view and test visual performance. Key points are:

1. New, more sensitive tests of visual performance need to be developed that capitalize on the visual system's sensitivity to contrast and phase.
2. With the advent of clinically practical wavefront sensing, the need to use measures of visual performance as a surrogate measure of retinal image quality will diminish.
3. Differences between retinal image quality and visual performance measures will be used to explore amblyopia.
4. Improvements in retinal image quality of the normal eye will not be reflected by large gains in traditional acuity tests.
5. New tests should allow full physiological pupil dilation.

Both retinal image quality and visual performance measures need to be reported as a function of pupil diameter.

ACKNOWLEDGMENTS

Preparation of this chapter was supported by National Institutes of Health (National Eye Institute) grants R01-EY08520 to Dr. Applegate, R01-EY05109 to Dr. Thibos, and an unrestricted grant from

Research to Prevent Blindness to the Department of Ophthalmology, University of Texas Health Science Center San Antonio. We thank Arthur Bradley for permission to reproduce Figures 7-7 and 7-8.

REFERENCES

1. Applegate RA. Limits to vision: can we do better than nature? *J Refract Surg.* 2000;16:5547-51.

2. Applegate RA, Howland HC, Sharp RP, Cottingham AJ, Yee RW. Corneal aberrations and visual performance after radial keratotomy. *J Refract Surg.* 1998;14:397-407.

3. Martinez CE, Applegate RA, Klyce SD, McDonald MB, Medina JP, Howland HC. Effect of pupil dilation on corneal optical aberrations after photorefractive keratectomy. *Arch Ophthalmol.* 1998;116:1053-1062.

4. Oliver KM, Hemenger RP, Corbett MC, et al. Corneal optical aberrations induced by photorefractive keratectomy. *J Refract Surg.* 1997;13:246-254.

5. Oshika T, Klyce SD, Applegate RA, Howland HC. Comparison of corneal wavefront aberrations after photorefractive keratectomy and laser in situ keratomileusis. *Am J Ophthalmol.* 1999;127:1-7.

6. Seiler T, Kaemmerer M, Mierdel P, Krinke HE. Ocular optical aberations after photorefractive keratectomy for myopia and myopic astigmatism. *Arch Ophthalmol.* 2000;118:17-21.

7. Liang J, Williams DR. Effect of higher order aberrations on image quality of the human eye. *Vis Sci Appl Tech Digest (OSA).* 1995;1:70-73.

8. Liang J, Williams DR, Miller DT. Supernormal vision and high resolution retinal imaging through adaptive optics. *J Opt Soc Am A.* 1997;14:2884-2892.

9. MacRae SM, Schwiegerling J, Snyder R. Customized corneal ablation and supervision. *J Refract Surg.* 2000;16:S230-S235.

10. Yoon GY, Williams DR. Visual benefits of correcting the higher order monochromatic aberrations and the longitudinal chromatic aberration in the eye. Paper presented at the 2000 Vision Science and its Applications Annual Meeting. Sante Fe, NM.

11. Woods RL, Bradley A, Atchison DA. Monocular diplopia caused by ocular aberrations and hyperopic defocus. *Vision Res.* 1996;36:3597-3606.

12. Woods RL, Bradley A, Atchison DA. Consequences of monocular diplopia for the contrast sensitivity function. *Vision Res.* 1996;36:3587-3596.

13. Owsley C, Ball K, McGwin G, et al. Visual processing impairment and risk of motor vehicle crash among older adults. *JAMA.* 1998;279:1083-1088.

14. Owsley C. Vision and driving in the elderly. *Optom Vis Sci.* 1994;71:727-735.

15. Applegate RA. Set shot shooting performance and visual acuity in basketball. *Optom Vis Sci.* 1992;69:765-768.

16. Bailey IL, Bullimore MA, Raasch TW, Taylor HR. Clinical grading and the effects of scaling. *Invest Ophthalmol Vis Sci.* 1991;32:422-432.

17. Elliott DB, Bullimore MA. Assessing the reliability, discriminative ability, and validity of disability glare tests. *Invest Ophthalmol Vis Sci.* 1993;34:108-119.

18. Raasch TW, Bailey IL, Bullimore MA. Repeatability of visual acuity measurement. *Optom Vis Sci.* 1998;75:342-348.

19. De Valois RL, De Valois KK. *Spatial Vision.* New York, NY: Oxford University Press; 1988:147-175.

20. Elliott DB. Contrast sensitivity and glare testing. In: WJ Benjamin, ed. *Borish's Clinical Refraction.* Philadelphia, Pa: WB Saunders; 1998:203-241.

21. Miller DT. Retinal imaging and vision at the frontiers of adaptive optics. *Physics Today.* 2000;53:31-36.

22. Regan D, Neima D. Low-contrast letter charts as a test of visual function. *Ophthalmology.* 1983;90:1192-1200.

23. Bailey IL, Lovie JE. New design principles for visual acuity letter charts. *Am J Optom Physiol Opt.* 1976;53:740-745.

24. Bailey IL. Visual acuity. In: WJ Benjamin, ed. *Borish's Clinical Refraction.* Philadelphia, Pa: WB Saunders; 1998:179-202.

25. Verdon W, Bullimore MA, Maloney RK. Visual performance after photorefractive keratectomy. *Arch Ophthalmol.* 1996;114:1465-1472.

26. Bullimore MA, Olson MD, Maloney RK. Visual performance after photorefractive keratectomy with a 6-mm ablation zone. *Am J Ophthalmol.* 1999;128:1-7.

27. Hilmantel G, Applegate RA, Tu EY, Starck T, Howland HC. Low contrast acuity: a substitute for contrast sensitivity? *Invest Ophthalmol Vis Sci.* 1999;40(Suppl):S534.

28. Rabin J, Wicks J. Measuring resolution in the contrast domain: the small letter contrast test. *Optom Vis Sci.* 1996;73:398-403.

29. Klein S. Personal communication. October 1999.

30. Smith WJ. *Modern Optical Engineering: The Design of Optical Systems.* New York, NY: McGraw-Hill, Inc; 1990:327-363.

31. Bradley A, Hong S, Chung L, Thibos LN. The impact of defocus-induced phase reversals on letter recognition is different for hyperopes and myopes. *Invest Ophthalmol Vis Sci.* 1999;40(Suppl):S35.

Chapter Eight

Optical Aberrations and Ablation Pattern Design

Jim Schwiegerling, PhD
Robert W. Snyder, MD, PhD
Scott M. MacRae, MD

INTRODUCTION

The evolution of excimer laser technology for refractive surgery has allowed for the correction or reduction of refractive errors. This technology sculpts the cornea of an ametropic patient to a new shape, thereby reducing the patient's required correction. Targeted shapes for ablation patterns in laser refractive surgery are typically based on the shapes seen in more traditional modes of refractive correction, namely spectacles and contact lenses. The laser ablation shapes take on a spherical pattern to correct spherical refractive error and/or a cylindrical shape to correct for regular astigmatism. However, lasers are not inherently limited to delivering only spherocylindrical ablation patterns. Furthermore, eyes not only suffer from spherical and cylindrical refractive error, but also from other errors usually lumped together under the term *irregular astigmatism*. Irregular astigmatism is caused by aberrations in the eye. Emerging laser technology allows for the treatment of the irregular astigmatic or aberrated portion of refractive error.

> Lasers are not inherently limited to delivering only spherocylindrical ablation patterns.

FEASIBILITY OF CORRECTING IRREGULAR ASTIGMATISM

Irregular astigmatism, or the component of refractive error that cannot be corrected with traditional spherocylinder lenses, has been largely ignored in the correction of ametropia. There are several reasons for ignoring this effect. First, the magnitude and form of irregular astigmatism varies greatly within the population, from almost nonexistent in the normal eye to highly irregular in eyes with distortions such as keratoconus. These variations cause traditional methods for measuring refractive error to become unmanageable. Typically, spherical and cylindrical refractive errors are measured by objectively or subjectively nulling the errors with a series of lenses. A finite number of spherical and cylindrical lenses can be used to rapidly assess spherical and cylindrical ametropia. Following the same procedure to measure irregular astigmatism would require an unwieldy, if not infinite, number of optical elements to account for all variations and levels of irregularity. Furthermore, a systematic method for isolating the degree and form of irregular astigmatism would be impractical or impossible using traditional methods.

The second reason for ignoring irregular astigmatism in the past is that in the majority of healthy eyes,

> Previously, it has not been possible to measure irregular astigmatism using the older traditional methods. Now it is possible to measure them.

this component is small and vision in these eyes can be corrected to 20/40 or better by conventional spherocylinder lenses. Finally, ignoring the irregular astigmatism portion of refractive error allows spectacles and contact lenses to be mass-produced, thereby driving down cost, minimizing delivery time, and facilitating quality control. Adding irregular astigmatism correction to conventional corrective lenses would force each lens to be custom made with complex manufacturing techniques and individually tested to ensure performance. Manufacturing these types of lenses is cost prohibitive.

Excimer laser refractive surgery coupled with wavefront sensing technology offers the potential to avoid the drawbacks of incorporating irregular astigmatism into the correction of refractive error. First, wavefront sensing techniques such as the Shack-Hartmann sensor, the Tscherning aberroscope, and the crossed-cylinder aberroscope offer a rapid means of measuring the aberrations of the eye in addition to spherical and cylindrical error. Aberrations are the cause of irregular astigmatism, and these devices quantify the magnitude and form of the aberration structure of the entire eye, allowing an ablation pattern to be predicted that would postoperatively minimize the aberration of the eye. Secondly, the cost associated with customizing ablation patterns is manageable. The primary cost for giving customized treatment of refractive error and aberrations is development of the technologies for measuring aberration structure and precisely delivering the customized treatment to the cornea (eg, Shack-Hartmann sensor linked to a scanning excimer laser with an eye-tracking system). Following the development of these systems, a wide array of complex ablation pattern

> Following the initial technological investment, cost and time for delivering customized treatment should be comparable and competitive to current noncustomized procedures.

shapes can be delivered without further cost. Following the initial technological investment, cost and time for delivering customized treatment should be comparable and competitive to current noncustomized procedures. Finally, by incorporating aber-

> Higher-order aberration correction should elevate our standards so that even less optimal outcomes still approach or achieve 20/20.

ration treatment into refractive surgery procedures, the overall quality of vision following surgery can be improved. Currently, "successful" outcomes are deemed as 20/40 vision or better uncorrected following surgery. Aberration correction may allow an improvement in visual acuity for patients pushing the theoretical limits of vision. However, more importantly, it should elevate the artificial 20/40 standard so that less than optimal outcomes still achieve 20/20 vision.

In this chapter, an introduction to aberrations is given. When viewing a star at night, in order for good vision to occur, the eye requires entering light to focus to a sharp point on the retina. Aberrations blur these star images. Different classes of aberrations will be identified based on how the image is blurred. Furthermore, familiar spherical and cylindrical refractive error will be shown to be only two of many classes of aberrations. Following this introduction, designs for ablation patterns that attempt to reduce aberrations in the eye will be reviewed. These patterns include current spherocylinder ablations, as well as proposed aspheric and customized ablations. The ensuing discussion will provide a foundation for understanding the challenges and goals of customized refractive surgery.

> The perfect eye would image every infinitesimal point in a scene to a corresponding infinitesimally small point on the retina.

ABERRATIONS

The perfect eye would image every infinitesimal point in a scene to a corresponding infinitesimally small point on the retina. In other words, no blurring would occur for every point in the scene. To accomplish this perfect imaging, the eye must capture the wavefronts emanating from a given point and perfectly focus them onto the retina. Figure 8-1 shows wavefronts emanating from an arbitrary point out in the world. The wavefronts are perfectly spherical and emanate outward or diverge from the point. As the waves propagate through space, they will remain perfectly spherical until they encounter the perfect eye. The perfect eye shown in Figure 8-1 converts

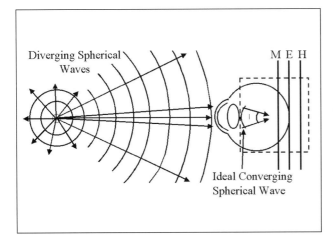

Figure 8-1. Light from a point source will radiate outward in perfectly spherical diverging waves until the waves encounter the eye. The eye ideally converts these waves to perfectly spherical waves converging to the retina. Three planes relative to the retina are shown: the myopic plane (M), the emmetropic plane (E), and the hyperopic plane (H).

these diverging spherical waves into converging waves. The converging waves now have two requirements in order for perfect imaging to occur. First, the converging waves must be perfectly spherical, because this is the only wavefront shape that will focus to a perfect point. Second, the wavefronts must converge to a point on the retina. If the point of convergence is on either side of the retinal point, then a blurred point is perceived.

Of course for real eyes, perfect imaging never occurs. The best possible scenario is that the imaging is limited by diffraction. In the diffraction-limited case, the converging wavefronts are perfectly spherical except at their periphery. Along the periphery, light interacts with the pupil margin, resulting in a slight distortion to the wavefront at its periphery. The diffraction-limited wavefront will converge to a small, but finite point known as an Airy disk. In general, the eye suffers from more severe errors than diffraction. The wavefronts converging toward the retina in a real eye are not spherical and therefore converge to a finite-sized blob on the retina, which is larger than the Airy disk. Blobs corresponding to different points in the outside world overlap on the retina and degrade the image formed on the retina. The size of these blobs determines the limit to resolution of fine detail. In general, the larger the blobs, the worse the resolution of the eye. The deviation of the converging wavefronts from perfect spheres is called aberration.

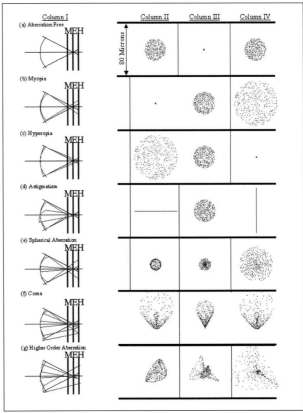

Figure 8-2. The lefthand side compares the shape of the actual wavefront (blue) to the ideal wavefront (black) for various types of aberrations. The righthand side shows spot diagrams on the myopic (column II), emmetropic (column III), and hyperopic planes (column IV). Spot diagrams illustrate the intensity distribution formed on each of these planes, where the intensity is proportional to the density of spots. a: ideal case; b: myopia; c: hyperopia; d: astigmatism; e: spherical aberration; f: coma; and g: higher-order aberration.

Monochromatic Aberrations

Monochromatic aberrations are for a specific wavelength of visible light and can be further classified into general categories. These classes of monochromatic aberrations are spherical refractive error (sometimes called defocus), cylindrical refractive error (astigmatism), spherical aberration, coma, and higher-order aberrations. Figure 8-2 illustrates the shape of the wavefront and the effects on an image of a point for the different classes of aberrations. The far lefthand column of Figure 8-2 shows how the aberrated wavefront converges toward the retina and corresponds to the region of the posterior segment outlined by the box in Figure 8-1. The righthand columns of Figure 8-2 show what the image of a point source would look like if an imaging screen is placed in front of the retina (II), at the retina (III), and behind the retina (IV). The point source images are depicted for three different positions of the imaging screen: in front of the retina, at the retina, and behind the retina. In Figure 8-1, the positions for these screens are labeled myopic plane, emmetropic plane, and hyperopic plane, respectively. In the case of perfect imaging, the far lefthand column of Figure 8-2a(I) shows perfectly spherical wavefronts converging toward the retina. In the three righthand columns of Figure 8-2a, the image of a point source on the myopic, emmetropic, and hyperopic planes are shown, respectively. Note that the images on the myopic and hyperopic planes, a(II) and a(IV) are out of focus, but the image formed in the emmetropic plane, a(III), is a perfect point. Therefore, the retina would need to be located at the emmetropic plane, a(III), in order for perfect imaging to occur.

Spherical Refractive Error (Defocus)

Figure 8-2b shows myopic spherical refractive error. The converging wavefront is again perfectly spherical but converges to a point on the myopic plane b(II) and is out of focus when it reaches the emmetropic plane b(III). Similarly, Figure 8-2c shows hyperopic spherical refractive error. In this case, the perfectly spherical waves converge to a point on the hyperopic plane c(IV), and the point image is out of focus on the emmetropic (c[III]) and myopic (c[IV]) planes. Aberrations have different classifications. Spherical and cylindrical refractive error are simple aberrations. Spherical aberration, coma, and higher-order aberrations are more complex.

Astigmatism

For cylindrical (astigmatic) refractive error, as shown in Figure 8-2d, the converging wavefront takes on a toric shape such that different meridians focus at different planes relative to the retina. The righthand side of Figure 8-2d shows a horizontal line focus on the myopic plane d(II), the circle of least confusion on the emmetropic plane d(III), and a vertical line image on the hyperopic plane d(IV). The orientation of the astigmatic axis can rotate these line images through various angles.

> Aberrations have different classifications. Spherical and cylindrical refractive error are simple aberrations. Spherical aberration, coma, and higher-order aberrations are more complex.

Spherical Aberration

For spherical aberration, as shown in Figure 8-2e, the converging wavefront looks spherical near the center of the pupil but changes its curvature toward the edge of the pupil. This aberration gives a continuum of foci and results in point images with halos.

Coma

Figure 8-2f shows comatic error. The wavefront is asymmetric about the perfectly spherical wavefront, producing a comet-shaped pattern on the emmetropic plane.

Higher-Order Aberrations

Finally, higher-order aberrations, as shown in Figure 8-2g, are an amalgam of all other deviations of the converging wavefront from perfect sphericity. The resulting point images can take on complex patterns (g[II] to g[IV]).

In general, the wavefronts formed by the eye will take on complex nonspherical shapes, and different wavelengths will have different wavefront shapes. To push the eye to its theoretical limits of performance, all of the monochromatic and chromatic aberrations would need to be corrected. In other words, the wavefronts converging toward the retina need to be perfectly spherical regardless of wavelength, and all of them must converge to a perfect point on the retina. In this manner, a point of white light out in the world is imaged to a point of white light on the retina.

Chromatic Aberrations

The eye also suffers from chromatic aberration, or aberration that depends upon the color or wavelength of light coming into the eye. In terms of foveal vision, the dominant chromatic aberration is longitudinal (or axial) chromatic aberration. This aberration is equivalent to spherical refractive error as discussed above. However, the degree of spherical refractive error depends on the color or wavelength of light. In general, when a subject views a point of white light, blue light focuses in front of the retina, green light focuses at the retina, and red light focuses behind the retina. The spectral sensitivity of the eye helps to reduce the effects of chromatic aberration by making the visual system more sensitive to the green light focused on the retina and less sensitive to blue or red light focused away from the retina.

The cause of chromatic aberration is dispersion in the cornea, aqueous, crystalline lens, and vitreous humor. Dispersion is simply a variation in index of refraction of a material with wavelength and causes white light to be dispersed into the various spectral colors, just as a prism disperses light into a rainbow. Refractive surgery techniques cannot correct chromatic aberration, since this error is inherent to the properties of the ocular materials and not to the shape of the ocular components.

A Mathematical Description of Aberrations

Aberrations are also classified in terms of orders, with first, second, third, fourth, and higher-order aberrations being the common classifications. As shown in Figure 8-2, the shape of the wavefront is, in general, a complex two-dimensional surface. To describe this surface mathematically, the wavefront is typically broken down into a combination of simpler surfaces. The shape and number of these simpler surfaces determines the order of the aberration.

Representing complex data with simpler mathematical expression is a common technique for managing and analyzing data. Consider a hypothetical example of measuring the attempted and achieved refractive correction on a group of 100 patients. Plotting this data gives a scattered distribution of points, which hopefully has correlation between the attempted and achieved correction. To simplify the analysis of this data, a linear regression is typically performed, or in other words, the straight line that "best fits" the data is found. The equation of a straight line is given by (equation 1):

$$y = mx + b$$

where m is the slope of the line and b is the intercept of the line with the y axis. The powers or exponents of the x variable in equation 1 can be written explicitly, such that an equivalent expression for equation 1 is given by (equation 2):

$$y = mx^1 + bx^0$$

since $x^1 = x$ and $x^0 = 1$. Recall that the definition of a polynomial is a linear combination of powers of x (eg, $y = A + Bx + Cx^2 + Dx^3 + \ldots$ is a polynomial). Equation 2 shows that a line is a polynomial with its highest power equal to one. A line, therefore, is called a first-order polynomial because its highest power is unity.

Taylor Polynomials: Defining the Order of a Polynomial

Suppose the data set in the preceding example was decidedly nonlinear. A line would not well rep-

resent this data, and a higher-order polynomial (higher powers of x) would be needed to adequately fit the data set. The order of the fit would be given by the highest power of x in the polynomial that adequately fits the data. The preceding example is one-dimensional since a curve is being the data, but the concepts can be extended to two dimensions for cases in which a surface, such as a wavefront, is being fit. In this case, the surface elevation z would need to be described by a two-dimensional polynomial at various Cartesian coordinates (x,y), such that (equation 3):

$$z = A + Bx^1y^0 + Cx^0y^1 + Dx^2y^0 + Ex^1y^1 + Fx^0y^2 + Gx^3y^0 + Hx^2y^1 + Ix^1y^2 + Jx^0y^3 + \ldots$$

where the values A through J are adjusted to fit a two-dimensional data set. The order of the polynomial is now given by the sum of the powers of x and y. For example, if the surface to be fit was adequately represented by a polynomial that included only the A through J terms in equation 3 and no additional terms, then the polynomial would be third order. The sum of the x and y exponents in the terms $Gx^3y^0 + Hx^2y^1 + Ix^1y^2 + Jx^0y^3$ all add up to 3. Second-order terms would be given by the terms $Dx^2y^0 + Ex^1y^1 + Fx^0y^2$, since the sum of the x and y exponents in these terms all add to 2. Similarly, the terms $Bx^1y^0 + Cx^0y^1$ are first order since the sum of the x and y exponents in these terms all add to unity. The preceding two-dimensional example is an example of a Taylor series. The Taylor series is a common representation of the wavefront shapes, such as the ones depicted in Figure 8-2.

Zernike Polynomials

An alternative representation of the wavefront shape can also be performed in polar coordinates (r,q), where r is the radial distance from the pupil center and q is the angle of the semimeridian for a given point on the wavefront. In this case, an expansion into Zernike polynomials is typically used. To determine the order of a surface fitted by Zernike polynomials, the highest power of r—the radial coordinate—is found.

Ordering of Aberrations

In Figure 8-2, the aberrated wavefronts can be examined to determine their order. The wavefront error, or the difference in shape between the aberrated wavefront and the ideal wavefront for myopia, hyperopia, and astigmatism in Figures 8-2b through 8-2d are well represented by a polynomial of second order. These aberrations are therefore called second-order aberrations. Coma, from Figure 8-2f, is a third-order aberration since its wavefront error is well fit by third-order polynomials. Spherical aberration, from Figure 8-2e, is a fourth-order aberration since its wavefront error is described by a polynomial with an order of four. In general, the actual wavefront in the human eye will have a complex shape, and many higher orders of aberration will exist.

Irregular astigmatism is the component of refractive error that is not correctable with a spherocylinder lens.

ABLATION OPTICAL ZONE DESIGNS

Munnerlyn, et al[1] derived ablation thickness profiles for myopic and hyperopic ablation patterns.

$$z_0 \text{ ablation depth (or height)} = \frac{\text{OZ diameter}^2 \text{ (diopter correction)}}{3}$$

This derivation assumes both thin lens theory and paraxial optics. Figure 8-3, adapted from Munnerlyn, et al[1] shows the preoperative corneal radius of curvature R_{pre}, the desired postoperative radius of curvature R_{post}, the ablation optical zone diameter D, and the central ablation depth z_o for a myopic ablation. The tissue in the region between the pre- and postoperative corneas can be considered a contact lens of diameter D. Removal of this tissue (height) is equivalent to adding a thin negative lens of power ϕ given by (equation 4):

$$\phi = (n-1) \left(\frac{1}{R_{post}} - \frac{1}{R_{pre}} \right)$$

where n = 1.3771 is the index of refraction of the cornea. It should be noted here that the actual index of the cornea is required in equation 4 and not the keratometric index of refraction, n_k = 1.3375, commonly used to represent corneal dioptric power or keratometric diopters. The thickness, z_o, of this contact lens is approximately

$$z_o = -\frac{D^2 \times \text{(dioptric correction)}}{8(n-1)}$$

where D is the optical zone diameter and n = 1.3771.

In the Munnerlyn derivation, the preoperative

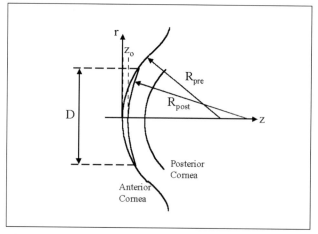

Figure 8-3. The pre- and postoperative cornea in refractive surgery. R_{pre} is the preoperative radius of curvature, R_{post} is the postoperative radius of curvature, z_o is the central ablation depth, and D is the diameter of the ablation zone.

cornea shown in Figure 8-1 is assumed to be a sphere. The elevation of the preoperative corneal surface z_{pre} is given by (equation 5):

$$z_{pre}(r) = R_{pre} - \sqrt{R^2_{pre} - r^2}$$

where r is the radial coordinate shown in Figure 8-3. Similarly, the elevation of the postoperative cornea is assumed spherical and is given by (equation 6):

$$z_{post}(r) = z_o + R_{post} - \sqrt{R^2_{post} - r^2}$$

where again z_o is the central thickness (height) of the ablation pattern. Equation 6 is only valid for the region inside the ablation optical zone (r < D/2). At the edge of the ablation optical zone, r = D/2, the elevation of the pre- and postoperative cornea must be equal. In other words, $z_{pre}(D/2) = z_{post}(D/2)$ at the edge of the treatment. Furthermore, equation 4 can be solved for R_{post} and the result substituted into equation 6. Using these two relationships, the ablation depth $z_{abl}(r)$ is then given by (equation 7):

$$z_{abl}(r) = z_{pre}(r) - z_{post}(r) = \left[R^2_{pre} - \frac{D^2}{4} \right]^{1/2} - \left[R^2_{pre} - r^2 \right]^{1/2} + \left[\left(\frac{(n-1) R_{pre}}{\phi R_{pre} + n-1} \right)^2 - r^2 \right]^{1/2} - \left[\left(\frac{(n-1)R_{pre}}{\phi R_{pre} + n-1} \right)^2 - \frac{D^2}{4} \right]^{1/2}$$

Equation 7 is equivalent to equation 2 in Munnerlyn, et al[1] except for a change in notation and sign convention. A negative value of z_{abl} represents the removal of corneal tissue is this case, whereas the

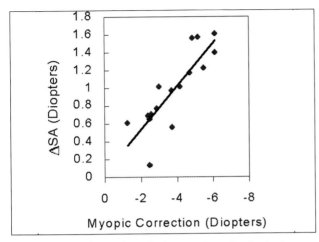

Figure 8-4. The induced change in spherical aberration (expressed in diopters) caused by PRK in 16 patients.

> The Munnerlyn pattern is designed to eliminate spherical and cylindrical refractive error. It does not address problems like spherical aberration.

preceding work had a positive value corresponding to tissue removal. Equation 7 can be extended to incorporate astigmatic correction by superimposing a cylindrical ablation pattern onto the rotationally symmetric pattern described above.

The Munnerlyn pattern is designed to eliminate spherical and cylindrical refractive error. The drawback to the Munnerlyn equation is that it really only targets correcting spherical refractive error while ignoring the other aberrations of the eye. In effect, the Munnerlyn equations work well in regions of the cornea where the surface is well represented by a sphere and the corresponding portion of the wavefront passing through this region is essentially spherical as well. This restricts the ability of the Munnerlyn formula to correcting aberrations in a small region around the visual axis. As shown in Figure 8-2e, wavefronts with spherical aberration look spherical in their center but deviate from a spherical shape in their periphery. The eye has inherent spherical aberration, and the Munnerlyn shape modifies the degree of spherical aberration in the eye in an uncontrolled fashion. Furthermore, imperfect delivery of the Munnerlyn pattern and the effects of healing can introduce large levels of spherical aberration. By not controlling the spherical aberration introduced by refractive surgery, detrimental effects such as glare and halos can be introduced, thus degrading postoperative visual performance. The

> By not controlling spherical aberration introduced by refractive surgery, detrimental effects such as glare and halos can be introduced.

righthand side of Figure 8-2e(III) shows the image of a point for an eye with spherical aberration. Note the halo around the tight spot in this diagram.

CLINICAL STUDIES ON SPHERICAL ABERRATION

Several researchers have shown elevated levels of spherical aberration in the eyes of photorefractive keratectomy (PRK) patients.[2-4] Schwiegerling, et al[4] examined the introduction of spherical aberration caused by PRK in 16 myopic patients. Each patient underwent PRK using a Summit OmniMed laser (Summit Technologies, Waltham, Mass). Each procedure had an OZ size of 6.0 mm and attempted corrections ranging from -1.25 to -6.12 D. Informed consent was obtained prior to the procedure and all institutional review board procedures were followed. Figure 8-4 shows the change in spherical aberration ΔSA at the edge of a 4.0-mm pupil for the 16 study patients. All postoperative data were obtained at least 9 weeks following the PRK procedure. Regression analysis was used to fit the data, and the fit has a correlation coefficient r^2 of 71% and is described by (equation 8):

$$\Delta SA = -0.242\phi + 0.052 \, D$$

where ϕ is the attempted spherical correction in diopters. The plot in Figure 8-4 demonstrates that spherical aberration is introduced by the PRK procedure above and beyond the inherent spherical aberration of the eye, and the magnitude of the aberration increases with attempted correction. Equation 8 suggests that for a 4.0-mm pupil, approximately 0.25 D of spherical aberration is added for each diopter of attempted correction. To control the spherical aberration introduced by refractive surgery, the asphericity of the postoperative cornea needs to be controlled.

A BICONIC ABLATION FORMULA

A biconic is a useful representation of an aspheric corneal surface with axial astigmatism. The surface elevation $h(r,\Theta)$ of a biconic is given by (equation 9):

$$h(r,\Theta) = \frac{r^2 \cos^2(\Theta-\Theta_o)/R_x + r^2 \sin^2(\Theta-\Theta_o)/R_y}{1+(1-[1-(K_x+1)r^2\cos^2(\Theta-\Theta_o)/R^2_x-(K_y+1)r^2\sin^2(\Theta-\Theta_o)/R^2_y]^{1/2}}$$

where, again, r is the radial position on the cornea and U is the azimuthal coordinate or angular position on the cornea. While equation 9 appears complex, it is simply a general description for a spherocylinder surface that can be aspheric. The equation describes a surface with an aspheric profile of radius of curvature Rx and conic constant Kx along one meridian. The profile along the perpendicular meridian is an asphere with a radius of curvature Ry and a conic constant of Ky. In the special case of Rx = Ry and Kx = Ky = 0, equation 9 collapses to an equation of a sphere. In this manner, equation 9 can be used as a generalization of the Munnerlyn spherical cornea such that the cornea can now be aspheric (ie, flatten toward its periphery), as well as contain corneal astigmatism. Schwiegerling, et al[5] have derived a generalization of the Munnerlyn ablation pattern such that spherical and cylindrical refractive error, as well as spherical aberration, can be corrected with the appropriate ablation. The biconic ablation pattern is designed to eliminate spherical aberration in addition to spherical and cylindrical refractive error.

> The biconic ablation pattern is designed to eliminate spherical aberration in addition to spherical and cylindrical refractive error.

The ablation pattern as a function of position on the cornea can be described in terms of the preceding relationships. The pre- and postoperative corneal shapes can be written as (equations 10 and 11):

$$z_{pre}(r,\Theta) = h_{pre}(r,\Theta)$$

and

$$z_{post}(r,\Theta) = z_o + h_{post}(r,\Theta)$$

respectively. The functions $h_{pre}(r,\Theta)$ and $h_{post}(r,\Theta)$ represent pre- and postoperative biconic surfaces described mathematically by equation 9. The value of z_o represents the central ablation depth. As in the case of the Munnerlyn ablation, equation 11 is only valid for the region inside the ablation optical zone (r < D/2). The ablation depth is given by the difference in shape between the pre- and postoperative corneas, or (equation 12):

$$z_{abl}(r,\Theta) = z_{pre}(r,\Theta) - z_{post}(r,\Theta)$$

for r < D/2. Equation 12 must be strictly less than or equal to zero (ie, only tissue can be removed from the cornea) for ablation processes, which sets a minimum for the central ablation depth z_o. The preceding biconic ablation patterns control for spherical and astigmatic refractive error, as well as spherical aberration. The next level of sophistication in ablation pattern design is to measure the aberration structure of a given individual and deliver a customized ablation based on this information.

A Customized Ablation Formula

To predict the shape of a customized ablation pattern, an accurate measurement of the aberration structure of an individual's eye is necessary. Current wavefront sensor technology indirectly measures the wavefront error of the eye. The wavefront error is simply the difference between the actual wavefront shape and the perfectly spherical wavefront. The shape of the actual wavefront changes as it propagates through space. For customized ablation, the wavefront shape at the anterior corneal surface is required. If the wavefront error at the anterior cornea is described in polar coordinates by $W(r,\Theta)$, then the customized ablation pattern required to correct is given by (equation 13):

$$z_{abl}(r,\Theta) = \frac{W(r,\Theta)}{n-1}$$

where n = 1.3771 is the index of refraction of the cornea. There are several assumptions implicit to equation 13. First, the wavefront error must be accurately described in the corneal plane. As the aberrated wavefront propagates through space, it changes shape. Measurement of the aberration structure at another plane requires the wavefront to be propagated to the corneal plane or an assumption of only small wavefront shape changes between the measurement and corneal planes. Second, the wavefront error measured with light coming from a distant point, as is the case with aberroscopes, will not be the same as wavefront error from a point source placed on the retina, as in the Shack-Hartmann sensor. In general, these differences will be small. Finally, as a given light ray passes through the unablated cornea, it follows a prescribed path as it passes through the other optical surfaces of the eye. The ray acquires aberration from each of the surfaces. The ablation pattern is designed to compensate the aberrations introduced by the posterior cornea and crystalline lens for this ray. Following ablation, the light ray will follow a slightly different path or optical path length through the surfaces of the eye, and the posterior cornea and crystalline lens contributions to aberrations will be slightly different than they were prior to treatment. Equation 13 assumes that the ablation pattern still compensates for the aberrations introduced into a given ray, even though it will take a slightly different path through the eye.

> The customized ablation pattern is designed to eliminate all of the significant aberrations of the eye.

The three different types of ablation patterns—Munnerlyn, biconic, and customized—described in this section illustrate different levels of sophistication. The Munnerlyn formula is designed to correct the spherical and cylindrical refractive error. The biconic ablation generalizes the ablation pattern to compensate for spherical aberration in addition to spherical and cylindrical refractive error. Finally, the custom ablation pattern accounts for the aberrations in the eye. The customized ablation pattern is designed to eliminate all of the significant aberrations of the eye.

> One cannot simply grind an optical design into the cornea without considering the importance of smooth transitions.

ABLATION TRANSITION ZONE DESIGN

We have reviewed the optics of customized ablation design and now would like to describe some principles of ablation design that are a practical concern. One cannot simply grind an optical design into the cornea without considering the importance of smooth transitions. Recall our previous discussion on ablation optical zone that stated at the edge of the ablation optical zone the elevation of the pre- and postoperative cornea must be equal (equation 7). This needs to be done with a smooth transition in curvature.

Conservation of Curvature

The concept of conservation of curvature is critical to understanding ablation designs. In general, if one steepens the cornea in one location, there will be a flatter area adjacent to this steepened zone to compensate for the steep curvature. This places constraints on how much curvature can occur over the diameter of the cornea. We can correct refractive errors in higher-order aberrations in the ablation optical zone, but we also need to consider how to smoothly blend this curvature to be continuous with the untreated peripheral cornea. This should also be done while minimizing excessive tissue removal (tissue conservation).

Corneal ablation is also constrained by the biologic and biomechanical reactions of the cornea. We have learned that one cannot simply perform a 6-mm, 60-micron deep plano lenticle (a crater) without having a significant filling by the epithelium and stroma in an attempt to smooth out the crater that has been created. This is essentially what one does in the flat meridian using a 4 D PARK cylindrical ablation pattern with no transition zone (Figure 8-5). One observes hypertrophic scar and excessive flattening (probably from tissue addition and biomechanical effect). This is not anticipated from optical and engineering perspectives. The biomechanical effect is described in Chapter Nine.

We can further improve on the design of this myopic astigmatic ablation by adding a transition zone that can blend out the steep curvature change to improve the biologic tolerance (Figure 8-6). A three-dimensional view of this is provided in Figure 8-7. The slope of this transition zone should be kept to a minimum to prevent regression and shrinkage of the effective optical zone. In general, the greater the correction attempted, the larger the required transition zone. One can also minimize excessive tissue removal by creating an elliptical transition zone, which is done by reducing the transition zone diameter in the steep meridian (Figure 8-8). Similar strategy can be used for hyperopic astigmatic ablation (Figure 8-9). We also see combinations of these strategies for cross cylinder ablation, as will be discussed by Drs. Chayet and Vinciguerra later in this book.

> **Conservation of curvature:** in general, if one steepens the cornea in one location, there will be a flatter area adjacent to this steepened area to compensate for the steep curvature. The same rule applies for flattening.

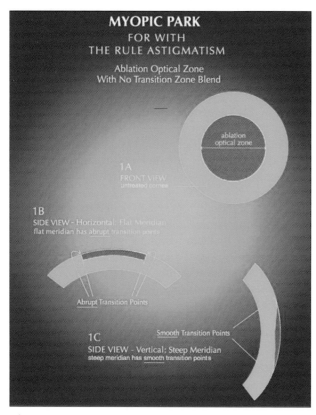

Figure 8-5. Astigmatic ablation pattern with circular optical zone. Note abrupt transition in the flat horizontal meridian.

TRANSITION POINTS

A transition point is where there is a change in curvature. Hyperopic treatments have three times as many transition points as do simple myopic ablations, which only have one transition point in each hemimeridian (Figure 8-10). For instance, myopic PARK treatments have one transition zone in the steep meridian and two transition zones in the flat meridian. The one transition zone in the steep meridian is at the junction of the ablated and nonablated zones. The two transition zones in the flat meridian with myopic PARK include one at the junction of the ablation optical zone and the transition zone. The second transition point is at the junction of the transition zone with the untreated cornea in each hemimeridian. Hyperopic treatments have three transition points in each hemimeridian.

This may explain why hyperopic treatments, which have three times as many transition points, can only treat one-third of the amount of hyperopia when compared to simple myopia. Typically, the highest treatments are roughly in the 4 to 6 D range

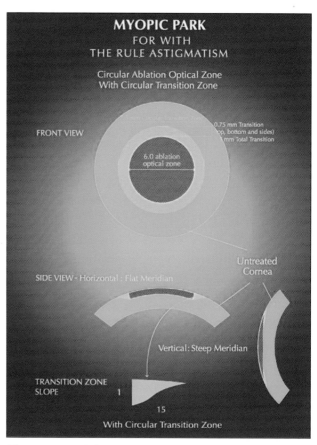

Figure 8-6. High astigmatism PARK myopic treatment with a 6.0-mm circular optical ablation zone and a 7.5-mm circular transition zone. The preoperative refraction on this eye is -4.00 -4.00 x 180 degrees. The slope of the transition zone is steep at 1/15. The treatment demonstrates a smoother transition, which is better tolerated than for Figure 8.5. This can be further improved or smoothed by increasing the transition zone in the flat meridian (and making it elliptical), as noted in Figure 8-8.

> Hyperopic ablations have three times as many transition points as myopic ablations. This may explain why we are only able to treat one-third the amount of hyperopia compared to myopia.

for hyperopia and 12 to 18 D for myopia. This may also explain why larger diameter transition zones are required when compared to myopic treatments. The typical myopic transition zone is approximately 1.0 to 1.5 mm compared to 2.0 to 3.0 mm for hyperopia.

Over the last several years, much attention has been paid to the critical nature of transition zones and how they may help create a smoother transition for the ablation optical zone. With customized abla-

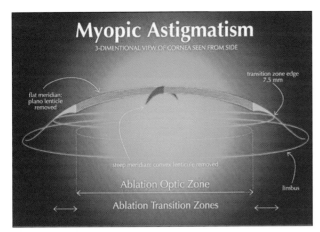

Figure 8-7. Three-dimensional view of PARK with a transition zone. In the flat meridian, a plano lenticle is removed. In the steep meridian, a convex lenticle is removed. Note the smooth transition points, which are well-tolerated biologically.

> Aberrations are inherent to any optical system, and their complexity ranges from a simple shift in focus from the retina to highly aberrated wavefronts, which form distorted images on the retina.

tion this will become even more critical. Since wavefront sensors only measure the area of the cornea within the pupil, they are not able to measure the transition zones outside of a widely dilated pupil. This is where corneal topography may be quite helpful in the future. By paying careful attention to transition zone design, one can obtain more effective improvement in the optics of ablations. One can also minimize unnecessary tissue removal while customizing the ablation design. This will continue to be critical for customized ablation.

> With customized ablations, smoother transition points and zones will be more important.

OVERVIEW

In this chapter, an introduction to aberration has been presented. Aberrations are inherent to any optical system, and their complexity ranges from a simple shift in focus from the retina to highly aberrated wavefronts, which form distorted images on the retina. Spherical and cylindrical refractive aberrations are basic because they are the most prevalent aberrations in the eye, and they can be corrected with conventional spectacles or contact lenses. However,

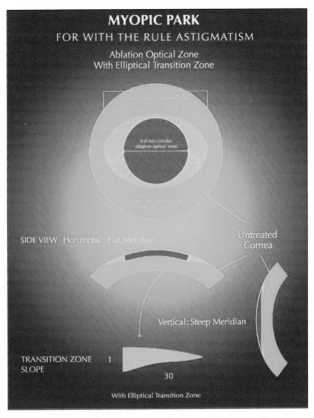

Figure 8-8. Higher astigmatism PARK myopia treatment with a 6-mm circular optical zone and a 9-mm elliptical transition zone. The slope of the transition zone is reduced to 1/30 in the flat meridian to treat a -4.00 -4.00 x 180-degree patient using a 6.0-mm ablation optical zone. The reduced slope makes the transition more gradual (than that noted in Figure 8-7) at the 3:00 and 9:00 positions, which is better tolerated biologically.

spherical and cylindrical refractive errors are only a portion of the possible aberrations in the eye. With the advent of new technology, it is now possible to measure and dramatically reduce aberrations in the eye. By accounting for these other aberrations inherent to the eye, visual performance following refractive surgery may be markedly increased.

Three different types of ablation patterns have been discussed. Each pattern accounts for higher degrees of aberration correction. The Munnerlyn formula corrects spherical and cylindrical error. However, it was shown that current treatments introduce large amounts of spherical aberration as they reduce spherical and cylindrical error. The biconic ablation gives a prescription for simultaneously controlling spherical and cylindrical error, as well as spherical aberration. Finally, the custom ablation

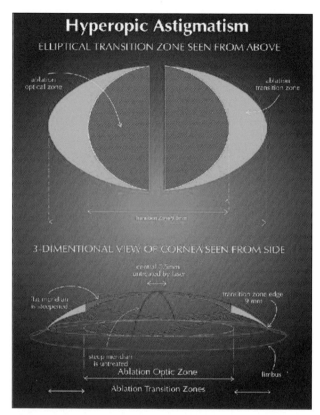

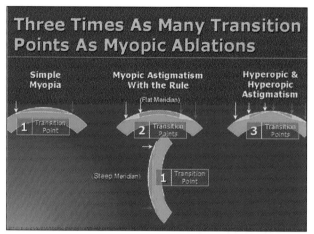

Figure 8-10. Transition points of the cornea demonstrating corneal ablation for simple myopia, compound myopia, as well as hyperopia and hyperopic astigmatism. The simple myopic ablation has one transition point on each side (semimeridian). Compound myopic treatment has two transition points in the steep meridian and one transition point in the flat meridian on each side. Hyperopic and hyperopic flat meridian ablation treatment has three transition points on each side.

Figure 8-9. The same principle of elliptical transition can be applied to hyperopic treatment. A: hyperopic PARK using an elliptical transition zone. The steep vertical meridian at 90 degrees and 270 degrees is untreated by the laser, while the flat meridian is steepened using the elliptical pattern. This same pattern may be used to treat mixed astigmatism. B: three-dimensional view of hyperopic astigmatism treatment.

allows for the correction of the measurable aberrations of the eye. Each successive ablation pattern accounts for more of the aberrations of the eye, and each should therefore offer improvements in visual performance. Accounting for more aberrations in the ablation patterns, however, also requires improvements in technology. The Munnerlyn formula requires knowledge of the patient's refractive error and K values. The biconic ablation requires knowledge of the patient's refractive error, K values, and an estimate of his or her spherical aberration. Finally, custom ablations require knowledge of the aberration structure of the entire eye. The laser technology to deliver these ablation patterns accurately is also required. The tolerances on placement and shape of the ablation pattern are much more critical when more aberrations are accounted for because of the

subtle features inherent in these patterns. This is particularly true for higher-order aberrations.

The ablation patterns outlined in this chapter are based upon optical principles. They represent the required shape of the cornea following surgery. In order for the cornea to match these shapes, the laser tissue removal must incorporate biological changes to the cornea, including biomechanical shape changes induced by weakening the framework of the cornea and the healing response. By only looking at the optical properties of the refractive surgery cornea, the boundary between the ablated and unablated regions has been ignored. In general, there should exist a smooth and continuous transition between these two regions to facilitate uniform healing. The shape of the transition regions will be largely dependent upon the shape and type of ablation pattern used for correction. For example, performing an ablation pattern to correct for cylindrical error requires the ablation pattern to be oval so that no discontinuities or steps in corneal tissue occur. Forcing this ablation pattern to be circular causes a step in the rim of the pattern everywhere except at the edge of the flat meridian. Figure 8-5 shows an example of an astigmatic ablation with a circular ablation optical zone. Along the flat meridian, the tissue in the ablated region blends perfectly with the tissue outside of the ablation pattern. However, along the steep meridian, there is a discontinuity or step in tissue height at the boundary of the ablation pattern. In this case, a well-designed transition zone is important to control the healing response of the cornea. One of the authors has suggested using an elliptical blending zone to alleviate the step problem. The blending zone would have the narrow portion of the ellipse along the flat axis of the ablation pattern. The narrow portion of the ellipse is almost the same size as the ablation pattern so that minimal additional tissue is removed outside of the ablation pattern along the flat axis. The long axis of the ellipse would lie along the steep axis of the ablation pattern. The long axis of the ellipse is larger than the ablation optical zone such that the step height is slowly blended back to the height of the cornea along the steep axis.

This chapter is meant to provide an overview of aberrations inherent to the eye and how ablation patterns are designed to correct for these aberrations. The tools to correct aberrations beyond spherical and cylindrical error were not feasible in the past. However, emerging technology now offers the potential to correct for aberrations in the eye. To correct simple spherical and cylindrical error, the Munnerlyn pattern is required. To further correct spherical aberration, biconic ablation patterns, which control the asphericity of the cornea, are required. To go further and correct even higher-order aberrations in the eye, the more complex shape of a customized ablation is necessary. Each of these steps in complexity of the ablation pattern forces the wavefront converging from the crystalline lens toward the retina to become closer to the ideal spherical shape. Therefore, each step in complexity offers a step toward improving visual performance toward the theoretical limit.

REFERENCES

1. Munnerlyn CR, Koons SJ, Marshall J. Photorefractive keratectomy: a technique for laser refractive surgery. *J Cataract Refract Surg*. 1988;14:46-52.

2. Oshika T, Klyce SD, Applegate RA, Howland HC, El Danasoury MA. Comparison of corneal wavefront aberrations after photorefractive keratectomy and laser in situ keratomileusis. *Am J Ophthalmol*. 1999;127:1-7.

3. Oliver KM, Hemenger RP, Corbett MC, et al. Corneal optical aberrations induced by photorefractive keratectomy. *J Refract Surg*. 1997;13:246-254.

4. Schwiegerling J, Snyder RW. Corneal ablation patterns to correct for spherical aberration in photorefractive keratectomy. *J Cataract Refract Surg*. 2000;26:214-221.

5. Schwiegerling J, Snyder RW. Custom photorefractive keratectomy ablations for the correction of spherical and cylindrical refractive error and higher-order aberration. *J Opt Soc Am A*. 1998;15:2572-2579.

6. MacRae S. Excimer ablation design and elliptical transition zones. *J Cataract Refract Surg*. 1999;25:1191-1197.

Chapter Nine

Corneal Biomechanics and Their Role in Corneal Ablative Procedures

Cynthia Roberts, PhD
William J. Dupps, Jr, MD, PhD

In the quest for the ideal corneal ablation, a major obstacle yet to be overcome is the inadequacy of current models for predicting the *corneal response* to ablation, which impacts the potential future success of both topography- and wavefront-guided customized procedures. In its current state, the process of ablation design relies on a "black box" approach, wherein enormous efforts are directed at linking "input" variables (the ablation algorithm) to "output" variables (refractive error, visual acuity, glare, aberration, patient satisfaction, etc), while the physical interface between input and output—the actual mechanisms of interaction between all relevant components—is largely neglected. Ablation and surgical outcome are ultimately linked on two levels: (1) a deterministic cause-effect relationship dictated by physical reality and (2) a statistical relationship rooted in probability and defined in retrospective regression analyses of the same variables in large-scale clinical trials. Initial attempts at photorefractive keratectomy (PRK) used a simple model presented by Munnerlyn, et al.[1] This "shape-subtraction" paradigm (to be described in the next section) is based on a logical geometric approach to tissue removal and secondary curvature change. When this approach failed to produce the expected refractive outcomes with consistency, it became clear that the model was incomplete. Growing appreciation for the complexity of the corneal response, coupled with a rapidly growing body of clinical experience, led to a more empirical approach to algorithm design. Ablation routines in widespread use today are derived from large statistical analyses in which a number of variables are evaluated for their ability to predict refractive outcome without an understanding of the physical response of the cornea to structural change secondary to tissue removal.

Among a large array of possible input variables, the ablation algorithm is the most exquisitely controllable. Consequently, it is often the sole focus of refractive control in developing sophisticated corneal ablation routines based on topographic and/or wavefront analysis. However, the components of corneal response that contribute to unpredictability in noncustomized procedures still influences the refractive outcome and overall visual performance. Although empirically modified ablation algorithms have produced reasonable results in many patients, they are unlikely to provide the individual predictability that physicians desire and patients increasingly demand. Algorithms derived from probabilistic models are optimized for the *mean population* response rather than that of the *individual*, and a certain degree of prediction error is inescapable. The current practical approach to refrac-

> Algorithms derived from probabilistic models are optimized for the *mean population* response rather than that of the *individual*, and a certain degree of prediction error is inescapable.

tive surgery has become one of iteration between ablation recipe and surgical response, with most surgical decisions being made at the empirical level and confounded by an incomplete working knowledge of the cornea's physical behavior during and after ablation. Individual surgeons use their own "fudge" factors, making systematic interpretation of results difficult. Thus, the fundamental challenge to the future of custom corneal ablation is to develop deterministic models that can be successfully applied to the individual patient, rather than relying heavily on empirical modification. This chapter addresses an important biomechanical determinant of the corneal response to ablation and presents a rationale for its inclusion in customized corneal ablation models.

CURRENTLY ACCEPTED "SHAPE-SUBTRACTION" MODEL OF LASER REFRACTIVE SURGERY

Munnerlyn, et al[1] described the equations that served as a starting point for developing current ablation algorithms. For a myopic ablation, the preoperative cornea is modeled as a sphere of greater curvature than the desired postoperative cornea, which is also modeled as a sphere. The apex of the desired postoperative cornea is displaced from the preoperative cornea by the maximal ablation depth, which is determined by the ablation zone size. The intervening tissue is simply removed or "subtracted" to produce the final result. This is illustrated in Figure 9-1 for a myopic, as well as a hyperopic, profile (which is similar in concept but with a different planned ablation profile that produces increased postoperative curvature). This concept will be referred to as the shape-subtraction model of refractive surgery and treats the cornea as if it were a homogeneous structure, like a piece of plastic. The shape-subtraction paradigm permeates current thinking in refractive surgery and forms the basis for both topography- and wavefront-guided procedures. Therefore, it is important to understand the weaknesses of the shape-subtraction model in order to move into the new arena of individual customization with greater demands for postoperative visual performance.

> There are three flawed assumptions inherent to the shape-subtraction model of laser ablation.

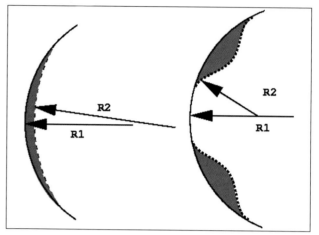

Figure 9-1. Schematic diagram of shape-subtraction model of refractive surgery for a myopic ablation (left) and hyperopic ablation (right). The preoperative radius of curvature is R1 and the desired postoperative curvature is R2. The maximum ablation depth is determined by the ablation zone size. The intervening tissue, shown in red, between the preoperative curve (solid) and postoperative curve (dashed/dotted) is "subtracted" with an excimer laser to produce the desired result (adapted from Munnerlyn CR, Koons SJ, Marshall J. Photorefractive keratectomy: a technique for laser refractive surgery. *J Cataract Refract Surg.* 1988;14:46-52).

There are three *flawed* assumptions inherent to the shape-subtraction model of laser ablation that may account for some of the outcome variability and visual aberrations produced by laser refractive surgery. They are:

1. The only part of the corneal shape affected by the procedure is within the ablation zone.
2. "What you cut is what you get."
3. Even if changes occur outside the ablation zone, they do not affect central shape or vision.

Each of these assumptions will be examined in turn for validity with both case reports and results from clinical studies.

Question #1. Are corneal shape changes confined to the ablation zone where laser energy is deposited?

The shape-subtraction model of refractive surgery allows for corneal shape changes only within the ablation zone, with some possible edge effects due to healing across the transition from ablated to unablated tissue. Yet, clinical data show substantial changes in curvature well *outside* the ablation zone where

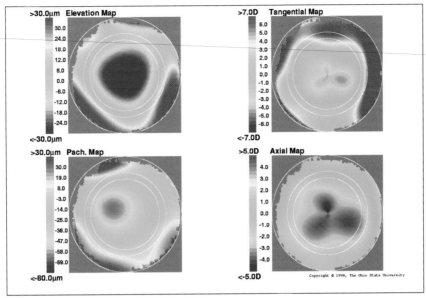

Figure 9-2. Postoperative minus preoperative difference maps from a -2.25 D LASIK correction with a 6-mm-diameter ablation zone. Topography was acquired using Orbscan and exported for analysis using custom software. The inner, middle, and outer white circles have radii of 2.75 mm, 3.25 mm, and 4.5 mm, respectively. The central zone within the inner circle lies within the ablation zone. The edge of the ablation zone is contained within the annulus between the center and middle circles. Expected central decreases in elevation, pachymetry, and curvature are seen as negative differences on the respective maps. However, unexpected increases in elevation, pachymetry, and curvature have occurred outside the ablation zone due to the biomechanical response of the cornea to a change in its structure. This is seen within the annulus between the middle and outer circles where the redder colors represent increases.

laser energy was *not* deposited. To investigate this phenomenon, a retrospective study was performed on a population of 19 eyes of 30 subjects who had Orbscan corneal topography (Orbscan, Salt Lake City, Utah), both pre- and postoperatively after laser-assisted in situ keratomileusis (LASIK) with a Technolas 217 (Munich, Germany) excimer laser. Curvature maps were exported to a custom analysis software tool[2] for processing. Average differences were calculated in two corneal regions, both inside and outside the ablation zone. The average curvature change was -2.62 diopters (D) within the ablation zone, and +5.42 D well outside the ablation zone to a diameter of 9 mm.[3] In addition, regression analysis between the central and peripheral curvature changes showed a significant negative correlation (p < 0.0053), indicating that greater central flattening produced greater peripheral steepening. The peripheral increase in curvature is a known consequence of laser refractive surgery but has never been fully explained other than as a "knee" at the edge of the ablation profile. If this were an accurate description, the change would be confined near the edge of the ablation zone, yet it extends well beyond that region. Additional data in the form of elevation and pachymetry maps from the same patient population also showed significant peripheral *increases* in both elevation and pachymetry *outside* the ablation zone, corresponding to the increase in curvature.[3] These paradoxical changes in elevation and pachymetry have been anecdotally attributed to measurement device errors without exploration of the responsible biomechanical mechanisms. Figure 9-2 shows four difference maps from a sample patient in this population with a 6-mm ablation zone, including elevation, tangential, axial, and pachymetry differences. The expected decreases in curvature, elevation, and pachymetry centrally within the ablation zone are noted. However, the maps also show unexpected *increases* in elevation, pachymetry, and curvature *out-*

Table 9-1

RMS Error Between Predicted and Measured Topography After LASIK

	ELEVATION MEAN (N = 10) RMS ERROR	CURVATURE MEAN (N = 10) RMS ERROR
Central 4 mm diameter	18 ± 14 microns	4.92 ± 1.89 D
4 to 9 mm diameter zone	23 ± 11 microns	8.06 ± 1.76 D
Overall	22 ± 11 microns	6.85 ± 1.50 D

side the ablation zone. Therefore, the results of this study challenge the validity of the assumption that corneal curvature changes are confined to the ablation zone. The proposed mechanism for the paradoxical changes in elevation and pachymetry will be given in the Biomechanical Model section of this chapter.

Question #2. Does the ablation profile alone define the resulting corneal shape?

The results of the analysis of question #1 demonstrated that shape changes occur well beyond the ablation zone. Question #2 can be examined more directly by comparing ablation profiles to actual corneal surface changes. A preliminary study was performed on 10 LASIK patients without astigmatism who had symmetric ablation patterns. Pre- and postoperative topography was obtained using an Orbscan I. LASIK was performed using a Technolas 217 excimer laser. Ablation algorithms were approximated using Munnerlyn's formulas.[1] The calculated ablation profile was subtracted from the preoperative topography to generate a predicted postoperative topography. Actual postoperative topography was compared to predicted postoperative topography and error maps generated. RMS errors were calculated within the central 4-mm diameter zone, outside the central zone, and over the entire map. Results averaged for all 10 subjects are given in Table 9-1 and demonstrate a larger error outside the 4-mm central zone than inside. A sample error map is given in Figure 9-3, which shows a pattern of positive error peripherally in elevation, pachymetry, and curvature with negative error centrally in elevation, pachymetry, and somewhat in curvature, although curvature is not consistently negative over the whole central region. These patterns of error cannot simply be attributed to using an estimated rather than known ablation profile since they are both nonrandom and nonlinear. Ideally, the actual ablation algorithms should be used in a study of this type rather than Munnerlyn's formulas, but they were not available due to their proprietary nature. However, despite using estimated ablation profiles, the evidence presented challenges the validity of question #2. These patterns of error are not consistent with a shape-subtraction model of ablation, but they are consistent with the biomechanical model to be proposed in the next section. In addition, further work has been done using actual proprietary ablation algorithms, demonstrating both central and peripheral error relative to predicted corneal shape.[4]

Question #3. Do corneal shape changes outside the ablation zone affect central shape and vision?

It has been known since the inception of refractive surgery that altering the corneal structure will alter the shape of the entire cornea, whether using an incisional or thermal mechanism. Fundamentally, if the cornea was a piece of plastic, radial keratotomy would not have worked! Yet, with the development of laser refractive surgery, the structural link between the central and peripheral cornea was ignored. The cornea was thought of quite simply as a homogeneous structure to be "sculpted" into a new shape. However, this conceptualization cannot account for all of the corneal shape changes that occur after an ablative procedure. An important component of the proposed biomechanical model of corneal response to laser refractive surgery, to be described in the next section, is peripheral stromal thickening or an *increase* in corneal elevation *outside* the ablation zone. Evidence that this occurs was pre-

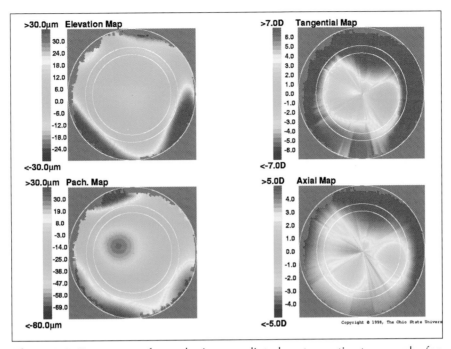

Figure 9-3. Error maps of actual minus predicted postoperative topography for the same subject as in Figure 9-2. Predicted postoperative topography was generated by calculating an estimated ablation profile using Munnerlyn's formulas[1] and subtracting it from the preoperative raw elevation. Predicted curvature was then calculated along corneal meridians. Note that both the elevation and pachymetry error maps demonstrate less than predicted central values (or greater than expected ablation depth), as indicated by negative numbers and blue color. However, both maps also paradoxically show greater than predicted differences outside the ablation zone. The tangential curvature error map also shows greater than expected curvature change outside the ablation zone. Centrally, the values range from less than predicted to greater than predicted, with overall less error than outside the ablation zone. These errors are consistent with the biomechanical model proposed in this chapter.

sented in the analysis of question #1. However, the question remains as to the linking of the central and peripheral corneal events. Is the peripheral increase in corneal elevation statistically correlated to central curvature changes or are they independent, unrelated occurrences? Regression analysis between central curvature change and peripheral elevation change from the 30 subjects presented under the analysis of question #1 demonstrated a significant positive correlation ($R^2 = 0.56$, $p < 0.0001$), indicating that the greater the increase in elevation outside the ablation zone, the greater the curvature change (flattening) centrally.[4] This provides evidence that the peripheral response of the cornea is linked to the central response, although it does not account for all the variance.

The following case study further illustrates how

central curvature changes can actually track peripheral thickness changes after ablation. The patient had 6-mm diameter PRK (VisX Star, Santa Clara, Calif) for a refractive error of -3.75 + 0.75 x 90, with Orbscan I topography pre- and postoperatively. Both superior and inferior corneal thicknesses were calculated by averaging a 1-mm diameter region in the pachymetry map along the vertical meridian at the edges of a 7.5-mm diameter circle centered on the ablation zone. Central curvature was calculated by averaging the curvature in the 3-mm diameter central region of the tangential map. The values as a function of time relative to surgery are given in Table 9-2. Note that both central curvature and peripheral thickness demonstrate postoperative fluctuation in opposite directions. Regression analysis of central curvature versus peripheral thickness was performed, and the

Table 9-2

Case Study of Curvature and Thickness Changes After 6-mm Diameter PRK

	SUPERIOR THICKNESS	INFERIOR THICKNESS	CENTRAL THICKNESS	CENTRAL CURVATURE
Preoperative	715 µm	682 µm	605 µm	41.55 D
30 minutes	770 µm	729 µm	710 µm	36.20 D
Day 4	727 µm	691 µm	589 µm	39.39 D
3 weeks	744 µm	701 µm	568 µm	38.81 D
3 months	722 µm	690 µm	570 µm	39.32 D

plots are given in Figure 9-4. Central curvature has a strong negative correlation with peripheral thickness, both inferior and superior, meaning the greater the peripheral thickness the flatter the central curvature. This provides further support that the central and peripheral changes are linked and assumption #3 is not valid.

Evidence has been presented challenging the inherent assumptions of the shape-subtraction model of refractive surgery. Clinical data indicate that substantial changes occur outside the ablation zone that are structurally linked to central curvature and may affect central vision. The proposed mechanism for the measured increases in elevation, thickness, and curvature that occur outside the ablation zone will be presented in the next section.

A BIOMECHANICAL MODEL OF KERATECTOMY-INDUCED CURVATURE CHANGE

In recent decades, a great deal of effort has been devoted to characterizing the cornea as a biomechanical entity. This work has included an *in vitro* measurement of key material properties such as the modulus of elasticity and shear modulus, and numerous computational models have been generated to approximate the structural response to simulated incisional keratectomy.[5-10] While these efforts have undoubtedly advanced the basic understanding of corneal behavior under certain specific conditions, less has been done relative to modeling the structural changes induced by laser keratectomy, and the predictive value of existing numerical models is limited by their implicit simplifications.

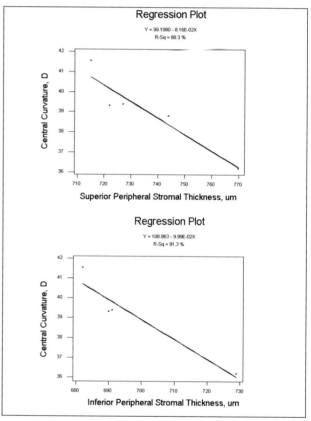

Figure 9-4. Regression analysis of peripheral stromal thickness of the superior region (upper plot) and inferior region (lower plot) against curvature in the central 3-mm region preoperatively and at four time points postoperatively after PRK in one patient. This demonstrates how central curvature for this patient closely tracked peripheral stromal thickness over time, also shown in Table 9-2.

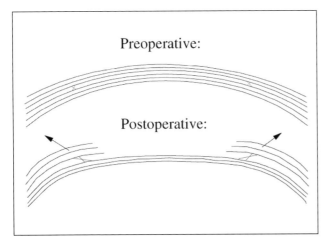

Figure 9-5. A biomechanical model for acute central flattening in photoablation. Preoperatively (top), the cornea is a layered structure consisting of many lamellae that stretch limbus to limbus and is loaded via the IOP. The interlamellar spacing is related to the tension carried in the individual lamellae. Postoperatively (bottom), a defined series of lamellae are circumferentially and permanently severed. Central ablation therefore reduces the tension in the remaining peripheral lamellar segments, analogous to cutting a stack of taut rubberbands with compressed sponges (matrix) in between each layer. The reduction of the "squeezing" force on the "sponges" allows expansion of the peripheral stromal matrix, indicated by arrows. Thickening generates an outward force that is communicated to the peripheral aspects of underlying lamellae through a network of lamellar interconnections (x). The postoperative lamellar interconnections are shown by blue x's, and the preoperative lamellar interconnections are shown by red x's. The result is flattening of the residual ablation bed and a refractive shift toward hyperopia independent of the ablation profile cut on the cornea.

> We have hypothesized that during PRK, PTK, and LASIK, central ablation causes an immediate circumferential severing of corneal lamellae under tension, with a subsequent relaxation of the corresponding peripheral lamellar segments.

The Biomechanical Theory

We have hypothesized that during PRK, PTK, and LASIK, central ablation causes an immediate circumferential severing of corneal lamellae under tension, with a subsequent relaxation of the corresponding peripheral lamellar segments. This causes a peripheral decompression of the extracellular matrix and an increase in stromal thickness outside of the ablation zone.[11,12] It is further hypothesized that this response has important effects on central curvature due mainly to the presence of interlamellar crosslinking, which predominates in the anterior one-third[13] and periphery[14] of the stroma and has been associated with significant lamellar shearing strength[15,16] and interlamellar cohesive strength.[17,18] Interlamellar stress is generated in the expanding stromal periphery and may be transferred through this network of crosslinks to the underlying lamellae, whose central portions comprise the postoperative anterior surface (Figure 9-5). The outward expansive force in the periphery causes the central cornea to flatten independent of the ablation profile. Thus, even in the absence of a myopic (centrally weighted) ablation pattern, biomechanical changes in the unablated peripheral cornea may produce an acute postoperative flattening of the central cornea and a refractive shift toward hyperopia. This response is perhaps most clearly demonstrated by the clinical phenomenon of unintended hyperopic shift in PTK, but its contribution to refractive variability in PRK and LASIK is also important since biomechanical central flattening will enhance a procedure to treat myopia and oppose a procedure to treat hyperopia. An additional feature of the model—an acute depth-dependent response—will also be discussed.

Essentials of Corneal Architecture and Mechanics

Of the five anatomic layers of the cornea, only Bowman's zone and the stroma contain collagen fibrils.[13] These layers are presumed to provide the majority of the cornea's tensile strength. Although tension in the superficial epithelial cells has been cited as a potential mechanism for maintaining a smooth optical surface in the presence of underlying stromal surface undulations,[19] removal of the epithelium causes little or no change in the anterior corneal curvature,[20] and the epithelium is generally attributed a minimal role in corneal tensile strength.

The mechanics of Descemet's layer—the 7-μm thick hypertrophied basil lamina of the underlying endothelium[21]—was studied in intact human and rabbit globes by Jue and Maurice[22] and compared to findings in stroma from the same species. Stress-strain investigations revealed that in the *in situ* human cornea, the stromal stress-strain curve is quite steep, corresponding to a high Young's modulus, while Descemet's layer is highly extensible. By superimposing the stress-strain curves for the two layers, Jue and Maurice demonstrated that Descemet's layer is essentially unstrained over a large range of intraocular pressures (IOPs) for which the stroma is simultaneously fully strained. This leads to the conclusion that, like the epithelium, Descemet's layer probably does not bear a significant proportion of the corneal tension over a physiologic range of pressures. Marked differences in the stress-strain relationships of rabbit and human stroma highlight the need for critical interpretation when using the rabbit as a model for corneal mechanical behavior in humans.

Structurally, Bowman's zone is little more than an acellular extension of the anterior stroma.[21] Relative to the stroma, the individual collagen fibrils are two-thirds smaller (20 to 25 nm in diameter) and more randomly oriented throughout the 8 to 12-μm thick sheet.[13] However, it has long been believed that Bowman's zone contributes a structural rigidity to the cornea that is distinct from that provided by the stroma.[23] Seiler, et al used a linear extensiometer to study a number of mechanical parameters in de-epithelialized corneal strips obtained from 10 fresh human cadaver eyes.[23]

> The stroma, which makes up about 90% of the total corneal thickness,21 is the layer thought to most significantly influence the mechanical response of the cornea to injury.

Finally, the stroma, which makes up about 90% of the total corneal thickness,[21] is the layer thought to most significantly influence the mechanical response of the cornea to injury. The stroma is approximately 78% water by weight, 15% collagen, and 7% other proteins, proteoglycans, and salts.[21] Three hundred to 500 lamellae—flattened bundles of parallel collagen fibrils—run from limbus to limbus without interruption.[21] In the posterior two-thirds of the stroma, the lamellae are successively stacked parallel to the corneal surface such that each lamellae has an angular offset from its anterior and posterior neighbors.[13] Anteriorly, the lamellae are more randomly oriented (often obliquely to the corneal surface), are more branched, and are significantly interwoven.[13] These regional differences correlate well with observations that shearing of the lamellae is generally difficult in the human stroma,[15] but particularly so anteriorly.[16] Collagen interweaving is also more extensive in the corneal periphery than in its center.[14]

Komai and Ushikis' observation under the electron microscope of collagen bundles extended between neighboring lamellae provides an important structural foundation for the transfer of tensile loads between lamellae. A review of investigations into the nature of interlamellar cohesive strength is important since the biomechanical model proposes that these interlamellar connections provide a mechanical link between peripheral stromal expansion and central flattening in photoablation. In 1990, Maurice and Monroe measured the force required to split a stromal sample along a plane parallel to the anterior and posterior surfaces at 50% of the stromal depth in rabbits.[24] The mean tearing strength in stromal strips did not vary significantly across the cornea and was calculated to be 0.098 N/mm. Smolek and McCarey performed similar experiments in the horizontal meridian of 16 human eye bank corneas[17] and found the central stroma (0.139 ± 0.0049 N/mm) to be weaker than the peripheral stroma (0.310 ± 0.036 N/mm). These measurements corresponded well to histological observations of collagen interweaving in the corneal periphery.

Though the interlamellar cohesive strengths of the temporal and nasal peripheries of the horizontal meridian were equivalent in the study referred to above, cursory studies of the vertical meridian revealed large and consistent differences between the strengths of the superior and inferior regions. These differences were confirmed in a 52-eye follow-up study by Smolek,[18] which revealed a mean central strength of 0.165 ± 0.0088 N/mm and mean peripheral strengths at 4 mm from the central cornea of 0.185 ± 0.0088 N/mm and 0.234 ± 0.0137 N/mm (p < 0.01) for the inferior and superior regions, respectively. Again, interlamellar cohesive strength in the human corneal stroma was shown to be greater in the periphery than in the center. Smolek also identified five distinct corneal patterns of cohesive strength that were largely asymmetric about the corneal center. The fact that strength distributions in eyes of the same donor were nearly identical may account for some intersubject differences in the mechanical response to refractive surgery and reinforces the importance of considering the fellow-eye

> Cohesive strength has been measured as the force required to separate a stromal sample along a cleavage plane parallel to the lamellar axes by pulling in a direction perpendicular to the cleavage plane (ie, like peeling a banana.

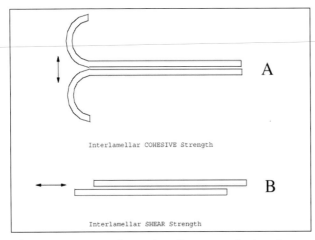

Interlamellar COHESIVE Strength

Interlamellar SHEAR Strength

Figure 9-6. A schematic diagram of the forces described by (A) the interlamellar cohesive strength and (B) the interlamellar shear strength.

response in laboratory and clinical studies of corneal mechanics.

It is important to distinguish between cohesive strength and interlamellar shear strength, as the two terms are frequently used interchangeably. Cohesive strength has been measured as the force required to separate a stromal sample along a cleavage plane parallel to the lamellar axes by pulling in a direction perpendicular to the cleavage plane (ie, like peeling a banana, as shown in Figure 9-6A). Thus, the cohesive strength is a measure of the interlamellar resistance to separation in the transverse direction and is expressed as a function of distance from the corneal center. Alternatively, the shear strength manifests as a resistance to shearing or sliding of one lamellae over another in the plane parallel to the lamellar axes (the longitudinal direction); as such, it is an integrated function of the connective forces across the entire lamellar interface and is therefore conceivably larger in magnitude (Figure 9-6B). Both forces are likely to contribute to the peripheral-to-central transfer of stress in the proposed biomechanical model of corneal response to laser ablation.

These studies provided anatomical and mechanical evidence of an interlamellar cohesion strength at 50% depth that is greater peripherally than centrally and greater superiorly than inferiorly. The predomi-

The shear strength manifests as a resistance to shearing or sliding of one lamellae over another in the plane parallel to the lamellar axes (the longitudinal direction).

nance of interlamellar binding in the anterior one-third of the stroma suggests that the magnitudes of these forces are even greater in that region. Whatever bearing these interlamellar relationships have on the shape of the structurally intact cornea, their importance is likely to increase considerably in the ablated cornea when a redistribution of tensile loading induces nonphysiological stresses between cut and uncut lamellae, as illustrated in Figure 9-5. Furthermore, the asymmetric distribution of cohesive strengths could be an important source of induced corneal astigmatism in keratorefractive procedures.

The lamellar organization of the stroma and the capacity of this collagenous network to bear tension is a natural starting point for biomechanical models of curvature change. A relationship that is generally neglected in this context, however, is that between the interfibrillary constituents of the stroma and water, the major component of the stroma. The collagen fibers are enmeshed in a ground matrix of glycosaminoglycans (GAG) such as keratan sulfate and chondroitin sulfates of varying degrees of sulfation.[25] Both substances, but particularly chondroitin sulfate, are markedly hydrophilic and contribute to a negative intrastromal fluid pressure under which the entire stroma is heavily compressed.[21] IOP further compresses the stroma through its direct effect at the posterior surface[26] and by its contribution to lamellar tension.[21] The intrastromal pressure, often called the "swelling" pressure because of its tendency to draw water into the stromal ground substance, has been measured as -50 to -60 mmHg through a variety of *in vitro* and *in vivo* techniques.[27-29] In one *in vivo* study, Klyce[30] measured this force with implanted hydrogel discs and confirmed that the intrastromal pressure caused a true physical compression of the stromal matrix.

In the normal physiologic state, this swelling tendency is resisted and relative dehydration is maintained by a combination of lamellar tension, anterior evaporation of the tear film,[31] low permeability of the epithelial and endothelial layers to water,[32] and active endothelial transport of bicarbonate.[33] During the act of central ablation, however, a number of lamellae proportional to the depth of ablation are obliterated centrally and tension is lost in their unablated peripheral segments. The resulting loss of compression introduces a hydrostatic disequilibrium, and the peripheral stroma thickens as it takes up fluid.[12] While tissue expansion is likely to occur within the ground substance rather than in the fibrils themselves,[34] the source of the fluid has not been discerned. Hedbys and Mishima[35] showed that local deficits in hydration were resolved by intrastromal fluid shifts in stromal strips immersed in oil to create a closed system with respect to the water balance. *In situ*, the cornea may imbibe additional water through the limbus as a result of the pressure difference between the perilimbal capillaries and the stromal interstitium.[36] As one would expect, the swelling pressure diminishes as stromal hydration and thickness increase[21] and a new steady state is established.

As stated earlier, the essential link between peripheral stromal thickening and central flattening is the existence of a mechanical relationship between disrupted and intact lamellae. On the contrary, if lamellae are assumed instead to be structurally and mechanically independent of neighboring lamellae (ie, arranged in layers without any interconnections), then the severed peripheral segments are unable to bear or transfer any tension. This is, in fact, a simplifying assumption incorporated into most numerical models of refractive surgery.[5-8] Within this scenario, the tensile load previously borne by the full complement of lamellae is shifted to the remaining posterior fibers, which now strain (stretch) slightly under the concentrated stress. If the limbal circumference is assumed to be fixed, the stretch may not be accomplished by an increase in corneal diameter and must therefore occur as central corneal bulging and anterior *steepening*. However, if the proposed peripheral response is considered, this occurs as a peripheral thickening and peripheral steepening with coincident central *flattening*. Although the latter scenario aptly describes the characteristic peripheral "knee" and central flat zone of PTK, PRK, and LASIK, finite element analyses of uniform thickness profiles have not incorporated the peripheral response and have predicted a corneal configuration opposite that produced clinically.[9] When a mathematical model by Pinsky and Datye[5] was refined to include the effect of shear transfer between cut and uncut lamellae, it was concluded that the role of corneal shear was indeed significant. In short, consideration of the proposed peripheral stromal response and its mechanical relationship to the central cornea may be critical not only for correctly predicting the *magnitude* of refractive correction, but in some cases, the *direction*.

SUPPORT FOR THE MECHANICAL MODEL IN EXPERIMENTAL LITERATURE

In this section, we will briefly review important cadaveric studies that address some of the mechani-

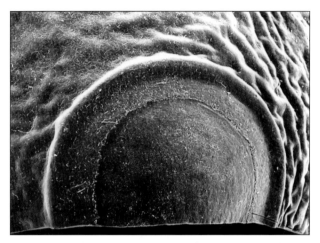

Figure 9-7. Electron micrograph illustrating peripheral lamellar relaxation after central ablation of a rabbit cornea. Note the visible "buckling" or "wrinkling" of the lamellae that is no longer held in tension outside the ablation zone (photo courtesy of John Marshall, PhD).

cal underpinnings of our proposed biomechanical model. The first is a 1985 study of corneal ultrastructure following slit-shaped ablations of rabbit corneas with an early model 193-nm excimer laser.[37] When Marshall, et al investigated wound morphology with the scanning electron microscope, they found that the incised stromal regions were swollen to between two and two and a half times the thickness of the unincised regions. Swelling was maximal immediately adjacent to the incision, where lamellae tended to be splayed and divergent and interlamellar separation was approximately doubled. Swelling was restricted to the interfibrillary ground substance, and the investigators speculated that thickening was caused by an acute change in stromal fluid relationships around severed lamellae. Although the thickening response may be less dramatic in humans due to greater interlamellar resistance to expansion, this study qualitatively illustrates the tendency of the cornea to thicken locally when lamellar continuity is disrupted. Also, peripheral lamellar relaxation has been documented via electron microscopy in the form of visible "buckling" or "wrinkling" of the lamellae that are no longer held in tension. This is illustrated in Figure 9-7 after central ablation of a rabbit cornea and lends further support to the model.

Central photoablation has multiple mechanical analogs in the incisional keratorefractive setting, with perhaps the best examples being corneal trephination and annular keratotomy. Despite differences in their intended effects, PRK, PTK, LASIK, trephination, and annular keratotomy all effectively produce a circumferential dissection of the stromal lamellae. Conflicting reports of both corneal steepening and flattening upon trephination of failed epikeratoplasty lenticles initially confused the issue of how such curvature changes came about, but a later series of studies highlighted the importance of treatment depth as a variable. Using a partial-thickness variation of trephination known as annular keratotomy, Gilbert, et al[38] induced 6 to 7 D of steepening in 12 donor eyes subjected to 85% depth treatments. In a follow-up report, the same group[39] investigated the effect of shallower trephination in human eye bank eyes. They noted that after restoration of IOP and partial reversal of post-mortem edema, 7-mm trephinations were performed to an approximate stromal depth of 150 µm. Central flattening—not steepening—was observed (-2.81 ± 2.28 D) with notable induced astigmatism (1.87 ± 1.62 D). Digital analysis of keratoscopic rings confirmed central corneal flattening and marked peripheral steepening. The authors acknowledged the marked impact of treatment depth on curvature change, and although steepening in deep treatments was attributed to weakening of the corneal cap, no explanation was offered for flattening of superficially incised corneas.

In a small but very important study, Litwin, et al addressed this depth-dependent curvature response by measuring the effect of successive 50-µm PTK ablations in four pressurized donor globes.[20] Photokeratoscopic data from the central 3 mm of the cornea revealed no curvature change after epithelial debridement but statistically significant flattening (3.09 D and 5.56 D) after ablation to 50 µm and 100 um, respectively. After ablation, corneal curvature ultimately steepened to a level actually exceeding preoperative curvature, presumably due to a loss of structural integrity. Although the purpose of the study was to determine how deeply the cornea could be ablated in therapeutic procedures without causing central ectasia, an unintended yet impressive demonstration of the stroma's nonlinear response to ablation depth was provided. A similar depth-dependent flattening response has been observed in several clinical series of PTK patients.[40-42]

This nonlinear depth dependence may be explained in terms of the biomechanical consequences of progressive central ablation. In the "shallow" phase of the response, flattening may increase with ablation depth due to exaggeration of peripheral thickening and its secondary effects on central curvature (ie, continued ablation yields continued peripheral thickening, which in turn yields more central flattening). When ablation extends into the deep stroma, however, peripheral thickening may become decoupled from central curvature due to the decreased presence of interlamellar connections in the posterior stroma (where the new interface between cut and uncut lamellae lies). At this transitional depth, the flattening response to peripheral thickening has likely reached a maximum and steepening secondary to central corneal weakening (ectasia) becomes increasingly important. Current clinical opinion presumes this transition level to correspond with 250 µm of intact residual stromal bed. Beyond this point, further ablative weakening of the central stroma is likely to result in isolated ectatic steepening. The interaction of these biomechanical effects and their dependence on treatment depth are clearly an important consideration in ablation profile design. The magnitudes of these responses in LASIK, PRK for high myopia, and PTK for deep stromal scarring are likely to be even greater due to the extent of stromal disruption involved, and the need to account for them is suggested by the relatively low predictive value of current surgical algorithms in high myopia.

TARGETED IN VITRO STUDIES OF THE BIOMECHANICAL MODEL

While the preceding studies indirectly supported the notion of a significant biomechanical response in central keratectomy, a prospective investigation of the proposed model had yet to be performed. In 1994, we launched a study of the etiology of unintended hyperopic shift in therapeutic photokeratectomy. Of the various forms of central photoablation, PTK has distinct advantages as a model for assessing biomechanical components of curvature change because the refractive contribution of the ablation profile is minimized. The clinical paradox of PTK-induced flattening arises from the expectation that a beam calibrated to remove a uniform depth of tissue across the ablation zone should not alter anterior curvature.[43,44] In the majority of patients, however, PTK causes significant flattening of the anterior corneal surface and a consequent refractive shift toward

> The clinical paradox of PTK-induced flattening arises from the expectation that a beam calibrated to remove a uniform depth of tissue across the ablation zone should not alter anterior curvature.[43,44]

hyperopia.[40,42-53] As previously noted, flattening typically occurs in proportion to the attempted stromal ablation depth[40,42,46,49] and, as in PRK, is characterized by some degree of postoperative regression. Residual hyperopic change is considered the principal complication of PTK.[42,45,46] Due to the practice of reporting hyperopic shift in terms of absolute rather than relative hypermetropia[45] and to the paucity of refractive data from the early postoperative period when flattening is generally most pronounced, the incidence and magnitude of induced corneal flattening may be significantly underestimated in the literature. In the context of customized corneal ablation, PTK-induced flattening is intriguing because it directly challenges a longstanding paradigm of how curvature change is achieved in all forms of central keratectomy, including PRK and LASIK.

Although hyperopic shift in PTK has been anecdotally attributed to systematic bias in the ablation pattern[44,48,49,54] or hyperopically biased tissue deposition in the postoperative phase,[42,55] no experimental work has clearly linked ablation pattern to hyperopic shift. Intrigued by the possibility that this clinical response represented a predominantly biomechanical phenomenon, we set out first to confirm that hyperopic shift could be reproduced in a donor model, then to investigate changes in peripheral stromal thickness as a potential correlate to hyperopic shift.[11,12] To characterize the ablation pattern and its role in acute hyperopic shift, we also calculated the potential curvature bias introduced by intraoperative thickness changes across the ablation zone. Fourteen de-epithelialized eye bank globes from seven donors were subjected in paired control fashion to either broadbeam ablation or sham photoablation. A Summit UVLA2000 excimer laser was used to deliver ~100-μm deep (400 pulse), 5-mm-diameter ablations with no programmed dioptric change, and anterior curvature and stromal thickness were measured by autokeratometry and corneal optical section image analysis (COSIA), respectively.[12] Relative to sham ablation, PTK resulted in a significant anterior flattening response (-6.3 ± 3.2 D, p = 0.002) on the same order of changes reported in PTK patients receiving treatments of comparable depth. Concomitant thickening of the peripheral stroma was also demonstrated (+57 ± 43 μm, p = 0.01), as illustrated in Figure 9-8. In an important validation of the biomechanical model, peripheral stromal thickening was found to be a significant predictor of acute hyperopic shift (r = 0.68, p = 0.047). Interestingly, estimates of curvature bias in the pat-

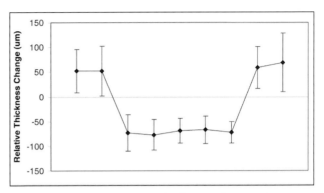

Figure 9-8. Intraoperative thickness changes in seven ablated (constant depth profile) donor eyes expressed relative to paired controls. Ablation zone diameter is 5 mm. Note central thinning and peripheral thickening.

One of the more important implications of this work is the notion that biomechanical changes measured *outside* of the ablation zone can have a significant impact on curvature changes *within* the ablation zone.

terns of central thickness change were not systematically skewed toward flattening; in fact, ablation zone bias could not, on its own, account statistically for actual anterior curvature change.

PERIPHERAL THICKENING MAY AFFECT CENTRAL CURVATURE

One of the more important implications of this work is the notion that biomechanical changes measured *outside* of the ablation zone can have a significant impact on curvature changes *within* the ablation zone. The ablation zone analysis demonstrated in a controlled fashion that central curvature change in refractive surgery is not solely a product of the ablation pattern. When peripheral thickness and ablation zone bias were both included in a regression model, over 83% of the variance in curvature response accounted for by the model was explained by peripheral thickening. Although the impact of ablation pattern on acute curvature change is likely to become increasingly influential when larger dioptric corrections are attempted, the associated increases in ablation depth would also be expected to further exacerbate the biomechanical response. Consequently, the utility of a pure shape-subtraction model is probably limited to cases involving only superficial ablation (ie, correction of low refractive error or astigmatism in PRK and removal of subepithelial scars in PTK). Finally, the argument for the role of lamellar interconnections playing an important role was bolstered by the correlations between central flattening and thickness changes in individual peripheral subregions. These correlations were strongest in the superior periphery, weakest in the inferior periphery, and strongest overall in the far superior periphery—a pattern that consistently reflects the strength distribution of interlamellar cohesive forces reviewed earlier in this chapter.[18]

As a more rigorous test of the hypothesis that peripheral thickening is a real mechanical stimulus for central flattening, we initiated a second study aimed at suppressing acute thickness changes in the stromal periphery and secondarily reducing the magnitude of acute central flattening during ablation.[56] In preliminary experiments in 16 donor eyes, a collagen crosslinking technique described by Spöerl, et al[57] was adapted for use in whole donor globes.[58] Twenty globes from 10 donors were used in the final experiments to measure the effect of preoperative pan-stromal crosslinking on keratectomy-induced thickness and curvature changes. One cornea from each donor was exposed to a topical 4% glutaraldehyde solution prior to surgery, and the other cornea served as a control for crosslinking effects. Each cornea then underwent sham photoablation followed by a 400-pulse, 5-mm-diameter PTK treatment performed with a Chiron Technolas Keracor (Claremont, Calif) system, and changes in thickness and curvature were measured with the Orbscan scanning-slit topography system.

Relative to same-eye sham treatments, central keratectomy in controls (ie, same-donor fellow corneas not pretreated with glutaraldehyde) produced significant peripheral stromal thickening and central flattening with correlated responses (r = 0.70, p = 0.02). The proposal that peripheral thickening is a biomechanical mediator of depth-dependent central flattening was supported by the additional finding that peripheral thickening occurred in proportion to the approximate depth of ablation (r = 0.69, p = 0.01). In corneas pretreated with the crosslinking reagent glutaraldehyde, partial suppression of the peripheral thickening response occurred and was associated with a 36% mean reduction in hyperopic shift relative to paired controls (r = 0.68, p = 0.03). Although the crosslinking procedure did not entirely eliminate the peripheral response and its effect on central sequelae, it did yield the most direct experimental

evidence to date of a causal relationship between peripheral expansion and hyperopic shift. The repeated demonstration of codependent peripheral and central corneal responses in these studies using different laser delivery systems and corneal imaging technologies than those described previously further suggests the existence of a true intrinsic mechanical response to ablation and not merely a device-dependent experimental artifact.

> The ability of PTK to produce acute refractive effects similar to those achieved with myopic ablation patterns of comparable depth is highly suggestive of an intrinsic stromal propensity to flatten with central ablation.

IN VIVO EVIDENCE OF BIOMECHANICAL REFRACTIVE CHANGE ACCORDING TO THE PROPOSED MODEL

Clearly, the ability of PTK to produce acute refractive effects similar to those achieved with myopic ablation patterns of comparable depth is highly suggestive of an intrinsic stromal propensity to flatten with central ablation. In a dramatic demonstration of biomechanical predominance over profile effects, Maloney, et al[59] investigated erodible masks as an alternative to diaphragm-based delivery systems. Two designs were tested: a convex mask, thicker centrally for correction of hyperopia, and a concave mask, thicker peripherally for correction of myopia (Figure 9-9). Thirty eyes of pigmented rabbits were treated, with five eyes in each of the following attempted correction groups: -5 D mask, -5 D diaphragm, -2.5 D mask, -2.5 D diaphragm, +2.5 D mask, and +5 D mask. Cycloplegic retinoscopic refractions 2 weeks after surgery revealed that ablation through convex masks designed to steepen the cornea actually produced the opposite effect: hyperopic shifts consistent with the proposed biomechanical model (Table 9-3). In fact, the magnitude of shift paralleled that achieved with mask and diaphragm techniques specifically designed to impose steepening profiles. What distinguishes this study from those previously discussed, apart from the limitations of the rabbit model, is the ability to confirm that paracentral cornea was indeed ablated to a greater degree than central cornea in attempted corrections of hyperopia. In other words, the paradoxical refrac-

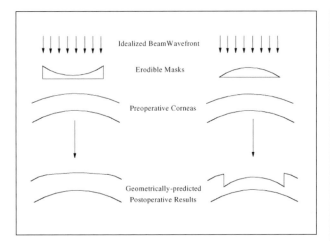

Figure 9-9. Approach to correction of myopia and hyperopia with erodible masks. Both mask types produced hyperopic shift in rabbits despite differences in ablation profile (adapted from Maloney RK, Friedman M, Harmon T, et al A prototype erodible mask delivery system for the excimer laser. *Ophthalmology.* 1993;100:542-549).

Table 9-3 **Ablation Through an Erodible Mask in Rabbits**	
ATTEMPTED CORRECTION (D)	*ACHIEVED CORRECTION (D)*
-5.0 (mask)	-2.60
-5.0 (diaphragm)	-3.90
-2.5 (mask)	-1.60
-2.5 (diaphragm)	-1.40
+2.5 (mask)	**-2.90**
+5.0 (mask)	**-1.40**

n = 5 eyes per attempted correction. Note that attempted hyperopic corrections designed to steepen the cornea in the last two groups paradoxically produced hyperopic refractive shifts rather than the attempted myopic shifts (adapted from Maloney RK, Friedman M, Harmon T, et al. A prototype erodible mask delivery system for the excimer laser. *Ophthalmology.* 1993;100:542-549).

tive effects cannot be simply attributed to an aberration in the beam profile. Corneal biomechanics offers an explanation not previously considered.

Following our early reports of the relationship between acute peripheral thickening and central flattening in ablated donor corneas,[11] Fahd, et al demonstrated a sustained peripheral thickening response after central ablation in living rabbits.[60] Although the relationship of peripheral thickness change to central curvature was not investigated, the study provided the first report of ablation-induced peripheral thickening in living corneas as well as an important step toward demonstrating a potential biomechanical influence beyond the perioperative period. In the next section, the model is explored in the context of clinical data from trials of PTK, PRK, and LASIK.

CLINICAL STUDIES SUPPORTING THE PROPOSED BIOMECHANICAL MODEL

Clinical studies have been reported in the literature and at scientific meetings that provide indirect support for the proposed biomechanical model of corneal response to laser refractive surgery. Critical features of the proposed model, including biomechanical flattening independent of ablation profile, as well as stromal thickening in the corneal periphery, will be addressed.

The potential for unexpected results when the ablation pattern is assumed to be the primary determinant of refractive outcome is illustrated in several clinical studies. In the first, a 2-year clinical follow-up of PTK,[42] Stark, et al presented results in 27 eyes treated with one of two variants of ablation: 4.0 or 4.5 mm single-aperture ablations bound by 0.5 mm concave (upsloping) peripheral tapers (n = 21), and 5.5 mm single-aperture ablations with a "modified" taper (n = 6)—an attempt to combat unintended hyperopic shift by overtreating the paracentral cornea as if one were attempting to treat primary hyperopia. Net hyperopic refractive shifts occurred in both groups, and the shift was actually more pronounced in the modified taper group at 1- and 3-month follow-ups (7.1 ± 2.3 D vs. 5.7 ± 1.1 D). The attempt to reduce hyperopic shift by steepening (and therefore deepening) the ablation profile actually produced more hyperopic shift at the stated intervals. These results support the previous discussion about the relative importance of shape-subtraction and biomechanical effects and the dependence of this relationship on ablation depth. From the standpoint of ablation pattern, the modified taper clearly introduces some bias toward a steeper corneal ablation profile. But for two treatments aimed at removing the same thickness of central tissue, the biomechani-

Table 9-4

Current Hyperopic LASIK Nomograms

| | *PRIMARY HYPEROPES* | | | *SECONDARY HYPEROPES* | |
| | *PREOPERATIVE MANIFEST SE* | | | | |
Age (years)	0 to 2 D	2 to 4 D	4 to 6 D	Post RK	Post LASIK
20 to 29	0%	+10%	+20%	-4%	-14%
30 to 39	+10%	+18%	+25%	-2%	-10%
40 to 49	+17%	+23%	+28%	-1%	-4%
50 to 59	+30%	+30%	+30%	0%	+4%
60 to 69	+35%	+32%	+31%	+2%	+8%

Represents percentage of preoperative manifest SE that is added to or subtracted from the spherical component of correction. Full cylinder to be treated is entered into the laser. For example, a +2 +2 refraction in a 35-year-old primary hyperope would be adjusted as follows: +3 (SE) x 0.18 = 0.54 for a correction of +2.54 sphere and +2 cylinder.

Adapted with permission from Lindstrom RL, Hardten DR, Houtman DM, et al. Six-month results of hyperopic and astigmatic LASIK in eyes with primary and secondary hyperopia. *Trans Am Ophth Soc.* 1999;XCVII:241-260.

cal implication of the taper is an increase in the maximum depth of ablation and exaggerated biomechanical flattening, which in this case turned out to be the dominant refractive determinant. Similar phenomena were reported in a 1991 phase II trial of the VisX LV 2000, in which attempts were made to minimize hyperopic shift by superimposing single-aperture PTK ablations and paracentrally biased ablations.[43]

Unintended hyperopic shift has also been clinically demonstrated in a myopic refractive surgery population using a large optical zone ablation and a Nidek EC-5000 laser. MacRae, et al reported hyperopic overcorrection with surface ablation (PRK and PARK), as well as a 70% hyperopic astigmatic coupling with astigmatic LASIK (A-LASIK). For A-LASIK procedures, a constant depth, PTK-type ablation is imposed on the flat meridian in an effort to leave it "untreated." However, according to the proposed model, a PTK ablation will produce biomechanical flattening. These investigators found marked overcorrection in the flat meridian consistent with both the model and clinical PTK results in the literature. In addition, they found significant coupling with the spherical component of the ablation. There were cases in which simply treating the astigmatism produced substantial overall corneal flattening, reducing the myopia enough that no further treatment was required.

HYPEROPIC VERSUS MYOPIC CORRECTIONS

The proposed biomechanical model predicts additional flattening over and above whatever ablation profile is programmed, whether myopic with an intent to flatten, hyperopic with an attempt to steepen, or nonrefractive PTK. This would theoretically make hyperopia a more difficult procedure since the biomechanical flattening would be in opposition to the ablation profile, thus requiring a deeper ablation to offset the biomechanical response. Clinical evidence for this prediction has been reported in the literature. Lindstrom, et al[62] reported prospective results of hyperopic LASIK using a VisX Star S2 from 46 eyes with primary hyperopia and 29 eyes with secondary hyperopia resulting from an overcorrected prior myopic refractive procedure. The nomogram derived from a regression analysis for trends is given in Table 9-4. There are several important features to note in the nomogram.

First, a primary hyperopic procedure requires a treatment of up to 35% greater than the spherical equivalent, meaning greater than expected depth must be ablated to achieve the desired correction. This is consistent with the proposed model predicting biomechanical flattening independent of the ablation profile. Greater depth must be ablated with

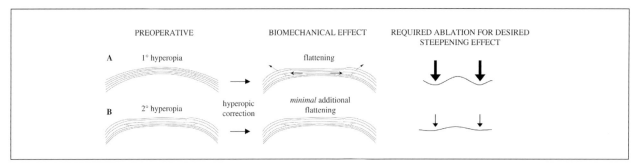

Figure 9-10. Proposed impact of biomechanics on LASIK nomograms for primary and secondary hyperopia. Biomechanical flattening opposes corneal steepening in attempted corrections of hyperopia. This effect is more pronounced in previously untreated corneas ±1 degree hyperopia (A) and requires compensatory enhancement of the ablation profile to achieve the desired steepening effect. Corneas of eyes that are hyperopic after previous surgical overcorrection (B) are less "loaded" biomechanically (ie, peripheral expansion [blue x's] and associated central flattening have already occurred). Accordingly, profile effects are opposed to a lesser degree and little or no enhancement of the ablation profile is required. Corneal geometry is exaggerated for illustrative purposes (based on data provided by R. Lindstrom, Table 9-4).

a hyperopic treatment to overcome the biomechanical flattening that creates a surface shape effect opposing that of the ablation profile.

Second, the secondary hyperopic group required substantially less depth of ablation to achieve the same level of correction as the primary hyperopia group. This is also completely consistent with the proposed biomechanical model. The secondary post-LASIK hyperopic group already had an altered corneal structure with an associated biomechanical response from the first refractive procedure. In other words, there was less biomechanical flattening to overcome in the second procedure, thus requiring less depth of ablation for the same correction since the biomechanical effect had already occurred in conjunction with the first procedure, as illustrated in Figure 9-10. Third, the secondary hyperopes had a more stable longer-term refraction, with the primary hyperopes exhibiting slight regression over the 6-month postoperative follow-up period. One possible explanation for this difference lies in the long-term healing related to the biomechanical effect, which would be exaggerated in the primary hyperopia group as opposed to the secondary hyperopia group where the biomechanical effects had already occurred and were thus reduced.

Additional evidence of the biomechanical response and the difference between hyperopic and myopic procedures lies in the first results from wavefront-guided ablations using the Autonomous CustomCornea system (Orlando, Fla), as described in Chapter Twelve. These data were reported at the First International Congress of Wavefront Sensing and Aberration-Free Ablative Corrections in February 2000.[63] The first five myopic cases treated with pure wavefront-guidance were generally overcorrected, and the first three hyperopic cases with pure wavefront guidance were generally undercorrected. Both myopic and hyperopic groups demonstrated additional flattening superimposed on the ablation profiles, which is consistent with the proposed biomechanical model. Following these results, the CustomCornea algorithms were empirically modified to account for the over-/undercorrections in subsequent ablations.

PERIPHERAL THICKENING AFTER LASER REFRACTIVE SURGERY IN VIVO

Indirect evidence of peripheral thickening after laser refractive surgery has been reported, which is consistent with the proposed model of biomechanical response. Munger, et al[64] presented clinical results using a VisX Star system on a total of 25 eyes from 25 patients with low astigmatism treated with myopic PRK. Corneal maps were acquired with PAR Corneal Topography System (CTS) at 2 hours before surgery, 2 to 3 minutes after surgery (Sx), on the day the bandage contact lens was removed, and 1 week, 3 months, and 6 months postoperatively. Ablation depth was defined as preoperative-postoperative, and epithelial depth was defined as Sx-postoperative, recognizing that edema may have been a factor in the immediate postoperative map. Munger reported epithelial thickening at the ablation edge. However, an increase in the calculated epithelial measurement outside the ablation zone may be due

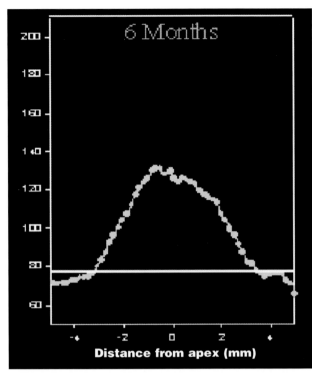

Figure 9-11. Sample ablation depth profile calculated at 6 months after PRK by subtracting preoperative minus postoperative height with an offset measured by a PAR corneal topography system. Maximal ablation depth is seen at the center of the profile near the apex. The edges of the ablation zone are seen as knees in the profile at approximately +3 mm from the apex at the intersection with the horizontal white line, which depicts a relative zero depth. Outside the ablation zone, the depth profile falls below the relative zero line, indicating a "negative" depth of ablation or increased elevation. Increased elevation of the unablated corneal periphery is consistent with the proposed biomechanical model (courtesy of Rejean Munger, PhD, slightly modified).

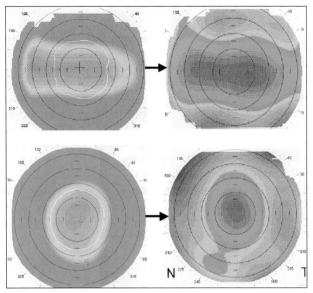

Figure 9-12. Comparison between planned ablation profiles using CIPTA (see Chapter Twenty-Two) on the left and measured topographic elevation difference maps on the right for two sample subjects. Topography was acquired using an Orbscan. Blue colors indicate a negative difference between postoperative and preoperative surfaces where tissue was removed, and yellow/red colors indicate a positive difference where tissue was "added" after surgery. Zero difference is displayed in green. Both planned profiles on the left are surrounded by green zones, indicating zero energy deposition. However, both elevation difference maps show positive elevation outside of the central ablation zone, indicating increase in elevation. This is consistent with the proposed biomechanical model, which predicts peripheral stromal thickening (planned profiles and topographic difference maps courtesy of Giovanni Alessio, MD).

to stromal thickening rather than epithelial, since the PAR CTS measures surface elevation and cannot distinguish between epithelial and stromal thickening. In addition, more convincing evidence lay in the ablation depth measurements as a function of distance from the apex at 6 months, an example of which is shown in Figure 9-11. Ablation depth is a more robust measurement than the much smaller epithelial thickness, and by 6 months the cornea should be relatively stable. Note that outside the ablation zone, there is negative ablation depth or increased elevation compared to the preoperative state. This provides indirect evidence of peripheral thickening, an important feature of the proposed

biomechanical model with a different laser/topographer combination.

Sborgia, et al[65] reported results of a corneal topography-guided system called Corneal Interactive Programmed Topographic Ablation (CIPTA), also described in Chapter Twenty-Two. A total of 28 eyes of 28 patients with irregular astigmatism were treated with a Laserscan 2000 and had pre- and postoperative topography with an Orbscan. Two examples of the planned ablation profile and actual elevation difference maps are shown in Figure 9-12. In both subjects, the left image is the planned ablation pattern, and the right image is the actual elevation difference map—note in both cases the large green area outside

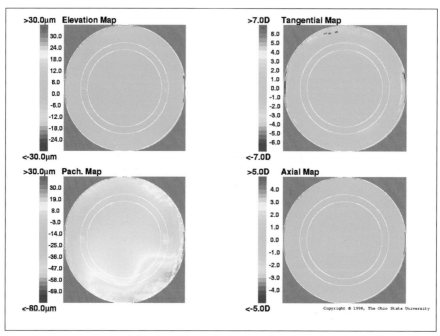

Figure 9-13. Average difference maps between repeated measures of 20 eyes of 10 normal subjects. The white circles define three corneal regions. The central region has radius 2.75 mm, the middle region has radius 2.75 to 3.25 mm, and the outer region has radius 3.25 to 4.5 mm. Elevation (upper left) differences were calculated by fitting the two surfaces in the middle region. Average tangential differences (upper right), average pachymetry differences (lower left), and average axial differences (lower right) are also given.

the ablation zone in the maps on the left, where the cornea will not be ablated. However, the elevation difference maps on the right demonstrate not only a decrease in central elevation (shown in blue) that matches the planned profile but are also accompanied by an unexpected increase in elevation outside the ablation zone (shown in red and yellow), again as predicted by the proposed biomechanical model.

CHARACTERIZATION OF THE BIOMECHANICAL RESPONSE

A prospective study is currently underway to characterize the biomechanical corneal response to LASIK and separate the resulting refractive effect from that produced by the ablation profile.[66] At the time of this writing, eight eyes of four subjects have been enrolled and partially analyzed. LASIK is performed with a Summit Apex Plus using a Krumeich-Barraquer microkeratome to make the flap. Corneal measurements are acquired pre- and postoperatively with optical coherence tomography and the following corneal topographers for validation of effect:

EyeSys, Humphrey Atlas, Keratron, Orbscan II, PAR, Technomed C-Scan, and TMS-1. Average preoperative refractive error of the small preliminary group is −6.875 ± 2.03 D sphere + 0.8125 ± 0.51 D cylinder. Only the Orbscan corneal topography data will be presented here. A comparison control group of 20 eyes of 10 subjects had repeated Orbscan I topography acquired at intervals from 1 to 2 days to establish baseline variations. The anterior tangential, anterior elevation, and pachymetry data were exported to the OSU topography tool[2] for analysis and the cornea was divided into three regions: central 2.75-mm radius (5.5-mm diameter), transition zone from a radius of 2.75 to 3.25 mm (5.5- to 6.5-mm diameter), and outside the ablation zone from a radius of 3.25 to 4.5 mm (6.5- to 9.0-mm diameter). The preoperative topography was subtracted from the postoperative topography for the surgical patients, and the repeated measurements were subtracted for the normal subjects. For the elevation maps, the two surfaces were fit within the 0.5-mm transition zone. For all maps, average regional differences were calculated over the normal and surgical populations, and statistical analysis was performed using the ANOVA procedure in the software package SAS.

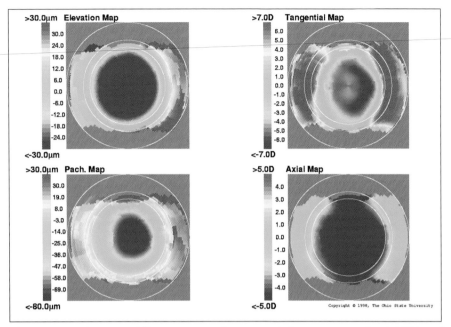

Figure 9-14. Average difference maps between 1 day postoperative LASIK and preoperative state for eight eyes of four patients. The white circles define three corneal regions. The central ablated region has radius 2.75 mm, the middle transitional region has radius 2.75 to 3.25 mm, and the outer nonablated region has radius 3.25 to 4.5 mm. Elevation (upper left) differences were calculated by fitting the two surfaces in the transitional region and demonstrate increased elevation in the outer zone. Average tangential differences (upper right) show increased curvature in the outer region. Average pachymetry differences (lower left) show increased pachymetry in the outer region after surgery. Average axial differences (lower right) are also given.

Figures 9-13 and 9-14 show the composite difference maps of all subjects for the normal and 1 day postoperative surgical groups, respectively. Significant (p < 0.05) decreases in elevation, pachymetry, and curvature in the central zone between normal and surgical subjects were demonstrated. In addition, significant (p < 0.05) increases in elevation, pachymetry, and curvature in the outer zone were found, as predicted by the proposed biomechanical model. These increases persisted at 1 month postoperatively, as seen in Figure 9-15.

WHAT IS THE IMPACT OF CORNEAL BIOMECHANICS ON CUSTOMIZED ABLATIVE PROCEDURES?

In vitro, in vivo, and clinical data have been presented using multiple laser systems and corneal measurement devices, demonstrating that unlike a piece of plastic, the cornea responds biomechanically

> Unlike a piece of plastic, the cornea responds biomechanically to the change in its structure imposed by laser refractive surgery.[4]

to the change in its structure imposed by laser refractive surgery.[4] This is a depth-dependent, nonlinear response that is a function of number of lamellae cut. It produces biomechanical flattening at levels that do not violate the accepted limit of structural integrity, which is 250 μm of intact stromal bed. How much of the final corneal shape is due to the biomechanical response, how much is due to healing, and how much is due to the ablation profile? These answers are not known and will come from future studies. However, the existence of important influences on corneal shape, other than the ablation profile, is critical to the development of customized ablative procedures. Both wavefront- and topography-guided ablations are built on the shape-subtraction model of refractive surgery, which is at best incomplete. The programmed ablations will not produce the expected

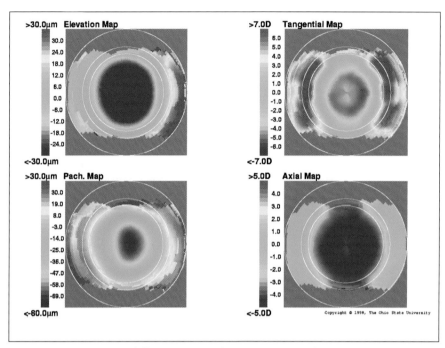

Figure 9-15. Average difference maps between 1 month postoperative LASIK and preoperative state for eight eyes of four patients. The white circles define three corneal regions. The central ablated region has a radius 2.75 mm, the middle transitional region has radius 2.75 to 3.25 mm, and the outer nonablated region has radius 3.25 to 4.5 mm. Elevation (upper left) differences were calculated by fitting the two surfaces in the transitional region and demonstrate persistent increased elevation in the outer zone. Average tangential differences (upper right) show persistent increased curvature in the outer region. Average pachymetry differences (lower left) show persistent increased pachymetry in the outer region. Average axial differences (lower right) are also given.

topographic or wavefront result. The algorithms can be "tweaked" empirically, similar to the development of current ablation algorithms. However, the goal of 20/10 vision with as aberration-free vision as possible cannot be consistently achieved without an understanding of the mechanisms involved that produce the discrepancy between planned and achieved results. Primary procedures may respond differently than secondary procedures, since the corneas are structurally and biomechanically distinct. Yet, secondary procedures are prime candidates for customization since they often have corneal irregularities that interfere with vision and cannot be treated with standard profiles. In addition, the corneal structure and biomechanics may impose limits on the shapes that will be accepted by the cornea following an ablative procedure. It may not be possible to produce an aberration-free profile on the corneal surface. A more realistic goal may be minimized aberrations. Many questions remain unanswered.

Where do we go from here? What is the solution to customization in laser refractive surgery? Many elegant techniques are described in this book to guide the laser in tissue removal. Yet, it is likely that the ultimate solution will rely on a combination of wavefront and topographic guidance. Corneal topography provides information on corneal shape but cannot account for aberrations that may be imposed by other important ocular structures like the crystalline lens. Wavefront analysis provides data on the entire eye's optical system, but it cannot measure the actual physical changes that occur during surgery to produce the final operative result. Corneal topography is a critically important tool to character-

> Corneal topography provides information on corneal shape but cannot account for aberrations that may be imposed by other important ocular structures like the crystalline lens.

ize and, hopefully through future research, predict the biomechanical response of the cornea. Neither device alone is sufficient. Utilized together, both devices may help to achieve the goal of 20/10 vision with minimized aberrations.

ACKNOWLEDGMENTS

The authors wish to acknowledge the technical support of Mr. Ashraf Mahmoud and Mr. Edward E. Herderick for customized topographic processing, statistical analysis, and figure generation; collaborating refractive surgeons Dr. Richard G. Lembach, Dr. Guy Chan, and Dr. David Castellano; the research support of the Ohio Lions Eye Research Foundation, Summit Technologies, and Zeiss Humphrey Systems; equipment loans from Humphrey, Orbscan, PAR, and Technomed; and the critical cooperation of the Central Ohio Lions Eye Bank. The authors also wish to acknowledge Rejean Munger, PhD and Giovanni Alessio, MD for supplying figures from their own research.

REFERENCES

1. Munnerlyn CR, Koons SJ, Marshall J. Photorefractive keratectomy: a technique for laser refractive surgery. *J Cataract Refract Surg.* 1988;14:46-52.

2. Mahmoud AM, Roberts C, Herderick EE. The Ohio State University corneal topography tool. Abstract. *Invest Ophthalmol Vis Sci.* 2000;41:S677.

3. Roberts C, Mahmoud A, Herderick EE, Chan G. Characterization of corneal curvature changes inside and outside the ablation zone in LASIK. Abstract. *Invest Ophthalmol Vis Sci.* 2000;41:S679.

4. Roberts C. The cornea is not a piece of plastic. *J Refract Surg.* 2000;16:407-413.

5. Pinsky PM, Datye DV. A microstructurally based finite element model of the incised human cornea. *J Biomech.* 1991;24:907-922.

6. Velinsky SA, Bryant MR. On the computer-aided and optimal design of keratorefractive surgery. *Refract Corneal Surg.* 1992;8:173-182.

7. Hanna KD, Jouve FE, Waring GO III. Preliminary computer simulation of the effects of radial keratotomy. *Arch Ophthalmol.* 1989;107:911-918.

8. Pinsky PM, Datye DV. Numerical modeling of radial, astigmatic, and hexagonal keratotomy. *Refract Corneal Surg.* 1992;8:164-172.

9. Bryant MR, Fredericks DJ, Campos M, McDonnell PJ. Finite element analysis of corneal topographic changes after excimer laser phototherapeutic keratectomy. *Invest Ophthalmol Vis Sci.* 1993;31(Suppl):804.

10. Pinsky PM, Datye DV. A microstructurally based mechanical model of the human cornea with application to keratotomy. *Invest Ophthalmol Vis Sci.* 1994;31(Suppl):1296.

11. Dupps WJ, Roberts C, Schoessler JP. Peripheral lamellar relaxation: a mechanism of induced corneal flattening in PTK and PRK? Abstract. *Invest Ophthalmol Vis Sci.* 1995;36:S708.

12. Dupps WJ. Peripheral stromal expansion and anterior corneal flattening in phototherapeutic keratectomy: an in vitro human study. Thesis. Columbus, Ohio: The Ohio State University; 1995.

13. Komai Y, Ushiki T. The three-dimensional organization of collagen fibrils in the human cornea and sclera. *Invest Ophthalmol Vis Sci.* 1991;32:2244-2258.

14. Polack FM. Morphology of the cornea. I: study with silver stains. *Am J Ophthalmol.* 1961;51:179.

15. Ehlers N. Studies on the hydration of the cornea with special reference to the acid hydration. *Acta Ophthalmol.* 1966;44:924-925.

16. Waring GO III. Corneal structure and pathophysiology. In: HM Leibowits, ed. *Corneal Disorders: Clinical Diagnosis and Management.* Philadelphia, Pa: WB Saunders; 1984:3-25.

17. Smolek MK, McCarey BE. Interlamellar adhesive strength in human eye bank corneas. *Invest Ophthalmol Vis Sci.* 1990;31:1087-1095.

18. Smolek MK. Interlamellar cohesive strength in the vertical meridian of human eye bank corneas. *Invest Ophthalmol Vis Sci.* 1993;34:2962-2969.

19. Dierick HG, Missotten L. Is the corneal contour influenced by a tension in the superficial epithelial cells? A new hypothesis. *Refract Corneal Surg.* 1992;8:54-59. Comments in: *Refract Corneal Surg* 1992;8:60 and 1993;9:147.

20. Litwin KL, Moreira H, Ohadi C, McDonnell PJ. Changes in corneal curvature at different excimer laser ablative depths. Letter. *Am J Ophthalmol.* 1991;111:382-384.

21. Maurice DM. The cornea and sclera. In: H Davson, ed. *The Eye. Vegetative Physiology and Biochemistry.* Vol 1b. Orlando, Fla: Academic Press; 1984:1-158.

22. Jue B, Maurice DM. The mechanical properties of the rabbit and human cornea. *J Biomech.* 1986;19:847-853.

23. Seiler TS, Matallana M, Sendler S, Bende T. Does Bowman's layer determine the biomechanical properties of the cornea? *Refract Corneal Surg.* 1992;8:139-142.

24. Maurice DM, Monroe F. Cohesive strength of corneal lamellae. *Exp Eye Res.* 1990;50:59-63.

25. Anseth A, Laurent TC. Polysaccharides in normal and pathologic corneas. *Invest Ophthalmol Vis Sci.* 1962;1:195-201.

26. Ehlers N. The fibrillary texture and the hydration of the cornea. *Acta Ophthalmol.* 1966;44:620-630.

27. Ytteborg J, Dohlman CH. Corneal edema and intraoc-

ular pressure. II. Clinical results. *Arch Ophthalmol.* 1965;74:375-381.

28. Hedbys BO, Dohlman CH. A new method for the determination of the swelling pressure of the corneal stroma in vitro. *Exp Eye Res.* 1963;2:122-129.

29. Hedbys BO, Mishima S, Maurice DM. The imbibation pressure of the corneal stroma. *Exp Eye Res.* 1963;2:99-111.

30. Klyce SD, Dohlman CH, Tolpin DW. In vivo determination of corneal swelling pressure. *Exp Eye Res.* 1971;11:220-229.

31. Mishima S, Maurice DM. The effect of normal evaporation on the eye. *Exp Eye Res.* 1961;1:46-52.

32. Mishima S, Hedbys BO. The permeability of the corneal epithelium and endothelium to water. *Exp Eye Res.* 1967;6:10-32.

33. Biswell R. Cornea. In: DG Vaughan, T Asbury, P Riordan-Eva, eds. *General Ophthalmology.* Norwalk, Conn: Appleton & Lange; 1992:125.

34. Kanai A, Kaufman HE. Electron microscopic studies of swollen corneal stroma. *Ann Ophthalmol.* 1973;5:178-190.

35. Hedbys BO, Mishima S. Flow of water in the corneal stroma. *Exp Eye Res.* 1962;1:262-275.

36. Maurice DM. The movement of fluorescein and water in the cornea. *Am J Ophthalmol.* 1960;49:1011-1019.

37. Marshall J, Trokel S, Rothery S, Schubert H. An ultrastructural study of corneal incisions induced by an excimer laser at 193 nm. *Ophthalmology.* 1985;92:749-758.

38. Gilbert ML, Roth AS, Friedlander MH. Human corneal steepening by annular keratotomy. *Invest Ophthalmol Vis Sci.* 1989;30(Suppl):186.

39. Gilbert ML, Roth AS, Friedlander MH. Corneal flattening by shallow circular trephination in human eye bank eyes. *Refract Corneal Surg.* 1990;6:113-116.

40. Rogers C, Cohen P, Lawless M. Phototherapeutic keratectomy for Reis Bucklers' corneal dystrophy. *Austral N Zealand J Ophthalmol.* 1993;21:247-250.

41. Amm M, Duncker GI. Refractive changes after phototherapeutic keratectomy. *J Cataract Refract Surg.* 1997;23:839-844.

42. Stark WJ, Chamon W, Kamp MT, Enger CL, Rencs EV, Gottsh JD. Clinical follow-up of 193-nm ArF excimer laser photokeratectomy. *Ophthalmology.* 1992;99:805-812.

43. Sher NA, Bowers RA, Zabel RW, et al. Clinical use of the 193-nm excimer laser in the treatment of corneal scars. *Arch Ophthalmol.* 1991;109:491-498.

44. Gartry D, Kerr Muir M, Marshall J. Excimer laser treatment of corneal surface pathology: a laboratory and clinical study. *Br J Ophthalmol.* 1991;75:258-269.

45. Campos M, Nielsen S, Szerenyi K, Garbus JJ, McDonnell PJ. Clinical follow-up of phototherapeutic keratectomy for treatment of corneal opacities. *Am J Ophthalmol.* 1993;115:433-440.

46. Starr MS, Donnenfeld E, Newton M, Tostanoski J, Muller J, Odrich M. Excimer laser phototherapeutic keratectomy. *Cornea.* 1996;15:557-565.

47. McDonnell PJ, Seiler T. Phototherapeutic keratectomy with excimer laser for Reis-Buckler's corneal dystrophy. *Refract Corneal Surg.* 1992;8:306-310.

48. Hersh PS, Spinak A, Garrana R, Mayers M. Phototherapeutic keratectomy: strategies and results in 12 eyes. *Refract Corneal Surg.* 1993;9(Suppl):S90-95.

49. Fagerholm P, Fitzsimmons TD, Örndahl M, Öhman L, Tengroth B. Phototherapeutic keratectomy: long-term results in 166 eyes. *Refract Corneal Surg.* 1993;9(Suppl):S76-81.

50. Hahn TW, Sah WJ, Kim JH. Phototherapeutic keratectomy in 9 eyes with superficial corneal diseases. *Refract Corneal Surg.* 1993;9(Suppl):S115-118.

51. Örndahl M, Fagerholm P, Fitzsimmons T, Tengroth B. Treatment of corneal dystrophies with excimer laser. *Acta Ophthalmol.* 1994;72:235-240.

52. O'Brart DPS, Gartry DS, Lohmann CP, Patmore AL, Kerr Muir MG, Marshall J. Treatment of band keratopathy by excimer laser phototherapeutic keratectomy: surgical techniques and long term follow-up. *Br J Ophthalmol.* 1993;77:702-708.

53. Seiler T. Der excimer-laser: ein instrument für die hornhautchirurgie. *Der Ophthalmologe.* 1992;89:128-133.

54. Azar D. Quoted by: Stark WJ, Chamon W, Kamp MT, Enger CL, Rencs EV, Gottsh JD. Clinical follow-up of 193-nm ArF excimer laser photokeratectomy. *Ophthalmology.* 1992;99:805-812.

55. Thompson VM. Excimer laser phototherapeutic keratectomy: clinical and surgical aspects. *Ophthalmic Surg Lasers.* 1995;26:461-472.

56. Dupps WJ, Roberts C. Suppression of the acute biomechanical response to excimer laser keratectomy. Abstract. *Invest Ophthalmol Vis Sci.* 1999;40:S110.

57. Spöerl E, Huhle H, Seiler T. The swelling behavior of the cornea after artificial cross-linking. ARVO abstracts. *Invest Ophthalmol Vis Sci.* 1997;38:S507.

58. Dupps WJ. Chemomechanical modification of the corneal response to photokeratectomy. Dissertation. Columbus, Ohio: The Ohio State University; 1998.

59. Maloney RK, Friedman M, Harmon T, et al. A prototype erodible mask delivery system for the excimer laser. *Ophthalmology.* 1993;100:542-549.

60. Fahd AK, Seitz B, Oliveira CBR, McDonnell PJ, Bryant MR. Effects of phototherapeutic keratectomy on peripheral corneal thickness. ARVO abstract. *Invest Ophthalmol Vis Sci.* 1996;37(3):S568.

61. MacRae SM, Durrie D, Rich LF, Shaw TL. Large opti-

cal zone ablation treatment of myopia in the Oregon-Kansas study. *Invest Ophthalmol Vis Sci.* 1999;40(4Suppl):S588. Abstract #3087.

62. Lindstrom RL, Hardten DR, Houtman DM, et al. Six-month results of hyperopic and astigmatic LASIK in eyes with primary and secondary hyperopia. *Trans Am Ophth Soc.* 1999;XCVII:241-260.

63. McDonald MB. Summit-Autonomous CustomCornea LASIK outcomes. *J Refract Surg.* 2000;16:S617-618.

64. Munger R, Jackson WB, Mintsioulis G. Ablation pro-file and epithelial regrowth after myopic PRK with the VisX Star. American Society of Cataract and Refractive Surgery Annual Meeting; 1999.

65. Sborgia C, Alessio G, Boscia F, Vetrugno M. Corneal interactive programmed topographic ablation: prelim-inary results. American Society of Cataract and Refractive Surgery Annual Meeting; 1999.

66. Roberts C. Future challenges to aberration-free abla-tive procedures. *J Refract Surg.* 2000;16:S623-629.

Chapter Ten

Technology Requirements for Customized Corneal Ablation

Ronald R. Krueger, MD, MSE

INTRODUCTION

With the recent surge of interest in wavefront sensing technology as a new diagnostic tool in refractive surgery,[1,2] the concept of wavefront customized correction has now come to the forefront.[3,4] Although customized corneal ablation refers to a broad view that encompasses the scope of this book, it includes both topographic-guided ablation and wavefront-guided ablation. The topographic-guided ablation, or TopoLink, was first conceptualized by Gibralter[5] and will be dealt with later in this book. Wavefront customization is the ultimate form of customization and the focus of this chapter.

Within the past year, there have been a number of different wavefront sensing devices placed on the market. With that, a number of different models of wavefront customized corneal ablation have been proposed. Each model, however unique, does have essential technology requirements that are necessary to properly correct refractive aberrations. Without the correction of these aberrations, true customized corneal ablation is not possible.

Aberrations have recently been reported to increase up to 17 times after laser vision correction.[6] Since all laser vision correction surgery to this point has been found to create aberrations, reduction of high-order aberrations with customized corneal ablation sets a new precedent. The technology required to achieve aberration-free laser vision cor-

rection may not be successfully implemented by every laser system's attempt in this area. Therefore, it is important to carefully consider the following requirements.

SCANNING SPOT DELIVERY

Spot Size and Shape

Although many of today's commercially available excimer laser systems have beam diameters that can decrease to as small as 1 mm, the shape of this small 1-mm beam varies according to its mode of formation being either a gaussian or top-hat pattern. A top-hat beam created by a concentric iris aperture produces sharp ablation edges that overlap in the laser vision correction profile. A gaussian beam allows for very uniform overlap in the creation of ablation profile (Figure 10-1). A truly customized profile can best be created by a gaussian beam with ideal spot overlap.[7]

The size of the beam also plays a factor when considering a top-hat or gaussian profile. In a study of small spot scanning, a 2-mm top-hat beam profile results in performance degradation of both low and

> A truly customized profile can best be created by a gaussian beam with ideal spot overlap.[7]

high spatial frequency during custom ablation.[7] This is in contrast to a 1-mm gaussian beam that shows good performance when treating both high and low spatial frequency aberrations.[7]

Finally, when implementing a gaussian pattern, the size of the spot must correspond to the resolution of aberrations being treated. As calculated and discussed in Chapter Five on custom ablation physics, an optical ablation zone diameter of 6 mm would require a spot size of ≤ 1 mm to correct fourth-order aberrations. Therefore, scanning spot lasers > 1 mm would not adequately treat the most common of higher-order aberrations, namely spherical aberration and coma.

This leads us to the question of which lasers provide a small, ≤ 1 mm spot. Table 10-1 lists seven excimer laser systems that attempt to provide a small scanning spot. The first four are used to correct refractive errors with a ≤ 1 mm spot during the entire treatment. Of the latter three, the Aesculap Meditec MEL 70 has a < 2 mm gaussian spot. The Bausch & Lomb Technolas 217 (Claremont, Calif) treats the cornea with a 2-mm top-hat truncated gaussian spot with a future implementation of 1-mm top-hat custom spot for treating aberrations. The VisX S3 uses a 2- to 3-mm smooth scan feature for the majority of the correction and then implements a 1 mm top-hat custom spot for aberration treatment. As discussed previously, a top-hat beam does not allow for the most smooth ablation profile due to overlap errors.

Spot Scanning Rate

Table 10-1 also identifies the spot frequency of each of the seven lasers listed. The majority of the small spot gaussian profile lasers use a spot scanning rate of approximately 200 Hz. The Alcon Summit Autonomous LADARVision laser, however, uses a spot scanning rate of only 60 Hz. Even though the spot frequency for the LADARVision system is considerably slower than the other small spot scanning lasers, the actual ablation time is shorter (8 seconds per diopter [D]) with the LADARVision than when using the Lasersight LSX system (Orlando, Fla). This is because of the slightly higher fluence and volume ablated per shot with the LADARVision system.

The frequency of spot placement is important with regard to hydration changes that occur over time, as treatments that take too long can adversely affect tissue hydration. The scanning spot, however, must not be more rapid than a rate that can be ade-

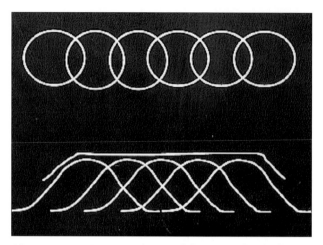

Figure 10-1. Gaussian beam delivery with ideal spot overlap to produce a very uniform, smooth ablation.

quately followed by the tracking system. This will be discussed in the next section.

Finally, a scanning spot must also be nonsequential in its pulse placement (one spot not directly placed next to the following spot), to avoid thermal buildup and improper plume evacuation during treatment. Figure 10-2 presents the nonsequential spot placement of the LADARVision system.

The Three S's of Scanning Spot

Steep Central Islands

When using a broadbeam laser, steep central islands have been found to occur in as much as 80% of eyes treated with photorefractive keratectomy (PRK)[8] (Figure 10-3). The unwanted formation of steep central islands led to the development of special ablation software to compensate for their formation. Yet even after implementing anticentral island software, they frequently occur.

The proposed mechanism for steep central island formation has been attributed to a micro explosion phenomenon on the corneal surface during photoablation. This occurs due to a central shielding of subsequent pulses from trapped particles within the center of the broadbeam, as well as the accumulation of central fluid.[9] Figure 10-4 demonstrates the ablation plume with a broadbeam, which causes a central vacuum (arrow) that traps the effluent and shields subsequent pulse placement. The narrow plume with a small spot laser does not show any central attenuation. Profilometry of broadbeam ablation in plastic demonstrates peripheral overcorrection with

Table 10-1
Comparison of Small-Spot Scanners

	LADARVision	*LASERSIGHT LSX*	*WAVELIGHT ALLEGRETTO*	*SCHWIND ESIRIS*	*MEDTEC MEL 70*	*B & L TECHNOLAS 217*	*VISX S3*
Spot size	0.8 mm	0.6 mm	0.95 mm	1 mm	1.9 mm	2 mm & 1mm custom	2 to 3 mm & 1 mm custom
Spot profile	Gaussian	Gaussian	Gaussian	Gaussian	Gaussian	Top-hat (truncated gaussian)	Top-hat
Spot frequency	60 Hz	200 Hz	200 Hz	200 Hz	35 Hz	50 Hz	≥10 Hz

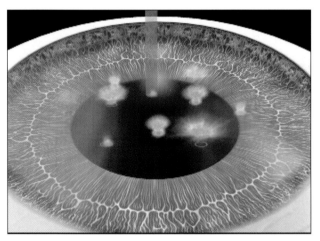

Figure 10-2. Nonsequential spot placement of the LADARVision system demonstrating adequate space to avoid interference with the plume evacuation and thermal build-up between pulses.

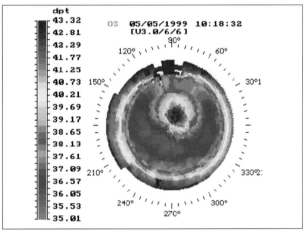

Figure 10-3. Steep central island following LASIK surgery with a broadbeam laser (VisX Star).

central undercorrection[10] (Figure 10-5). Since this profilometry was performed in plastic, the total explanation of central islands being due to accumulation of fluid would be unsubstantiated.

Basically, the formation of steep central islands does show the presence of macro irregularities with broadbeam treatment. These macro irregularities are not present when using a scanning spot.

Surface Smoothness

Concern over microscopic smoothness of the beam has been a long-standing issue. Broadbeams are noted as having a variety of inhomogeneities and hot spots within the beam. Scanning spot ablation

with perfect overlap when using eye tracking demonstrates no inhomogeneities or hot spots (see Figure 10-1). This results in the greater smoothness of scanning electron microscopy (SEM) after LADARVision treatment versus that of a broadbeam laser (VisX 20/20B), as noted in Figure 10-6. Recently, unpublished studies by Yee, et al confirm this observation (Richard Yee, MD, ASCRS, 2000). Smoother surfaces are believed to result in better healing and outcome, but this idea has not been substantiated. Smoother surfaces, however, would certainly be predictive of greater precision in wavefront customization, which is another benefit of scanning spot delivery.

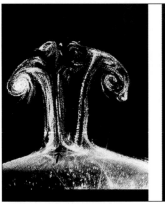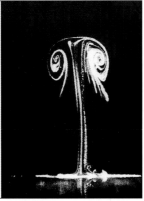

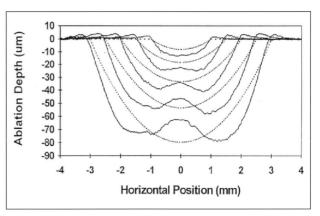

Figure 10-4. Left: Ablation plume with a broadbeam laser delivery demonstrating a central vacuum (arrow) that traps the effluent and shields the subsequent pulse. Right: Ablation plume with scanning spot laser delivery that does not trap particles or shield subsequent pulse placement (reprinted with permission from Krueger RR. Steep central islands: have we figured them out? *J Refract Surg.* 1997;13:215-218).

Figure 10-5. Profilometry of broadbeam ablation in plastic (PMMA) demonstrating peripheral overcorrection and central undercorrection leading to the formation of a steep central island (reprinted with permission from Shimmick JK, et al. Corneal ablation profilometry and steep central islands. *J Refract Surg).* 1997;13:235-245).

Stress Waves

The impact of excimer laser photoablation on the cornea produces a stress wave that propagates through the eye[11] as well as an ablation plume projected away from the eye.[12] The energy and speed of particulate ejection from the cornea is matched by an equal but opposite energy directed into the eye.

The magnitude of this excimer laser-induced stress wave is approximately 40 atmospheres at the plane of the cornea.[11] With a small spot ablation ($\leq$ 1.5 mm), this energy quickly dissipates beyond the corneal endothelium. However, for larger spots ($\geq$ 3 mm), a pressure focus is found 7 to 8 mm behind the corneal endothelium at the level of the posterior lens or anterior vitreous (Figure 10-7). For a 6-mm diameter beam, the magnitude of the pressure focus is approximately 80 atmospheres.[11] This additional acoustic stress at the anterior vitreous and lens may lead to vitreoretinal or lens abnormalities. Although the incidence of retinal detachments after PRK or LASIK is no greater than the general population,[13] a case of bilateral giant retinal tears with detachment has been recently reported after bilateral LASIK, bringing the impact of this acoustic effect into question.[14] Once again we see the benefit of scanning spot delivery.

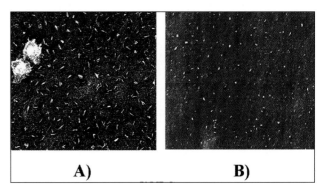

Figure 10-6. Scanning electron micrographs (SEM-1000X) of the ablated surface of paired fresh human cadaver eye corneas treated with A: VisX 20/20B; B: Alcon Summit Autonomous LADARVision laser. Note the smoother surface when using the scanning spot laser in comparison with the broadbeam delivery.

VERY FAST EYE TRACKING

Fixation-Related Eye Movements

During patient fixation, frequent saccadic eye movements have been recorded. They are:
1. Random
2. About 5 times per second
3. At a rapid rate proportional to distance traversed[15]

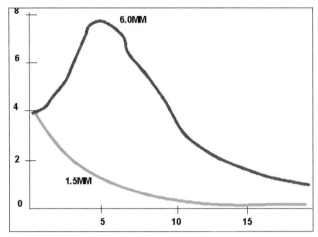

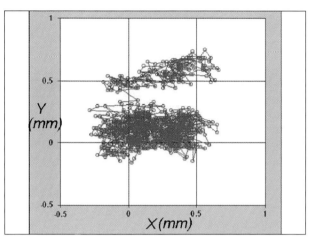

Figure 10-7. Stress wave amplitudes as measured with a hydrophone within a porcine eye treated with differing excimer laser beam diameters (1.5 mm to 7.5 mm). Note that with a 1.5-mm beam, the stress wave quickly dissipates as it travels through the eye, while the beams > 3 mm develop a pressure focus. This pressure focus is 7 to 8 mm posterior to the cornea (posterior lens/anterior vitreous) in human eyes.

Figure 10-8. Recorded tracing of fixation-related eye movement during LADARVision tracking, which demonstrates multiple saccades extending > 0.7 mm both horizontally and vertically from the point of fixation.

At present, LADARVision is the only tracker in which the sampling rate (4000 Hz) exceeds 10 times the optimal tracker bandwidth.

These characteristics of fixation-related saccadic eye movements make careful treatment of patients requiring laser vision correction impossible without the aid of a sophisticated eye tracking system. Typical fixation-related saccades traverse a distance of 1 to 10 degrees (0.1 to 2.0 mm) at a rate of 100 to 800 degrees/second (22 to 170 mm/second).[15] An example of the extent of random movement noted with fixation during laser vision correction is shown in Figure 10-8. This figure shows translational movements extending > 0.7 mm in both the x and y direction from the point of original fixation. The fastest saccadic eye movements are recorded and measured at greater than 10 degrees (2.0 mm) at a rate of up to 800 degrees/second (170 mm/second).[15,16] The speed of this movement is fast enough to allow the globe to rotate greater than twice within the orbit for each 1 second. Only a very fast eye tracking system can follow this type of movement during laser vision correction.

Eye Tracking of Significant Eye Movements

In order to adequately follow and track saccadic eye movements during fixation, a 100 Hz closed-loop bandwidth tracker is required. To understand what this means in relation to the tracker sampling rate, the closed-loop tracking frequency (sampling rate) must be approximately 10 times the desired tracker bandwidth (10 x 100 = 1000 Hz).

At present, LADARVision is the only tracker in which the sampling rate (4000 Hz) exceeds 10 times the optimal tracker bandwidth. LADARVision tracking compensates for saccadic eye movements by laser radar. This works by implementing two subsystems:

1. Detection
2. Response

The detection subsystem utilizes a 905-nm diode laser signal, which is transmitted and received 4000 times each second, locating the position of the dilated pupil margin. This detection subsystem is intimately connected to the tracking servomirrors, which are quickly repositioned in < 10 milliseconds. Hence, the closed-loop bandwidth response time of the tracker mirror assembly combined with the laser radar signal is > 600 radians/second or about 100 Hz.[18,19]

The laser radar device senses the position of the pharmacologically dilated pupil margin and centers it relative to capturing the position of the undilated pupil, relative to the limbus using the graphical user interface of the laser's computer. Figures 10-9a and b demonstrate the centration step outlining the undilated pupil in reference to the limbus (Figure 10-9a), as well as the alignment step redefining the position of the limbus on the graphical user interface prior to

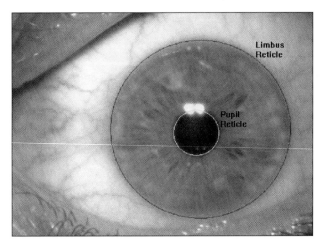

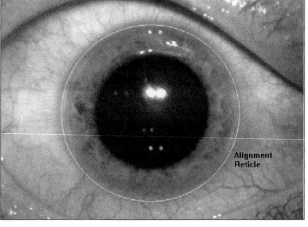

Figure 10-9a. Centration step outlining and recording the undilated pupil (yellow circle) relative to the limbus (red circle).

Figure 10-9b. Alignment step, overlaying the limbus reference mark (green circle) over the actual limbus during laser radar eye tracking. Centration from the undilated pupil relative to the limbus is achieved by tracking the dilated pupil margin relative to the limbus.

engaging the eye tracker (Figure 10-9b). Once engaged, the eye tracker locks onto the dilated pupil margin and the tracked image verifies that the laser sees an unwavering image of the eye even during fixation-related saccades and nystagmus.

Comparison of Laser Radar and Video Camera Eye Tracking

The closed-loop bandwidth tracking frequency of 100 Hz achieved by the LADARVision system can be compared with various infrared video camera tracking systems only in part because most video camera tracking systems are described as open-loop when considering their bandwidth frequency. This means that for each observed change in the position of the pupillary reflex in the video camera-based tracker, the servomirrors have an opportunity to respond or not respond to that change. For many of these systems, the scanning rate of the laser matches or is slightly faster than the tracking frequency. The most frequently used video camera tracking rate has been 60 Hz, limited by the frame rate of the camera. Faster, more sophisticated video camera technology has allowed this to be expanded up to 120, 250, and 300 Hz in some systems (Table 10-2). When considering that a tracker sampling rate needs to be 10 times the actual tracker bandwidth frequency, these video camera-based trackers at best achieve a 6 to 30 Hz tracker bandwidth frequency.

Although the VisX SmoothScan is considered a broadbeam laser with modified scanning features, it is considered in Table 10-2 for comparison. Although the table makes a comparison of the tracker detection frequency and bandwidth frequency, this only applies if the eye tracker is a closed-loop system. Open-loop systems can only respond to an individual sample without truly locking on to the position of the eye. Many video camera-based tracking systems are only available internationally outside the United States, and even in these locations, are intermittently used or not used at all.

In a study of ablation centration after active eye tracking during PRK and LASIK, a mean decentration of 0.33 mm (PRK) and 0.35 mm (LASIK) was consistently observed despite the use of an eye tracker (50 Hz Schwind Multiscan, Kleinostheim, Germany). The conclusion was that active eye tracking alone did not ensure good centration and that patient cooperation and fixation were important. This conclusion, however, does not consider the magnitude and frequency of fixation-related eye movement found despite the cooperation of the patient, nor does it consider the limited tracking frequency studied and the need to evaluate a more sophisticated eye tracker.

Clinical Benefit of Very Fast Eye Tracking

The laser associated with the fastest eye tracking system (LADARVision) has recently also demonstrated the fastest and most broad-ranging US Food

	LADARVision	*Video Camera*
Laser system	Autonomous	Technolas (120)
		Nidek, VisX (60)
		Lasersight (60)
		Wavelight (250)
Method	Laser radar	CCD/infrared
Transmittal signal	905 mm diode laser	None
Detection frequency	4000 Hz	60, 120, 250 Hz
Response time	3 ms rise time	50 ms rise time
	(100 Hz bandwidth)	(6 Hz bandwidth)

Table 10-2
Comparative Features of Eye Tracking in Scanning Excimer Lasers

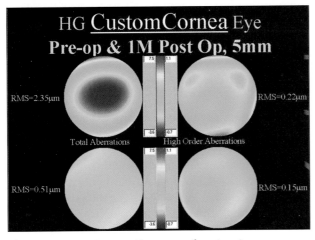

Figure 10-10. CustomCornea refractive image maps (two-dimensional) demonstrating a reduction in the RMS error after tracker-assisted CustomCornea LASIK for both the total refractive profile, including sphere and cylinder (left: preoperative above; postoperative below), as well as just the higher-order aberration including coma, spherical aberration, etc (right: preoperative above; postoperative below). The reduction of aberrations substantiates the benefit of very fast eye tracking (LADARVision) in performing CustomCornea LASIK.

and Drug Administration (FDA) approval rate. FDA approval for myopia, myopia with astigmatism, hyperopia, hyperopia with astigmatism, and mixed astigmatism have all been recently granted with outstanding clinical outcomes during the US investigational clinical trials. These approvals have all been granted exclusively for use with the laser radar eye tracking system, which is an essential component to the LADARVision laser treatment.

At present, the LADARVision system is under US FDA investigation of CustomCornea with the goal of reducing ocular aberrations, which are typically greatly increased during conventional LASIK.[6] Figure 10-10 illustrates the wavefront sensing map of a patient treated with CustomCornea. On the left you can see that the total aberrations, including sphere and cylinder, are markedly reduced after surgery. On the right, the high-order aberrations are shown and are also notably reduced after surgery—the first time that laser vision correction has not created an increase in aberrations.[4] This reduction of ocular aberration improves not only the uncorrected (UCVA) but also best-corrected visual acuity (BCVA) after surgery.

The improvement of best-corrected vision and reduction of ocular aberrations, however, has not been exclusively observed with the Autonomous LADARVision system. Reports using the Wavelight Allegretto laser (Erlangen, Germany) and its 250 Hz video tracker system have also demonstrated an improvement in the root mean square (RMS) wavefront error in isolated individuals. Approximately 20% of the custom treated patients achieve a "super vision" outcome of 20/10 BCVA or better. (Theo Seiler, ASCRS, Boston, Mass; 2000). The improvement in vision and higher-order RMS wavefront error has been recorded in peer-reviewed literature in three patients treated with the Wavelight

Allegretto laser.[3] The 250 Hz tracking system used by this laser verifies that video-based tracking systems can also be used to effectively perform wavefront customized corneal ablation in selected cases. But once again, very fast eye tracking is required.

A final example of the success and utility of very fast eye tracking with laser radar is demonstrated in two patients with congenital nystagmus. Each patient had a preoperative BCVA that was limited because of both amblyopia and refractive error limitations in fixating with glasses. In each case, the postoperative UCVA at 1 day was better than the preoperative best-corrected vision by at least one to five lines of visual acuity (personal communication, Brian Will MD, May 2000). Here, even during random large amplitude eye motion such as nystagmus, sophisticated eye tracking with LADARVision successfully follows nystagmus saccades to produce a good outcome. Very fast eye tracking is an important requirement for achieving the full potential for improved visual acuity with wavefront customized corneal ablation.

WAVEFRONT MEASUREMENT DEVICE

Corneal Topography versus Wavefront

Customized corneal ablation in refractive surgery has come to mean one of two things: topography-guided custom ablation or wavefront-guided custom ablation. The former utilizes information presented by computerized corneal topography instruments to change irregularities in the corneal shape into a smoother, more uniform pattern that improves the UCVA or BCVA. Although it was first proposed by Gibralter and Trokel approximately 4 years ago, widespread adaptation has been limited due to difficulty in registry of the topographic information with the laser. Attempts have been made at topographic guidance by TopoLink, as well as other methods described later in this book.

The second meaning for customized corneal ablation has been more recently adapted in wavefront-guided ablations. The essential components we have

> The wavefront pattern measured by such a device gives a two-dimensional profile of refractive error much in the same way as computerized corneal topography gives a two-dimensional mapping profile of keratometry.

been discussing have been for a wavefront-guided customized ablation, and this third, most vital component is a wavefront measurement device. The wavefront pattern measured by such a device gives a two-dimensional profile of refractive error much in the same way as computerized corneal topography gives a two-dimensional mapping profile of keratometry. Implementing the wavefront measurement device in customized ablation can be much more precise than corneal topography by attempting to achieve not just a smooth corneal surface, but a sharp focus of all corneal points on the retinal fovea.

Principles of Wavefront Measurement Devices

Much the same way that a number of computerized corneal topography devices became available during the past decade, there are now a number of different types of wavefront measurement devices being made available on the market. Although it is often difficult to adequately categorize new products in an understandable fashion, there appears to be three different principles by which wavefront aberration information is collected and measured.

Outgoing Reflection Aberrometry (Shack-Hartmann)

At the turn of the past century, Hartmann first described the principles by which optical aberrations in lenses could be characterized.[21] This was later modified by Shack and found practical application in adaptive optics telescopes to eliminate the aberrations of the earth's atmosphere for the past 20 years. It was finally introduced into ophthalmology by Liang and Bille in 1994.[2] The Shack-Hartmann wavefront sensor was used to objectively measure the wave aberrations of the human eye. Adaptive optics to eliminate the aberrations of the human eye were first used in viewing retinal structures with greater detail than ever before. In 1996, images of cone photoreceptors were viewed in the living human eye by adaptive optics defined by a Shack-Hartmann wavefront sensor.[22] This first attempt at customizing the optics of the eye to increase the resolution of structures within it defined the need for measurement specificity in achieving better resolution when viewing structures outside of the eye.

A typical Shack-Hartmann wavefront sensor utilizes > 100 spots, created by (> 100) lenslets that focus the aberrated light exiting the eye onto a CCD detection array. The distance of displacement (dx) of the focused spot from the ideal very accurately defines

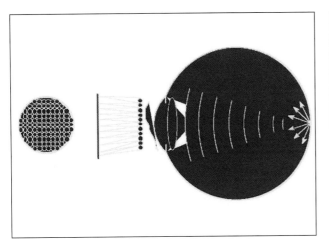

Figure 10-11. Principles of Shack-Hartmann wavefront sensing: low energy laser light reflecting off the retinal fovea passes through the optical structures of the eye, creating an outgoing wavefront. The wavefront passes through the lenslet array to define the deviation of focused spots from their ideal, which mathematically characterizes the wavefront pattern (courtesy of Raymond Applegate, PhD).

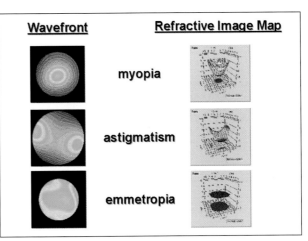

Figure 10-12. Wavefront fringe pattern and refractive image maps (three-dimensional) of myopia, astigmatism, and emmetropia. The refractive image map demonstrates the shape of the wavefront coming out of the eye (bottom to top direction). In this figure, myopia is bowl shaped (rays perpendicular to wavefront converge to a focus) and emmetropia is flat (rays perpendicular to wavefront are parallel, extending to infinity).

the degree of ocular aberration. Figure 10-11 demonstrates the principles of Shack-Hartmann wavefront sensing. Figure 10-12 demonstrates the wavefront fringe pattern and corresponding refractive image map for myopia, astigmatism, and emmetropia using the CustomCornea Measurement Device (CCMD).

The limitations of this type of wavefront sensing may include multiple scattering from choroidal structures beneath the fovea as well as an interference echo. However, this is likely to be insignificant in comparison to the axial length. The speed of capture helps to make this a suitable form of wavefront sensing.

Retinal Imaging Aberrometry (Tscherning and Ray Tracing)

The next type of wavefront sensing was first characterized by Tscherning in 1894 when he described the monochromatic aberrations of the human eye.[23] Tscherning's description, however, was not supported by the leaders of ophthalmic optics, including Gullstrand, and was not favorably accepted. It was not until 1977 that Howland and Howland used Tscherning's aberroscope design together with a cross cylinder lens to subjectively measure the monochromatic aberrations of the eye.[24] This same concept was more recently modified by Seiler using a spheri-

cal lens to project a 1-mm grid pattern onto the retina. This, together with a para-axial aperture system, could visualize and photographically record the aberrated pattern of up to 168 spots as a wavefront map.[1] Figure 10-13 demonstrates the schematic layout of the modified Tscherning aberrometer demonstrating its principles of retinal imaging and image capture.

The limitation of this type of wavefront sensing is the use of an idealized eye model (Gullstrand model eye) to perform the ray tracing computation. The model, however, is modified according to the patient's refractive error to maintain an accurate assessment of the axial length.

In the past several years an alternate form of retinal imaging has been introduced with Tracey retinal ray tracing. This form is slightly different in that it uses a sequential projection of spots onto the retina that are captured and traced to find the wavefront pattern. Sixty-four sequential retinal spots can be traced within 12 milliseconds.

Ingoing Adjustable Refractometry (Spatially Resolved Refractometer)

The final method of wavefront sensing is based on the 17th century principles of Scheiner and described by Smirnov in 1961 as a form of subjectively adjustable refractometry.[25] Peripheral beams of

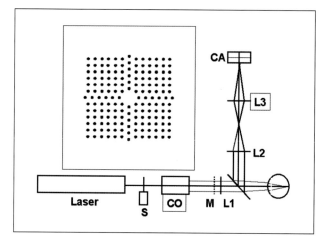

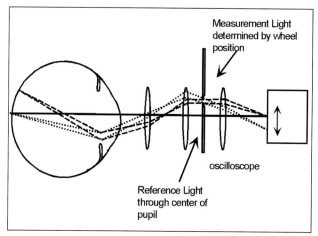

Figure 10-13. Principles of modified Tscherning aberrometry: low energy laser light is collimated and passed through a 13 x 13 spot grid mask to project a laser grid pattern into the eye and retina. The aberrated laser grid pattern can then be photographed through a small para-axial aperture and used to mathematically characterize the wavefront pattern (courtesy of Theo Seiler, MD, PhD).

Figure 10-14. Principles of spatially resolved refractometry: a peripheral measurement light source projected through a wheel (mask) can be subjectively redirected by moving a joystick to overlap a reference light in the center of the pupil. The movement varies the angle of light entering the eye without changing its location and hence can be used to mathematically characterize the wavefront pattern at that point. Rotating the wheel aperture to a new peripheral position can test multiple points (courtesy of Stephen Burns, PhD).

incoming light are subjectively redirected toward a central target to cancel the ocular aberrations from that peripheral point.[25] This was then modified by Webb and Burns in 1998 as a subjective form of wavefront refractometry of the human eye.[26] Figure 10-14 demonstrates the principles of the spatially resolved refractometer (SRR), which measures the wavefront pattern according to these principles. A SRR utilizes approximately 37 testing spots that are manually directed by the observer to overlap the central target in defining the wavefront aberration pattern. The limitation of this technique is the lengthy time required for subjective alignment of the aberrated spots.

An objective variant of this method is based on a form of slit retinoscopy (skioloscopy), which is rapidly scanned along a specific axis and orientation. The fundus reflection is then captured to define the wavefront aberration pattern. Although this latter technique is also sequential at various axes, the objective capture of the reflex makes it possible to acquire this information in a rapid sequence.

Practical Aspects of Wavefront Measurement Devices

Table 10-3 outlines the categorical listings of commercially available wavefront devices. The three main categories of wavefront measurement principles each have a representation by several commercial companies. Each company has made its own proprietary modifications to provide a practical device for clinical use. Careful comparison of these various wavefront measuring principles and their specific devices has not yet been performed clinically. The practical utility of one device versus another still remains to be seen and will continue to be the subject of future investigation.

In the next section of the book, each of the devices listed will be discussed in more detail. Their respective categories will be once again outlined as an introduction to the measuring principle utilized by each wavefront device.

Careful comparison of these various wavefront measuring principles and their specific devices has not yet been performed clinically.

Table 10-3

Categorical Listing of Commercial Wavefront Devices

OUTGOING REFLECTION ABERROMETRY	RETINAL IMAGING ABERROMETRY	INGOING ADJUSTABLE REFRACTOMETRY
Shack-Hartmann principles	**Tscherning principles**	**Scheiner principles**
Alcon Summit/Autonomous CustomCornea measurement device	Wavelight wavefront analyzer	Emory Vision spatially resolved refractometer
VisX/20/10 Perfect Vision Wavescan	Schwind wavefront analyzer	Nidek (slit skioloscopy) OPD Scan
Bausch & Lomb Zyoptics	Tracey retinal ray tracing	
Aesculap Meditec WOSCA		

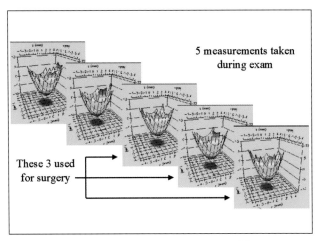

5 measurements taken during exam

These 3 used for surgery

Figure 10-15. Capture and comparison of five consecutive wavefront maps in a myopic eye before CustomCornea laser surgery. The three in closest agreement were used to generate a composite profile map to be used in creating the wavefront-guided laser ablation profile.

Laser/Wavefront Interface

Capture and Comparison

The first step to properly linking up the wavefront device and measurement with the actual laser treatment is to ensure that the most accurate and reproducible wavefront has been captured and implemented. In the US FDA trials of CustomCornea using the Alcon Summit Autonomous LADARVision laser and the CustomCornea measurement device (CCMD), the first step to this process of the laser/wavefront link-up is the capture of five consecutive wavefront measurements on the day of surgery. These five wavefront maps are then compared

statistically and the three in closest agreement are used to generate a composite profile (Figure 10-15). This new composite wavefront map is then used to create the wavefront-guided laser ablation profile and spot pattern. Whether all wavefront laser link-ups require a composite map to be created is not the point of this example, but rather that a very reproducible and accurate map be used when planning the wavefront-guided laser ablation.

Conversion to the Ablation Profile

The next step in the process is converting the wavefront measurement into an actual ablation profile of tissue that needs to be removed from the cornea to correct the refractive error and high-order aberrations. When implementing the step, it is important to have a wavefront measurement that has been captured through at least a 7-mm diameter pupil. To achieve a pupil diameter of this size, pharmacological dilation is necessary. However, subtle variations in the wavefront pattern have been demonstrated with the use of pharmacologic agents and this needs to be considered when forming the wavefront composite to be used during surgery.[27]

Using the Tscherning wavefront aberrometer, testing the reproducibility in 300 eyes by capturing five measurements in each eye with a pupil size of > 7 mm demonstrates a reproducibility of sphere and cylinder to be a standard deviation of ± 0.08 D. The reproducibility of the measured RMS wavefront error for the total refraction and high-order aberrations are a standard deviation of 0.04 mm and 0.02 mm, respectively (see Table 14-1). This high resolution and reproducibility brings into question whether a composite wavefront map needs to be formed in every situation.

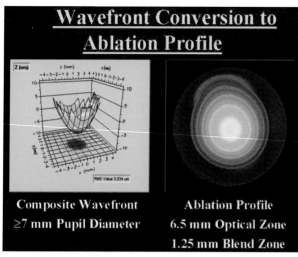

Composite Wavefront
≥7 mm Pupil Diameter

Ablation Profile
6.5 mm Optical Zone
1.25 mm Blend Zone

Figure 10-16a. Conversion of the CustomCornea wavefront map (left) into the ablation profile represented by interference fringes (right).

> In every instance of wavefront customized ablation, a blend zone is necessary to produce a smooth transition between the correction of high-order aberrations at the edge of the optical zone and the residual unablated cornea.

The conversion of the measurement profile into an ablation profile is a complex mathematical inversion of the three dimensional profile (see Figure 14-8). The ablation profile used by the Summit Autonomous LADARVision laser is defined by a 6.5-mm optical zone together with a 1.25-mm lens zone for a total ablation diameter of 9 mm. Figures 10-16a and b demonstrate the conversion process for the Summit Autonomous CustomCornea interface. Here the wavefront composite with a > 7-mm pupil is converted into an ablation profile as demonstrated by the interference fringes and two-dimensional profile of ablation depth.

In every instance of wavefront customized ablation, a blend zone is necessary to produce a smooth transition between the correction of high-order aberrations at the edge of the optical zone and the residual unablated cornea. With the Tscherning aberrometer link-up to the wavelight laser, a blend zone of at least 0.5 mm is added to the calculated ablation zone. In cases where the residual stromal thickness after LASIK makes it unsafe to treat with a full 7-mm optical zone, a slightly smaller optical zone diameter is implemented.

Before transferring the ablation profile to the laser, a final step is determining the excimer laser shot pat-

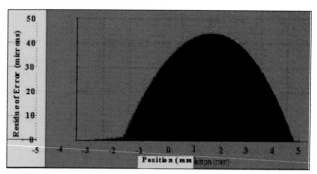

Figure 10-16b. CustomCornea wavefront map ablation depth.

tern. The ablation profile map, which measures the depth or elevation of corneal tissue that needs to be removed, must be broken down into a calculation of the position of each excimer laser pulse to achieve the ablation profile. This step requires knowledge of the fluence and approximate ablation depth for each pulse, as well as the proper gaussian overlap to achieve a smooth uniform ablation profile.

Transfer, Tracking, and Alignment

The next step in linking up the wavefront with the laser is the actual transfer of the wavefront ablation information to the computer-assisted input of the laser. At the present time, the link-up is achieved by a computer disk that downloads the information from the wavefront device and a computer that calculates the excimer laser spot pattern to the computer interface of the excimer laser. This transferred information includes the orientation data gathered during the wavefront measurement.

The excimer laser tracker can then be engaged to align the laser pulse positioning with the movement of the eye, but more importantly, a step of XYZ alignment is necessary to ensure that the wavefront-determined pulsing sequence corresponds with the exact position of the aberrations as seen at the level of the cornea. The Summit Autonomous LADARVision laser has eye tracking that is maintained by locking onto the edge of the dilated pupil but aligned by the position and landmarks of the limbus. For the CustomCornea study, specific markings are made along the limbus in four quadrants using a dye or light thermal cautery for orientation of the wavefront map with the eye during surgery. The graphic user interface on the LADARVision system demonstrates the alignment of the limbus and overlap of the orientation marks while the tracker follows the movement of the dilated pupil margin.

Further steps to ensure proper centration beyond just the center of the pupil, as well as accurate alignment to include cyclotorsion and tilt, will be necessary as wavefront technology further advances.

The issue of proper ocular alignment is an important one. Further steps to ensure proper centration beyond just the center of the pupil, as well as accurate alignment to include cyclotorsion and tilt, will be necessary as wavefront technology further advances. The previously used steps required for centration and alignment when treating only spherocylindrical error may not be adequate when considering the subtle deviations of higher-order aberrations. Since the true visual axis, which connects the fovea with a fixation target, goes through the nodal point of the eye, centering based on the center of the entrance pupil may introduce a slight error (see Figure 14-6). Small decentrations in alignment would allow for incorrect registry of the wavefront ablation pattern onto the cornea.

Algorithm Development

Finally, the last step of interfacing the wavefront ablation profile to the laser requires understanding the variables of the ablation process. Just as current excimer laser correction procedures utilize a carefully developed nomogram for the optimal visual outcome; complex nomograms—considering the multiple variables associated with wavefront-guided treatment—need to be developed and refined in order to successfully reduce the ocular aberrations. Attempts at wavefront-guided LASIK with the Wavelight laser and Tscherning aberrometer have so far shown only 40% reduction of the ocular aberrations in the best case scenario. Complex ablations need to be considered in order to try to improve upon these results. The following parameters outline a preliminary menu of variables that need to be further considered with wavefront-guided laser vision correction.

Corneal Topography (Shape)

Even though the wavefront map fully character-

Just as current excimer laser correction procedures utilize a carefully developed nomogram for the optimal visual outcome; complex nomograms will need to be developed and refined in order to successfully reduce the ocular aberrations.

izes the aberrations within the optical system of the eye, subtle shape changes in corneal topography may have a bearing on the proper placement of pulses onto the cornea.[28] Corneas that are unduly flat or steep may impact the way in which the wavefront-guided ablation pattern successfully remolds the cornea.

Corneal Biomechanics (Structure)

Besides the shape issues defined by corneal topography, there are also structural issues regarding the individual biomechanics of the cornea during laser vision correction. Corneas of differing thickness and corneal elasticity will likely have a different biomechanical impact on ablation. Chapter Nine outlines the issues regarding corneal biomechanics and how this changes with laser vision correction.

Flap Biomechanics (Surgery)

The wavefront measurement profile, which is highly sensitive to the structure and orientation of the cornea, will likely change after making a corneal flap. The biomechanical changes of the cornea secondary to flap creation and positioning of the hinge are not thoroughly understood. Initial studies with the CCMD have demonstrated induced coma along the axis of the hinge after making a corneal flap (personal communication, Christy Stevens, OD, June 2000). Further analysis of wavefront profiles after making a flap alone will need to be analyzed and factored into the ablation nomogram.

Healing Process (Remodeling)

Another very large variable in the ablation considerations is the healing of the corneal stroma and epithelium following wavefront-guided laser vision correction. The correction of subtle aberrations can, in part, be undone by filling in epithelium or remodeling the stroma. The biologic variability of laser vision correction makes it very difficult to achieve full optical quality when performing laser vision correction, and attempts at controlling wound healing have already been an important area of research in refractive surgery. Pharmacological or gene manipulation of biologic processes such as keratocyte apotosis may help us to reduce the wound healing response after refractive surgery and thereby further control our outcome.[29] Ablation algorithms and nomograms will need to be developed to consider the wound healing aspect of wavefront-guided laser vision correction in its current state as well as with our further control of wound healing in the future.

Environmental Issues (Humidity, Temperature, etc)

Another large variable that we currently face with laser vision correction is the hydration of the cornea, which is in part dependent on the humidity, temperature, technique, and length of treatment time. Uniform corneal hydration will be an important consideration in order to get a uniform pattern that fully corrects the wavefront error.

As with all complex systems, appropriate algorithms or nomograms will need to be developed to achieve the optimum optical result. Wavefront-guided customized corneal ablation offers a unique new application to refractive surgery that will hold a great deal of research interest and attention in the years to come. Potential to correct not only the refractive error but the higher-order aberrations has already been well demonstrated in physical applications such as the Hubble telescope and even of correcting the ocular aberration pattern when viewing cone photoreceptors in the retina. The promise of perfect optical quality after laser vision correction would be a well-received addition to our current techniques of laser vision correction. As we further explore this technology, its requirements will likely be expanded upon. Nonetheless, the technology requirements outlined here serve as a foundational basis in our current attempts to provide wavefront-guided customized corneal ablation.

REFERENCES

1. Mierdel P, Wiegard W, Krinke HE, Kaemmerer M, Seiler T. Measuring device for determining monochromatic aberrations of the human eye. *Ophthalmology.* 1997;6:441-5.
2. Liang J, Grimm W, Geolz S, Bille JF. Objective measurement of the wave aberrations of the human eye using Shack-Hartmann wavefront sensor. *J Opt Soc Am A.* 1994;11(7):1949-57.
3. Mrochen M, Kaemmerer M, Seiler T. Wavefront-guided laser in situ keratomileusis: early results in three eyes. *J Refract Surg.* 2000;16:116-21.
4. McDonald MB. Summit Autonomous custom cornea LASIK outcomes. *J Refract Surg.* 2000;16:S617-618.
5. Gibralter R, Trokel S. Correction of irregular astigmatism with the excimer laser. *Ophthalmology.* 1994;101:1310-15.
6. Seiler T, Kaemmerer M, Mierdel P, Krinke HE. Ocular optical aberrations after photorefractive keratectomy for myopia and myopic astigmatism. *Arch Ophthalmol.* 2000;118:71-21.
7. Campin JA, Pettit GH, Gray GP. Required laser beam resolution and PRK system configuration for custom high fidelity corneal shaping. *Invest Ophthalmol Vis Sci.* 1999;38:S538.
8. Krueger RR, Saedy NF, McDonnell PJ. Clinical analysis of steep central islands after excimer laser photorefractive keratectomy. *Arch Ophthalmol.* 1996;114:377-81.
9. Krueger RR. Steep central islands: have we finally figured them out? *J Refract Surg.* 1997;13:215-18.
10. Shimmick JK, Telfair WB, Munnerlyn CR, Bartlett JD, Trokel SL. Corneal ablation profilometry and steep central islands. *J Refract Surg.* 1997;13:235-45.
11. Krueger RR, Seiler T, Gruchman T, Mrochen M, Berlin MS. Stress wave amplitudes during laser surgery of the cornea. *Ophthalmology.* In press.
12. Puliafito CA, Stern D, Krueger RR, Mandel ER. High speed photography of excimer laser ablation of the cornea. *Arch Ophthalmol.* 1987;105:1255-59.
13. Arevalo JF, Ramirez E, Suarez E, Morales-Stopello J, et al. Incidence of vitreoretinal pathologic conditions with 24 months after laser in-situ keratomileusis. *Ophthalmology.* 2000;107:258-62.
14. Ozdomar A, Aras C, Sener B, et al. Bilateral retinal detachment associated with giant retinal tear after laser-assisted keratomileusis. *Retina.* 1998;18:176-7.
15. Bollen E, Bax J, Van Dijk JG. Variability of the main sequence. *Invest Ophthalmol Vis Sci.* 1993;34:3700-04.
16. Boghea D, Troost BT, Daroff RB, Dell'osso LF, Birkett JE. Characteristics of normal human saccades. *Invest Ophthalmol Vis Sci.* 1974;13:619-23.
17. Bahill AT, Clark MR, Stark K. Glissades eye movements generated by mismatched components of the saccadic motorneural control signal. *Mathematical Biosciences.* 1975;26:303-18.
18. McDonald MR, Vanhorn LC. Autonomous T-PRK. In: JH Talamo, RR Krueger, eds. *The Excimer Manual: A Clinician's Guide to Excimer Laser Surgery.* Boston, Mass: Little, Brown & Co; 1997:355-68.
19. Krueger RR. In perspective: eye tracking and Autonomous laser radar. *J Refract Surg.* 1999;15:145-9.
20. Yi-Yu Tsai, Jame-Ming Lin. Ablation centration after active eye tracker-assisted photorefractive keratectomy and laser in situ keratomileusis. *J Cataract Refract Surg.* 2000;26:28-34.
21. Miller DT, Williams DR, Morris GM, Liang J. Images of cone photorecptors in the living human eye. *Vision Res.* 1996;36(18):1067-79.
22. Hartmann J. Bemerkungen uber den bau die justierung von spektrographen. *Zeitschrift fuer Instrumenterkinde.* 1900;20:47.
23. Tscherning M. Die monochromatischen aberrationen des menschlichen auges. *Z Psychol Physiol Sinn.* 1894;6:456-71.
24. Howland HC, Howland B. A subjective method for

the measurement of monochromatic aberrations of the eye. *J Opt Soc Am A.* 1977;67:1508-18.

25. Smirnov HS. Measurement of the wave aberration in the human eye. *Biophys.* 1961;6:52-66.

26. He JC, Marces S, Webb RH, Burns S. Measurement of the wavefront aberration of the eye by a fast psychophysical procedure. *J Opt Soc Am A.* 1998;15(9):2449-56.

27. Fankhauser F, Kaemmerer M, Mrochen M, Seiler T. The effect of accommodation, mydriasis and cycloplegia on aberrometry. *Invest Ophthalmol Vis Sci.* 2000;41(4):S461.

28. Mrochen MC, Kaemmerer M, Riedel P, Seiler T. Why do we have to consider the corneal curvature for the calculation of customized ablation profiles? *Invest Ophthalmol Vis Sci.* 2000;41(4):S689.

29. Wilson SE. Programmed cell death, wound healing and laser refractive surgical procedures: molecular-cell biology for the corneal surgeon. *J Refract Surg.* 1997;13:171-75.

Chapter Eleven

Eye Tracking and Refractive Surgery

Michael Huppertz
Eberhard Schmidt, MBA
Winfried Teiwes, PhD

With the increasing demands of customized corneal ablation—smaller beam sizes, faster repetition rate, and greater precision of correction—exact positioning of each laser shot onto the eye becomes increasingly more important. This need for greater positioning accuracy has provided the impetus for several refractive laser companies to implement eye tracking as the "target acquisition system," to position the ablation beam accurately onto the corneal surface and compensate for patient head and eye movements during the surgery procedure. As the sophistication of the laser delivery systems and the whole treatment process increases, so do the requirements of the eye tracking system until it becomes part of a closed loop system in which each laser shot is guided to its precalculated ablation position on the eye. To meet these requirements, certain considerations of the physiological parameters of eye movements and the methodological aspects of the measurement technique are needed.

Furthermore, new techniques are providing online measurement of eye position not just in horizontal and vertical coordinates of the pupil center but also in torsion, a necessity to perform nonspherical ablations on the eye (ie, astigmatism correction). In addition, an estimation of rotation versus translation of the eye with respect to the laser system is needed to control ablation intensity as a function of the distance between laser and ablation zones.

In refractive laser systems, the laser operates in fixed space coordinates. The patient's eye is mostly stabilized by voluntary visual fixation of a visual target. However, eye movements cannot be eliminated completely by voluntary fixation; furthermore, slower head movements still occur during the surgical procedure, changing the eye's position relative to the laser. This already provided the impetus for several laser manufacturers to measure the eye position and stabilize the laser on the eye by means of controlled mirror system.

EYE MOVEMENTS

This section will first describe eye movements in general, then more specifically as they occur during the laser surgery as well as to some extent during the diagnostic procedure. For correct measurement of eye movements, it is essential to understand the principles of the static and dynamic behavior of the eye's high performance "actuator system"—the muscular structure that holds and controls the eye and its movements—and the neurological and vestibular control system that controls the "actuator system."

Kinematics of Eye Movements

The eye can be modeled as a ball and socket-mounted rigid spherical body and eye movements can be described as a series of infinitesimal rotations around three orthogonal axes that intersect in the

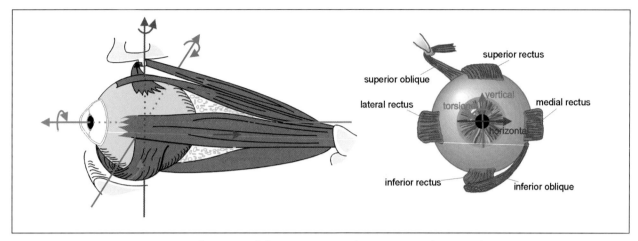

Figure 11-1. Eye movement coordinates and their generation from extraocular muscles.

center of the sphere. Three pairs of extraocular muscles, acting according to the push-pull principle, rotate the eye around these three axes, therefore performing eye movements in three dimensions of rotation: horizontal rotation around the vertical axis, vertical rotation around the horizontal axis, and torsional rotation around the line of sight (Figure 11-1). Eye movement coordinates are normally described in an eye-fixed coordinate system (Euler angles).

The necessity to also control torsional eye position becomes clear if we consider the same horizontal and vertical rotation of the eye but in different sequence results in a different torsional eye position in space (rotations are not commutative). For example, rotation of first 45 degrees up, then 45 degrees right results in a counter clockwise rotated retinal image; rotation first 45 degrees to the right, then 45 degrees up results in a clockwise rotation of the retinal image. A corrective torsional movement of the eye is therefore required to provide the same orientation of the image on the retina independent from the sequence. As identified more than 100 years ago by Donders and Listing,[1,2] all eye positions during a fixation may be described as a rotation around a single axis from a primary eye position (approximately straight ahead). All rotation axes are lying in a single plane perpendicular to the primary position of the eye (Listing's law; Figure 11-2).

Dynamics of Eye Movement

Eye movements are needed for five main purposes and are performed at different velocities and angular ranges (Table 11-1).

Saccades: The eye normally performs fast eye movements (saccades) to jump from one target posi-

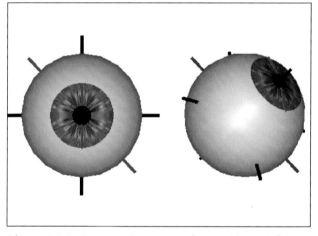

Figure 11-2. Eye rotations according to Listing's law.

tion to another (fixation). Peak velocities of saccades are somewhat proportional to the amplitude of the saccade, ranging from 10 deg/s (2 mm/s) to 800 deg/s (170 mm/s) (Figure 11-3).[3] The duration of saccades depends on the amplitude, ranging from 30 ms for small saccades of 5 degrees to 100 ms or even more for 20 degrees and above.

Vestibular eye movement stabilizes the retinal image to avoid blurring due to head movements. Linear (translatory) and rotational acceleration of the head is measured by the vestibular system in the inner ear and leads to slow compensatory eye movements up to approximately 100 deg/s (21 mm/s),[4] which are often compensated by faster saccades in the range of 100 deg/s to 400 deg/s (84 mm/s) in the opposite direction if the amplitude of the movement reaches a certain limit (nystagmus). Also, static rotations are introduced: different orientation of the head

Table 11-1

Eye Movements and Corresponding Dynamics

TYPE OF MOVEMENT	VELOCITY RANGE	ANGULAR RANGE
Saccades	10 to 800 deg/s (2 to 170 mm/s)	0.1 to 100 degrees
Vestibular eye movements	<100 deg/s (21 mm/s) or 100 to 400 deg/s (21 to 84 mm/s)	1 to 12 degrees
Pursuit and optokinetic movement	<40 deg/s (8 mm/s)	>1 degree
Vergence eye movements	10 deg/s (2 mm/s)	~15 degrees
Miniature movements	10 to 300 min/s (0.03 to 1 mm/s)	10 min to 10 sec (0.003 to 0.2 degrees)

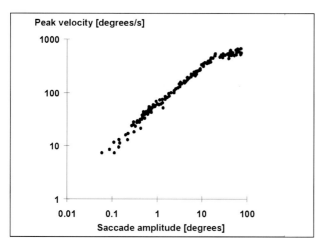

Figure 11-3. Peak saccade velocity as a function of the saccade amplitude.[3]

toward gravity results in a different torsional eye position (ocular counter-roll) in the order of ± 7 degrees.[5]

Pursuit and optokinetic movement stabilizes the retinal image due to moving objects relative to the eye. A retinal image slip creates a pursuit eye movement of up to 40 deg/s (8 mm/s) to follow the target and minimize retinal slip.[6] Movements with larger amplitudes also create fast saccades in the opposite direction, resulting in an optokinetic nystagmus.

Vergence eye movement removes retinal disparity introduced by looking at objects at different distances and by accommodation (retinal blur).[7] In humans, these are slow eye movements in the order of 10 deg/s (2 mm/s) and are mainly horizontal with amplitudes up to 15 degrees; however, vertical and torsional vergence can be observed by introducing prisms.[8]

Miniature movements occur while the subject is

trying to maintain fixation on a stationary target. These movements consists of three components: (a) tremor, a high frequency movement with a bandwidth up to 90 Hz[9] that introduces retinal image movement with velocities in the range of 10 min/s[10] in the range 10 to 40 sec[11] and comparable in size to the smallest cones on the retina (some 24 sec), (b) comparatively large but slow drift movement with amplitudes in the range of 5 min and velocities in the region of 4 min/s,[12] and (c) microsaccades in the range of 10 min and peak velocity in the order of 300 min/s.[10]

Therefore, even during perfect fixation, humans perform eye movements at least within a range of approximately 0.2 degrees (corresponding to 45 µm on the cornea) and peak velocities of around 5 deg/s (corresponding to 1000 µm/s on the cornea).

Eye Movements During Refractive Surgery

Within the refractive surgery procedure all eye movements except miniature movements may be reduced using voluntary fixation of the patient. One may argue that these movements (below 50 µm) on the cornea can be neglected. However, some of the above described components cannot be eliminated, and several residual unintentional eye movements may occur:

1. Saccadic square wave jerks within a range of 0.5 to 3 degrees occur during fixations.[13]

2. Vestibular ocular reflex may be suppressed by fixation and fixed head position, but the torsional eye position is changed through different head orientation with gravity between the diagnostic measurement and treatment process.

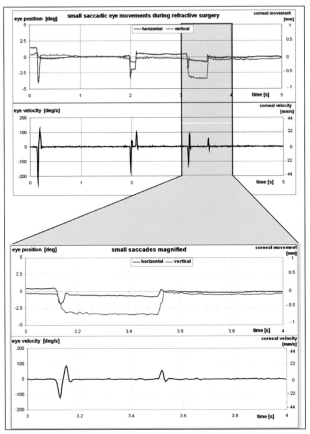

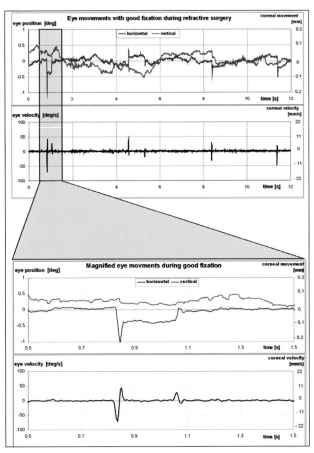

Figure 11-4. Typical saccadic eye movements during a refractive surgery procedure while fixating on a single target. Horizontal and vertical eye movements are sampled with 250 Hz temporal resolution. The first diagram shows a sequence of 5 seconds of horizontal and vertical eye movement: left ordinate in degrees of eye rotation, right ordinate in terms of corneal movement (mm). The second diagram shows the resultant eye movement velocity in rotational velocities (deg/s) and corresponding corneal movement velocity derived from the trajectory of both eye movement components. The lower pair of the diagram shows eye position and eye movement velocities within a magnified section of 1 second between 3 and 4 seconds.

Figure 11-5. Eye movements within a period of 12 seconds of good fixation during a refractive surgery procedure while fixating on a single target. Horizontal and vertical eye movements are sampled with 250 Hz temporal resolution. The first diagram shows a sequence of 12 seconds of horizontal and vertical eye movements and the diagram below shows the resultant eye movement velocity. The lower pair of diagrams shows eye position and eye movement velocities within a magnified section of 1 second between 0.5 and 1.5 seconds.

3. Optokinetic movements are reduced by fixations and by eliminating moving targets within the visual field, but movements such as the surgeon perceived by the patient within the highly motion-sensitive peripheral vision may occur and stimulate nystagmus.

4. Vergence movements are controlled by viewing a target at a fixed distance, but movements may occur due to temporary changes of the dominant viewing eye looking at the target, especially since the visual performance of the operated eye is changing during the procedure.

The surgeon may also introduce movements while trying to correct the patient's drifting eye movements. In addition, the mental state of the patient together with auditory cues of the laser during the procedure create distractions from the fixation task.

All of this results in a significant amount of fast saccadic and slower eye movements during surgery, as shown in Figure 11-4. Eye movement velocities of up to 100 deg/s, corresponding to a corneal movement of approximately 21 mm/s, can be clearly observed. Even during good fixation, as shown in

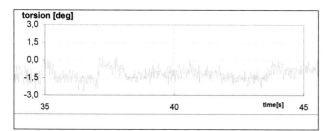

Figure 11-6. Torsional eye movements sampled at 50 Hz relative to the subject head while the subject is lying horizontally, facing the ceiling, and fixating on a single target in a 30-cm distance. Note the torsional shift of eye position relative to the head of -1 degree relative to the reference position for ocular torsion relative to the head before the measurement in head erect position.

Eye movement velocities of up to 100 deg/s, corresponding to a corneal movement of approximately 21 mm/s, can be clearly observed.

Figure 11-5, small square wave jerks occur with eye movement velocity up to 50 deg/s and a corresponding corneal movement velocity of 10 mm/s.

Torsional eye movements do not show such dynamic changes, as their amplitudes are limited at least in the controlled configuration with less dynamic movements of the head during the surgery procedure. Typical torsional eye movements while viewing a frontal target in the horizontal head position (similar to during a laser procedure) are shown in Figure 11-6. However, a possible torsional eye position change may occur between the diagnostic measurements of the eye (commonly performed with the head upright) and the laser surgery procedure (commonly performed in horizontal head position). This type of eye movement can easily amount to 1 degree or even more.

Furthermore, vertical and horizontal eye movements are associated with torsional eye movements as previously described, and the eye is viewed from the laser system as projection. Both effects, even within a restricted area of eye movement (±10 degrees or ±2 mm of corneal movements), may result in torsional differences of ± 2 degrees.

Knowing the type of eye movements to take into account, the question is what are the necessary requirements—sampling rate and delay—for measuring them in the context of refractive surgery? For this purpose we look at the power spectral density[14] of eye movements (Figure 11-7) already converted

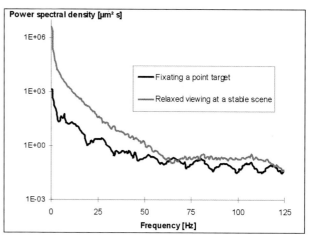

Figure 11-7. Power spectral density of 60-second recordings of horizontal eye movements fixating on a point target (black) and observing a fixed scene image similar to the scene during refractive surgery (gray) (sampling frequency 250 Hz, binwidth 0.49 Hz, 256 bins using Parzen windowing). Standard deviation of horizontal eye movement was 66 µm during fixation and 2.7 mm viewing the visual scene.

into movement of the cornea while a subject fixates for 60 seconds either on a single target or viewing relaxed at a fixed picture similar to the scene observed during surgery—the extreme situations for eye movements during refractive surgery. (Note: the power spectral density quantifies the size and amount of eye movements within a certain frequency range, calculated via a transformation from time to frequency domain of the recorded eye position data. The unit of the power spectral density is, in our case, microns[2] per second or microns[2] per Hertz, thus giving a measure for the uncertainty (hence variance) of the eye position related to a given frequency range.)

Figure 11-7 shows that if fixation cannot be performed accurately, then the main energy of eye movements is found below 60 Hz. The above power spectrum also demonstrates that for being able to perform accurate reconstruction and analysis of eye movements and avoid aliasing,[3] sampling rates of 200 Hz and above (at least four to five times higher than the significant power spectrum bandwidth) should be used.

However, this is not necessarily the only critical requirement for the refractive surgery application. During refractive surgery, the eye is ablated only during a very short period of time (approximately 10 ns for a single laser shot). If the eye position is obtained immediately preceding the laser shot, any

Eye movements need to be sampled at the same frequency as the laser Hertz rate but synchronous to the specific laser shot with a minimum of delay between measurement of eye position and laser treatment.

further movements of the eye during this shot may be neglected. For example, if it is assumed that the laser shot occurs during a saccade of 500 deg/sec—corresponding to a movement of the cornea of approximately 100 mm/s—the movement during this ablation pulse would be below 1 nm.

The dynamics of eye movements described above and current laser repetition rates from less than 50 to 200 Hz mainly result in the requirement that eye movements need to be sampled at the same frequency as the laser but synchronous to the specific laser shot with a minimum of delay between the measurement of the eye position and the corresponding laser shot.

PRINCIPLES OF LASER SURGERY AND THE NEED TO MAINTAIN ALIGNMENT

Laser refractive surgery has become widespread since the first procedure was preformed on a sighted patient in 1990. During this time, laser refractive techniques and technology have improved considerably. The first generation of laser systems used large beam or broad spot lasers with an effective laser spot size on the cornea of about 2 mm in diameter (not to be confused with the treatment zone of approximately 6 mm in diameter in these lasers). These systems could correct spherical error (myopia and hyperopia) but were limited in their ability to correct astigmatism and irregular topography. As a result of their limitations, while reducing the spherical or cylindrical error of the patient, these older laser systems introduced higher-order aberrations into the patient's optical path.[14,15] For example, decentration of the ablation zone reduces night time vision and contrast sensitivity, and increases higher-order aberrations.[16,17] Figure 11-8 illustrates the effect of a decentered ablation zone. Light passes through both the corrected and uncorrected sections of the cornea and focuses at different points on the retina, resulting in coma. (Note: aliasing is the effect of measuring power components of higher frequency components in lower frequencies. This occurs due to the limitation of measurement frequencies. In order to avoid

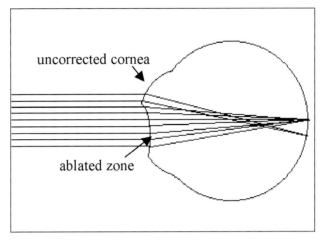

Figure 11-8. Rays from infinity entering an unaccommodated eye with a decentered ablation.

aliasing, all significant power spectrum components of the signal (eye position data) should be at frequencies significantly below the measurement frequency.)

Why Small Spot Scanning and CustomCornea Requires Even Better Alignment

Second- and third-generation refractive laser systems are based on low energy lasers with spot sizes below 1 mm. These "small spot" lasers "fly" over the cornea, guided by scanning mirror systems. The curvature of the optical correction is formed by a constant repositioning of the beam on the cornea. Small spot size and a flexible scanning system allow sophisticated higher-order aberration treatments like lower astigmatism (< 0.5 diopter [D]) correction that is customized to the specific cornea of the patient.

As lasers move to smaller spot sizes the sensitivity to error in the positioning of the laser increases, as shown in Figure 11-9. An error in position of 0.1 mm, for example, means for a 2-mm broadbeam spot profile, approximately 10% of the energy of a single shot was applied to the wrong area, whereas for a Gaussian small spot with standard deviation of 0.4 mm, the same error means approximately 20% in mislead energy.

In addition to the planar position requirements, more focused laser beams with smaller effective spot sizes also require a precise distance control of the target surface, as their focal depth is getting ever shorter. This adds another dimension—distance control of the eye to the laser head—to be monitored and controlled. Thus, to achieve a predictable result in more

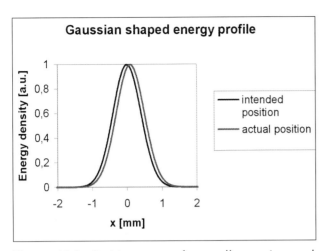

Figure 11-9. Position errors for small gaussian and broad constant energy profile. Two-dimensional representation and calculation for both profiles. Gaussian profile with standard deviation of 0.4 mm; constant profile with 2-mm width. Error calculation in two dimensions for 0.1-mm lateral offset of beam.

demanding procedures, a real-time alignment of the laser with the reference coordinate system of the eye is key.

Methods of Maintaining Alignment

There are several methods used to maintain alignment between the patient's eye and the laser beam. They range from completely subjective to fully automated measurement and control systems.

Passive Fixation

The simplest method of alignment requires the patient to fixate on an alignment light controlled only by the surgeon through either the microscope or an independent video monitor. This method is completely noninvasive and gives all control to the surgeon. It is, however, completely subjective and is not capable of eliminating involuntary eye movements or controlling them. A major systematic risk with this method is that the patient may change the leading eye used for fixation during the process, thus creating a significant offset. The surgeon minimizes decentration by suspending and recentering when large movements cause noticeable decentration.

Suction Rings

Alignment may be improved by a suction ring fixed onto the cornea and held in place by the clinician. Suction rings are effective in taking out a significant portion of the high frequency end of the eye

movement spectrum during surgery just by virtue of the additional mass fixed to the eyeball and the additional holding force of the surgeon. However, suction rings may be decentered, lose suction during the procedure, distort the cornea, and interfere with airflow around the cornea.[18]

To overcome these problems, suction rings can be combined with eye tracking techniques to provide additional objective measurement and control of the remainder of eye movements.

Eye Tracking

The third technique—eye tracking—may be harder to implement but has the advantages of being nonintrusive and, depending on the implementation, completely independent of subjective influences by the patient and doctor. For eye tracking, a sensing device such as a camera or photodiode (or a combination) acquires an image of the patient's eye. A processing subsystem calculates the position of the eye (usually defined as the center of the pupil or the center of the limbus) from that image, and a control system moves the laser beam to compensate for any change in eye position, thereby maintaining alignment. The disadvantages of eye tracking include the necessity of a specific illumination system (eg, infrared diodes or lasers) and the sensitivity to changes in pupil size, corneal surface, and illumination characteristics during the course of the treatment. In some cases, eye tracking systems "lose tracking" due to these complexities, thus relying solely on patient fixation during parts of the treatment. With improved sensor and processing technology, more robust systems are being developed that are capable of dealing with all patients throughout the whole treatment.

EYE TRACKING FOR LASER REFRACTIVE SURGERY

Eye tracking has been used in a variety of applications, but the requirements for laser refractive surgery are quite particular. The eye tracker must be fast, reliable, nonintrusive, work on all iris colors, and be insensitive to alignment lights and to removal of tissue from the cornea. The main techniques applied in refractive surgery are photoelectric and video-based eye tracking. Electro-oculography (EOG), briefly described below, is not useful for refractive surgery.

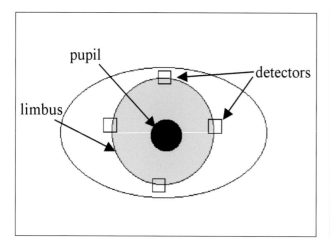

Figure 11-10. Detector array for limbus tracking used in IRVision AccuScan 2000 (Columbus, Ohio).

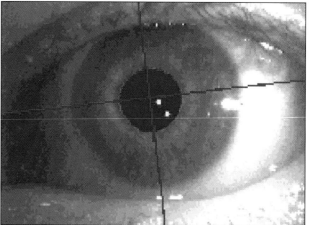

Figure 11-11. Tracked eye with dark pupil tracker for x,y coordinates and ocular torsion using SensoMotoric Instruments´ 3D VOG system (Berlin, Germany).

Electro-Oculography

EOG is one of the oldest and most common techniques for measuring eye movements in research and clinical environments and for measuring impedance changes using electrodes mounted around the eye on the skin. The advantage of EOG is its processing speed with high frequencies (> 1 kHz) and extremely short delay times (< 1 ms) from signal acquisition to data availability. However, this technique does not allow an accurate absolute measurement of the eye position due to the large drift of the corneal-retinal potential. Furthermore, it provides only a measurement of the eye position relative to the head, and a further head movement measurement would be needed to apply this technique in refractive surgery. Muscle artifacts from the eyelid also influence the eye position, and a resolution of better than 2 degrees can only seldom be obtained.

Photoelectric Techniques

Photoelectric techniques detect eye movement from changes in reflected light. Either focused spots, slits, or rings of light are projected onto the cornea and the response from multiple light detectors is analyzed using analog signal processing techniques. Figure 11-10 shows the configuration of one such tracker detector array.[19] Either the pupil/iris border or the limbus is monitored. If the pupil is tracked, it is generally backlit to maximize contrast and dilated to minimize interference from the procedure itself.[20] The limbus does not suffer these limitations, as it is located further away from the surgical zone. This technique may be sensitive to iris colorization, can-

not measure torsion, and can "lose track" during large head movements. However, because analog methods are used, the frequency response is high (4 kHz).

Video Eye Tracking

In video eye tracking, infrared (IR) light illuminates the eye and IR-sensitive cameras acquire the eye image. If the axis of the illumination and camera differ significantly, the pupil is a sink for IR light and appears dark on the image. (If the IR illumination and camera are close to or on the same optical axis, the IR light is reflected by the retina and the pupil appears light on the image.) The dark pupil approach is more commonly used in refractive surgery, since it is more robust in illumination set-up. Figure 11-11 shows a typical dark pupil tracking situation with crosshair overlay for pupil centering and tilt of crosshair for torsion of the eye around the visual axis.

With more powerful imaging sensors and processing units and more sophisticated algorithms for determining the pupil center and the limbus, video eye tracking is becoming increasingly robust and insensitive to a broad range of disturbances, changes in illumination, and image quality during refractive surgery. Figure 11-12 shows an example of a partly occluded eye in which the pupil is still detected.

Critical Issue for Laser Control: Delay in Determining Eye Position and the Laser Shot

All eye movement measurement techniques for laser refractive surgery have a critical side effect that

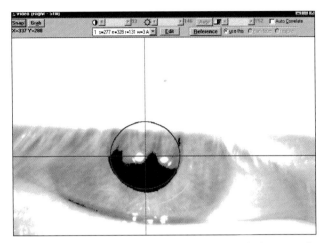

Figure 11-12. Detection of a partly occluded eye with image processing using SensoMotoric Instruments´ 3D VOG system.

is often underestimated. A processing delay is introduced when the eye position is obtained, which leads to delayed control of the mirror system that compensates for the eye movement. Furthermore, the positioning of the scanning mirrors to correct the eye movement introduces another delay until the "corrected" stable position is obtained. During these delays, the eye can continue to move significantly from the original detected eye position, resulting in an inaccurately positioned ablation.

Different eye tracking techniques have different problems in generating a correct fast measurement:

- The laser scanning eye tracking method like Summit/Autonomous' LADARVision needs to scan the eye to find several contrast boundaries of the pupil and/or iris to allow for robust and accurate eye tracking. Only after several boundaries are identified, an accurate center of the eye can be calculated. Servo loop response is also a consideration, with response times of some systems ranging from 0.04 seconds for small corrections to up to 10 ms for large corrections (to 3 mm).[19]

- Video-based techniques require an image of the eye to first be integrated on the image sensor. Using standard video cameras, this process alone requires 16.67 ms (NTSC)[12] or 20 ms (PAL). Once the image is acquired, the image information needs to be transferred (by means of a video signal or digital data signal) from the camera to an image processing unit, which digitizes and processes incoming information. The transfer of the image requires another 16.67 ms (NTSC) or 20 ms (PAL). Even if the image is processed during this transfer, the eye position can only be provided with a delay of 32 ms (NTSC) or 40 ms (PAL) to

NTSC and PAL are video standards used in the United States and Japan (NTSC) as well as in most European countries (PAL) using 60 Hz (NTSC) and 50 Hz (PAL) image refresh frequencies.

control the mirror system. During the delay time, the eye continues to move and, depending on the current velocity of the eye, a significant tracking error—or positioning error of the laser onto the eye, occurs (Figure 11-13).

In order to quantify the tracking error introduced by the processing delay, the following time series analysis was performed: A sequence of 60 seconds of eye movements were recorded during simulated surgery conditions with a high speed eye tracking system at a 250 Hz sampling rate (4 ms sampling interval). The sampling frequency of 250 Hz allows accurate reconstruction of all eye movement components, as previously shown. These recorded eye movements were used as "simulated real-time" eye position information in the subsequent simulation analysis.

In order to simulate the delay of 32 ms of a typical NTSC system or a delay of 8 ms of a custom high-speed system, the "simulated real-time" data sets were shifted by the amount of processing delay. Then, the difference between the "simulated real-time" and processing delayed data set was calculated for each 4 ms sampling interval, resulting in a simulated position error signal. A histogram analysis was performed for both 32 ms and 8 ms delay tracking errors over the full eye movement recording.

Figure 11-14 shows the accumulated frequency of positioning errors of the laser during the "simulated ablation" introduced by the 32 ms delay of a standard video system and 8 ms delay of a high speed system.

According to this analysis, a standard NTSC-based eye tracking system (32 ms processing delay) would position 5% of all laser shots with an error larger than 70 μm and 2% of all laser shots will have an error of larger than 400 μm.

With shortened processing delay of 8 ms, the frequency of laser shots with a positioning error larger than 400 μm can be reduced by 90% down to 0.2% of all laser shots.

With shortened processing delay of 8 ms, the frequency of laser shots with a positioning error larger than 400 μm can be reduced by 90% down to 0.2% of all laser shots.

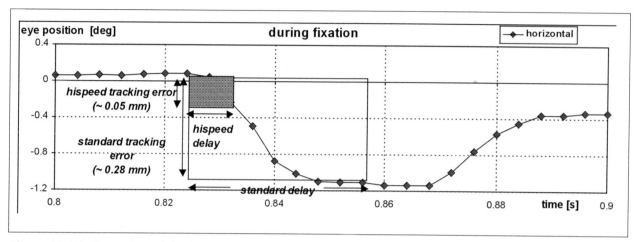

Figure 11-13. Illustration of the laser positioning error due to the processing delay for obtaining the eye position.

SUMMARY AND FUTURE WORK

During the refractive laser surgery procedure, a significant amount of slow and fast eye and head movements occur that need to be compensated for by an accurate eye tracking system to stabilize the laser at the planned ablation position. The sampling rate of the required eye tracking system is primarily determined by the repetition rate of the laser and should provide synchronous measurements with minimum processing delay. The processing delay creates a laser positioning error on the cornea, and this amount is determined by the speed of the current movement and the delay time of the eye tracking and laser positioning systems. In this context the often discussed "high speed" requirement should be interpreted as "high speed processing" or rather "short processing delay" to reduce the total processing delay. The errors for laser positioning with different processing show that processing delays under 8 ms should be achieved. One currently available video-based system may be able to measure eye movements with 6 ms processing delay.

Sophisticated future eye tracking technologies will consider several criteria in parallel to determine the pupil position, such as the pupil, limbus, and iris structures. Technologies for increasing the speed of video-based technology up to 250 Hz full frame are available, and current developments are targeting high resolution and high-speed processing up to 500 Hz full frame, with processing delays under 6 ms.

Although misalignment in laser refractive surgery is primarily caused by horizontal and vertical eye movements during the procedure, a torsional tilt of the visual axis may also occur between the alignment

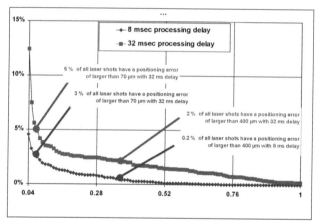

Figure 11-14. Accumulated frequency histogram showing the relative frequency of laser shots (vertical axis) having a laser positioning error shown on the horizontal axis.

axis of the diagnostic topography and aberrometry measurements and the subsequent laser treatment. This torsional tilt is caused by the different head orientations and the vestibular ocular reflex (ocular counter-rolling). For accurate customized ablation in the future, especially for astigmatism and higher-order aberrations, a torsional eye position measurement should be integrated. Furthermore, a common coordinate reference system linked to the eye should be provided and used in the different diagnostic and treatment machines and over all process steps from diagnostics over treatment to postoperative measurement. This is necessary to eliminate offsets between these steps and machines that cannot even be accurately compensated for by the surgeon.

With higher accuracy requirements for customized ablations, accurate centration becomes more critical. Up to now, the centration during the procedure was based on the center of the determined pupil area with an optional manually adjustable offset to this position to compensate for the shift of the visual axis. However, pupil size changes are not symmetrical to the center of the pupil nor to the center of the visual axis, which creates a shift of the treatment center. To ensure that the alignment axis during laser refractive surgery is consistent throughout the procedure and with the axis used during diagnosis, a landmark independent of pupil dilation should be used. Tracking algorithms is therefore required to provide independent eye tracking using the iris, sclera border, or artificial marks.

In the future, faster sensor technology and more powerful and robust processing should allow target acquisition systems to measure and control more parameters (x, y coordinates, z distance to laser, φ-rotation around the visual axis, and d pupil diameter) with higher frequency and lower delay time. This will be a necessary basis for high-precision laser vision correction with high reliability.

ACKNOWLEDGMENTS

We would like to acknowledge the cooperative work of our clients, especially within the eye movement research field, who made this work possible, as well as all our colleagues at SensoMotoric Instruments.

REFERENCES

1. Donders FC. Beitrag zur Lehre von Bewegungen des menschlichen Auges, Holländische Beiträge zu den anatomischen und psychologischen Wissenschafte. 1847;1,101-145, 384-386.

2. Listing JB. *Beitrag zu Physiologischen Optik.* Göttingen, Germany: Vandenhoeck & Ruprecht; 1845.

3. Bahill AT, Clark MR, Stark L. Glissades-eye movements generated by mismatched components of the saccadic motoneuronal control signal. *Mathematical Biosciences.* 1975;26:303-318.

4. Young LR, Meiry JL. A revised dynamic otolith model. *Aerospace Medicine.* 1968;39(6).

5. Miller EF. Counter-rolling of the human eyes produced by head tilt with respect to gravity. *Acta Otolaryngol.* 1962;54:479-501.

6. Honrubia V, Scott BJ, Ward PH. Experimental studies on optokinetic nystagmus. I. Normal cats. *Acta Oto-Laryngol.* 1967;65L:441-448.

7. Müller J. *Zur Vergleichenden Physiologie des Gesichtssinnes.* Leipzig, Germany: C Cnobloch; 1826.

8. von Helmholtz H. Handbuch der Physiologischen Optik. 3rd ed. Hamburg, Germany: Voss; 1867. Translated by J. P. C. Southall for the Optical Society of America (1924).

9. Findlay JM. Frequency analysis of human involuntary eye movement. *Kybernetik.* 1971;8:207-214.

10. Ditchburn RW. The functions of small saccades. *Vision Res.* 1980;20:271-272.

11. Yarbus AL. *Eye Movements and Vision.* New York, NY: Plenum; 1967.

12. Ditchburn RW. *Eye Movements and Visual Perception.* Oxford, England: Clarendon Press; 1973.

13. Feldon SE, Laneston JW. Square wave jerks: a disorder of microsaccades? *Neurology.* 1977;27:278-281.

14. Applegate RA, Howland HC. Refractive surgery, optical aberrations, and visual performance. *J Refract Surg.* 1997;13:295-299. Erratum in *J Refract Surg.* 1997;13(6):490.

15. Martinez CE, Applegate RA, Klyce SD, et al. Effect of pupillary dilation on corneal optical aberrations after photorefractive keratectomy. *Arch Ophthalmol.* 1998;116:1053-1062.

16. Maloney RK. Corneal topography and optical zone location in photorefractive keratectomy. *Refract Corneal Surg.* 1990;6:363-371.

17. Uozato H, Guyton DL. Centering corneal surgical procedures. *Am J Ophthalmol.* 1987;103:264-267.

18. Hall RW. Image processing algorithms for eye movement monitoring. *Computers and Biomedical Research.* 1983;16:563-579.

19. Telfair WB, Yoder PR, Bekker C, Hoffman HJ, Jensen EF. Scanning mid-IR laser apparatus with eye tracking for refractive surgery. Proceedings of the International Society for Optical Engineering. 1999;3591:220-228.

20. Pallikaris I, McDonald MB, Siganos D, et al. Tracker-assisted photorefractive keratectomy for myopia of -1 to -6 diopters. *J Refract Surg.* 1996;11:240-247.

BIBLIOGRAPHY

Aktunc R, Aktunc T. Centration of excimer laser photorefractive keratectomy and changes in astigmatism. *J Refract Surg.* 1996;12:S268-S271.

Buquet C, Charlier JR, Paris V. Museum application of an eye tracker. *Medical & Biological Engineering & Computing.* 1988;26:277-281.

Charlier JR, Hache J. New instrument for monitoring eye fixation and pupil size during the visual field examination. *Medical & Biological Engineering & Computing.* 1982;20:23-28.

Ebisawa Y, Amano M. Examination of eye detection technique using two light sources and the image difference method. Proceedings of the Society of Instrument and Control Engineers 33rd Annual Conference, Tokyo. 1994;985-990.

Gonzalez RC, Wintz P. *Digital Image Processing.* 2nd ed. Boston, Mass: Addison-Wesley Publishing Company; 1987.

Groen E, Bos JE, Nacken PF, de Graaf B. Determination of ocular torsion by means of automatic pattern recognition. *IEEE Transactions on Biomedical Engineering.* 1996;43:471-479.

Hatamian M, Anderson DJ. Design considerations for a real-time ocular counterroll instrument. *IEEE Transactions on Biomedical Engineering.* 1983;30:278-288.

Hutchinson TE, White KP, Martin NW, Reichert KC, Frey LA. Human-computer interaction using eye gaze input. *IEEE Transactions on Systems, Man, and Cybernetics.* 1989;19:1527-1534.

IEEE Service Center. Video eye tracking system based on a statistical algorithm. Piscataway, NJ: Author; 1993;1:438.

Kabuka M, Desoto J, Miranda J. Robot vision tracking system. *IEEE Transactions on Industrial Electronics.* 1988;35:40-51.

Kostrzewski A, Vasiliev AA, Kim DH, Savant GD. High-resolution ultra-fast eye tracking system. *SPIE.* 1907;3173:249-261.

Lam KM, Yan H. Locating and extracting the eye in human face images. *Pattern Recognition.* 1996;29:771-779.

Mulligan J. Image processing for improved eye tracking accuracy. *Behaviour Research Methods & Instrumentation.* 1997;29:54-65.

Murray RB, Loughnane MH. Infrared video pupillometry: a method used to measure the pupillary effects of drugs in small laboratory animals in real time. *Journal of Neuroscience Methods.* 1981;3:365-375.

Myers GA, Sherman KR, Stark L. Microcomputer-based instrument uses an internal model to track the eye. *Computer.* 1991;14-21.

Nixon M. Eye spacing measurement for facial recognition. *SPIE.* 1985;575:279-285.

Ober J, Hajda J, Loska J, Jamicki M. Application of eye movement measuring system OBER 2 to medicine and technology. *SPIE.* 1997;3061:327-336.

Razdan R, Kielar A. *Eye Tracking for Man/Machine Interfaces. Sensors (September).* Peterborough, NH: Helmers Publishing Inc; 1988.

Sliney D, Wolbarsht M. *Safety with Lasers and Other Optical Sources.* New York, NY: Plenum; 1980.

Tomono A, IIda M, Kobayashi Y. A TV camera system which extracts feature points for non-contact eye movement detection. *SPIE.* 1989;1194:2-12.

Xie X, Sudhakar R, Zhuang H. On improving eye feature extraction using deformable templates. *Pattern Recognition.* 1994;27:791-799.

Young LR, Sheena D. Survey of eye movement recording methods. *Behaviour Research Methods & Instrumentation.* 1975;7:397-429.

Wavefront-Guided Custom Ablation

CLINICAL SCIENCE SECTION

Overview of Wavefront Measurement Devices

Ronald R. Krueger, MD

This section of the book turns from reviewing the basic science issues of wavefront-guided custom ablation to practical applications of this technology in measuring and correcting ocular aberrations. The chapters that follow in this section are industry specific, as they deal with the commercial products developed or acquired by most of the major ophthalmic companies that are involved in refractive surgery. The commercial products include wavefront measurement devices that comprise a chapter for each device available in the field. Each chapter covers the principles by which a device operates, as well as the early clinical experience in using the device to measure and correct ocular aberrations. The chapters are not random in their order of presentation but rather follow a categorical structure, which defines the optical principles used to capture and define the ocular wavefront. For the sake of simplicity, the categories have been limited to three, which are represented by the three following subsections:

Outgoing Optics Aberrometry

The main differentiating feature of outgoing optics aberrometry is that the wavefront error pattern is defined by the slope of the rays **exiting** the eye, hence the word "outgoing." This form of wavefront sensing is uniquely characterized and described by the principles of Shack-Hartmann.

To best understand these principles in more detail, let us begin by reviewing the history of this form of wavefront sensing. Its earliest application was in the early 1900s when Hartmann first described these principles, which were later used in the form of a Hartmann screen in optical metrology.[1,2] In the early 1970s, Shack modified the Hartmann technique,[3] which was then used extensively by astronomers for measuring the optical aberrations of the atmosphere with telescopes. More recently, in 1994, Liang used these principles to measure refractive errors and higher-order aberrations of the eye.[4]

The principles of operation of the Shack-Hartmann wavefront sensor is based on the reflection of a narrow (approximately 1 mm) laser beam, which is focused onto the fovea by the eye's optical system. The reflected light then exits the eye to define the wavefront aberration pattern captured at the level of the entrance pupil by a CCD camera. The wavefront pattern is defined by a micro lenslet array that partitions the reflected wavefront of light emerging from the eye into

> The wavefront pattern is defined by a micro lenslet array that partitions the reflected wavefront of light emerging from the eye into a larger number of smaller wavefronts, each of which is focused into a small spot.

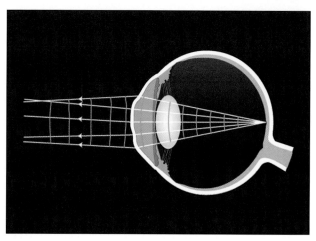

Figure I. Principles of "outgoing optics aberrometry" (Shack-Hartmann). Rays of light exit the eye and are deviated to define the wavefront aberration pattern (photo courtesy of D. Huang).

a larger number of smaller wavefronts, each of which is focused into a small spot. The spatial displacement of the spot, relative to the optical axis of the corresponding lenslet, directly measures the local slope of the incident wavefront and hence the shape of the wavefront profile.

These simple principles of "outgoing optics" aberrometry are shown in Figure I, which demonstrates the outgoing direction of the rays of light and how their angle of deviation and slope can be used to define a wavefront aberration pattern.

The commercial systems described in the chapters that follow include the Alcon Summit Autonomous CustomCornea measurement device (Chapter Twelve) and the VisX 20/10 Perfect Vision wavefront analyzer (Chapter Thirteen). In addition to these two chapters, a third and fourth could be included discussing the Bausch & Lomb Zyoptics system and Aesculap Meditec WOSCA; however, for the sake of brevity and timing, these are not included in this text. Additionally, in the future, other excimer laser providers and ophthalmic companies will likely provide this type of wavefront sensor. LaserSight, which currently uses topographic techniques and is designing a prolate ablation pattern, plans to implement Shack-Hartmann-style wavefront sensing as well (personal communication, Mike Farris, May 2000).

References

1. Hartmann J. Bemerkungen uber den bau und die jurstirung von spektrographer. *Zeitschrift fuer Instrumenterkinde*. 1900;20:47.
2. Hartmann J. Objektuventersuchungen. *Zeitschrift fuer Instrumenterkinde*. 1904;24:1.
3. Shack RV, Platt BC. Production and use of a lenticular Hartmann screen. *J Opt Soc Am A*. 1971;61:656.
4. Liang J, Grimm W, Goelz S, Bille JF. Objective measurement of the wave aberrations of the human eye using Hartmann-Shack wavefront sensor. *J Opt Soc Am A*. 1994;11(7):1949-57.

Chapter Twelve

CustomCornea Using the LADARVision System

George H. Pettit, MD, PhD
John A. Campin, BSc

INTRODUCTION

Autonomous Technologies has defined the term CustomCornea to refer to wavefront-guided refractive laser surgery. The Autonomous LADARVision system combines "flying spot" excimer laser technology, high-speed eye tracking, and sophisticated software algorithms to reshape the corneal surface with high accuracy.[1] This treatment device is well suited to the task of correcting both low- and higher-order visual aberrations. The goal of the CustomCornea program has been to develop the appropriate technology to provide the LADARVision system with patient wavefront data so that optimal vision correction can be achieved.

As discussed elsewhere in this book, wavefront sensing can be accomplished in several different ways.[2-4] The method used by the CustomCornea Measurement Device (CCMD) is shown in Figure 12-1. A narrow laser beam is directed into the eye to illuminate a small spot on the fovea. Light scattered from that spot exits the eye in the form of re-emitted wavefronts. For a perfectly emmetropic eye, each re-emitted wavefront will take the shape of a perfect plane wave. Optical aberrations in a real eye will distort the re-emitted wavefront from the ideal plane wave. Removing these distortions from the wavefront is the task of refractive laser surgery.

In our opinion, this measurement approach has three key advantages. First, the total aberration profile of the eye is obtained in a single pulsed measurement. Second, no assumptions are required regarding the eye's physical dimensions or optical properties—the re-emitted wavefront tells the whole story. Third, the optical design of the apparatus can be made to provide high accuracy and a large instantaneous dynamic range so that minimal adjustment is required to examine each patient.

A number of steps must be accomplished in order to carry out the customized refractive surgery. The patient must be positioned properly for the wavefront examination at the CCMD, and this orientation must be recorded for later reference in the surgical treatment. The patient's pupil must be large and the lens as relaxed as possible to obtain valid wavefront data over a large corneal region. Once the wavefront data were obtained, they must be analyzed to remove spurious signals and to confirm that the wavefront is appropriate for this particular patient. After a valid wavefront exam is performed, the wavefront and eye orientation data must be transferred to the LADARVision system. The treatment device must then calculate the appropriate excimer laser treatment profile to correct the aberrations detected in the wavefront exam. Finally, this ablation profile must be accurately delivered to the right location on the corneal surface. Each of these steps is considered in the following sections.

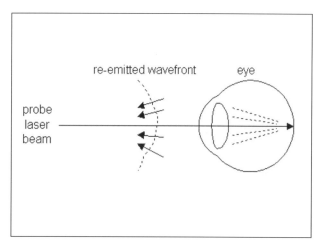

Figure 12-1. Essentials of the wavefront measurement approach used by the CustomCornea Measurement Device (CCMD). A small-diameter incident laser beam illuminates a small retinal area. Light scattered from the retina exits the eye as a series of re-emitted wavefronts. Each wavefront is distorted from the planar ideal shape by the aberrations present in the eye. In this example, the general myopic error of the eye produces a curved wavefront propagating to the left of the figure. The complex curvature of the myopic wavefront is due to additional higher-order aberrations in the eye.

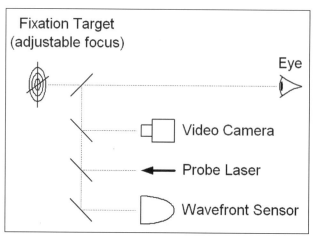

Figure 12-2. Principal optical pathways of the CCMD. One path allows the patient to fixate on a simple target, which is properly "fogged" to inhibit accommodation. A second path provides the system operator a video image of the eye at the examination plane for alignment purposes. A third optical pathway directs the probe laser beam into the eye. The final path conveys the re-emitted wavefronts to the entrance face of the wavefront sensor.

WAVEFRONT EXAMINATION

Patient Alignment

The basic optical layout of the CCMD is shown in Figure 12-2. The patient seated before the device looks into the instrument at a fixation target, which is mounted as part of an adjustable focus mechanism to correct for the patient's defocus error. At the same time, a video camera path monitors the position of the eye at the examination plane. When the patient is properly aligned, the probe laser is fired and the wavefront that is re-emitted from the eye is conveyed to the wavefront sensor. All four optical paths within the CCMD are bore-sight aligned to each other.

Clearly the patient must also be properly aligned to this assembly. The eye's line of sight is the chosen reference axis.[5] This is the line from the center of the natural entrance pupil to the point of fixation. If the patient is properly fixating on the target, then centering the natural pupil in the CCMD image will ensure proper alignment. However, at the time of wavefront measurement it is desirable to have the largest diameter pupil possible, and the center of the natural (daytime) pupil often does not coincide with the dilated pupil center.

This problem is addressed as follows. Before wavefront examination, the patient sits at the CCMD and views the fixation target. A still video image is obtained of the eye, with the pupil in the natural (daytime illumination) state. This video snapshot is displayed on the CCMD graphical user interface, as shown in Figure 12-3. Onscreen circular reticles are aligned to the natural pupil boundary and to the limbus. This information is then saved in memory. Later, when the patient returns for the actual examination with the pupil dilated by pharmacological means or dark adaptation, the CCMD software redisplays the limbal reticle in the live video display of the eye. The software displays this reticle at an appropriate offset location; positioning the limbus at the indicated position will place the natural pupil center in the middle of the field of view. This will align the patient's line of sight to the instrument's optical axis.

Eye Dilation

At the present time we are dilating each eye pharmacologically for wavefront examination. This method is chosen for two reasons. First, the LADARVision treatment is performed immediately after the wavefront exam. The eye tracking system in

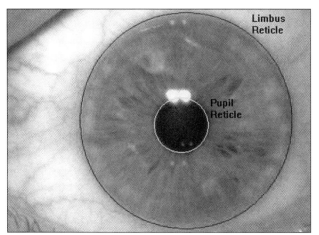

Figure 12-3. Video image of an eye during the "centration" step. Prior to eye dilation, the patient views the fixation target and a video snapshot of the eye is taken. Onscreen reticles aligned by the operator to the pupil and limbal margins tell the CCMD software the anatomical location of the natural pupil center with respect to the limbus.

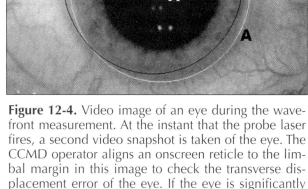

Figure 12-4. Video image of an eye during the wavefront measurement. At the instant that the probe laser fires, a second video snapshot is taken of the eye. The CCMD operator aligns an onscreen reticle to the limbal margin in this image to check the transverse displacement error of the eye. If the eye is significantly displaced from the desired location for proper alignment, then the wavefront data are rejected and the measurement repeated.

the treatment device utilizes the pupil margin as the anatomical reference and therefore requires a stable pupil boundary. Second, dilating agents such as 1% tropicamide have a marked cycloplegic effect. This helps in minimizing patient accommodation during the wavefront exam.

Wavefront Measurement

Preparing the patient for the actual wavefront exam takes only a moment. The patient again views the fixation target, which is now "fogged" or positioned optically just beyond the patient's most relaxed focal point. This further inhibits accommodation. The live video image is used to align the eye at the examination plane. Immediately prior to firing the probe laser beam, the clinician operator asks the patient to blink several times. An intact tear film is crucial to obtain an accurate wavefront image.

Once the operator fires the probe laser, the video image of the eye is frozen, as shown in Figure 12-4. At this point, the operator repositions the limbus reticle to identify the actual eye location at the time of measurement (labeled "A" in the figure). The CCMD software checks the displacement between the desired limbal location (labeled "B" in the figure)

and the actual location. This corresponds to the displacement of the natural pupil center (labeled "A'B'" in the figure). The measurement is rejected if this displacement is excessive. On surgery day, the operator also aligns linear reticles to ink marks applied to the eye outside the limbus to identify the cyclotorsional orientation.

In our prototype, CCMD design the probe laser produces an eye-safe < 10 µW, 670 nm pulse. These beam characteristics were chosen to produce satisfactory return signals at the wavefront sensor and still be acceptable to the patient. The patient perceives the pulse as a bright red flash originating at or near the center of the fixation target. Wavefronts re-emitted from the eye are conveyed by optics within the CCMD to the entrance face of the wavefront sensor. The sensor samples the local slope of each wavefront at 100 or more transverse locations. (The exact number is dependent on the pupil diameter.)

> Wavefronts re-emitted from the eye are conveyed by optics within the CCMD to the entrance face of the wavefront sensor. The sensor samples the local slope of each wavefront at 100 or more transverse locations. (The exact number is dependent on the pupil diameter.)

Wavefront Analysis

The CCMD software reconstructs the wavefront from the measured sensor slope data. Currently, we have chosen to represent the wavefront using fourth-order Zernike polynomials. This choice is conservative, given the large number of sample points. The 14 terms in the fourth-order Zernike expansion are sufficient to describe higher-order aberrations such as spherical aberration and coma, as well as conventional low-order aberrations (eg, defocus and astigmatism). Limiting the reconstruction to fourth order minimizes the error due to noise on the individual slope measurements. In the future we may add additional terms to our wavefront description.

We have conducted numerous tests to determine the wavefront measurement accuracy of the CCMD unit. In many of these tests a reference lens assembly is placed in front of the device at the nominal patient eye location. The assembly contains a precision-manufactured commercial lens with well-characterized optical properties. A synthetic scattering surface is mounted behind the lens at a distance that can be varied using a translation micrometer. Changing this spacing will alter the aberration content of the re-emitted wavefront, most significantly the defocus term. Wavefront data is obtained as the spacing is varied over some range of interest (eg, the expected range of myopic/hyperopic defocus error to be encountered in a clinical trial). In all testing to date, utilizing various lens geometries and orientations with respect to the CCMD optical axis, the worst case error has been < 0.2 µm over an 8 mm circular test region. This is significantly smaller than the root mean square (RMS) errors we have measured for patients with exceptional uncorrected visual acuity (eg, 20/16 or better). We believe, therefore, that the CCMD has ample measurement accuracy to guide the customized refractive correction.

The CCMD software also uses the wavefront reconstruction to calculate the effective clinical prescription. This allows the wavefront measurement to be cross-checked against the conventional clinical exam prior to the customized laser surgery. The plot in Figure 12-5 shows a comparison of the CCMD-calculated spherical prescription to the spherical error determined by phoropter exam for 79 eyes enrolled in a diagnostic clinical trial of the wavefront sensing technology. The agreement between the two measurement techniques is excellent.

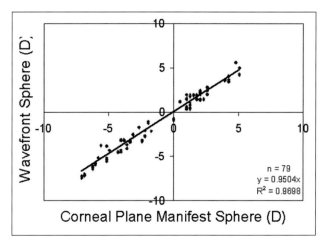

Figure 12-5. Comparison of spherical refractive error calculated from wavefront data (vertical axis) to the spherical error determined by phoropter exam (horizontal axis). The individual data points are for 79 patients prior to refractive laser surgery. The line in the figure indicates a least-square-error linear fit to the data. The fit has a linear slope close to one and an R^2 value of 0.97, indicating excellent agreement between these two clinical methods of determining defocus error.

LADARVISION TREATMENT

Wavefront Data Transfer

For patients undergoing conventional LADARVision surgery, all required patient information (ie, name, medical record number, etc) is to be entered by the operator into the LADARVision system. The alignment of reticles to the limbus and natural pupil is then performed on the LADARVision system prior to the pharmacological dilation of the pupil.

With CustomCornea procedures, all required patient and geometry information is entered or computed on the CCMD and then transferred electronically, along with the wavefront measurement information to the LADARVision system. These data transfer can be achieved via floppy disk or other electronic transfer means, such as over a local area network (LAN).

Treatment Profile Calculation

The data transferred to the LADARVision system contain all information necessary to fully define a

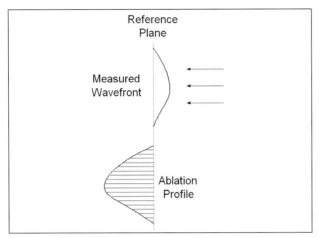

Figure 12-6. First-order approach in determining the appropriate ablation profile from the wavefront shape. The difference between the measured wavefront and the plane wave ideal is calculated at each point in the examination plane. This OPD profile is then multiplied by –1 and then divided by the refractive index difference between cornea and air. In actuality, additional factors must be included in determining the correct ablation profile (see text).

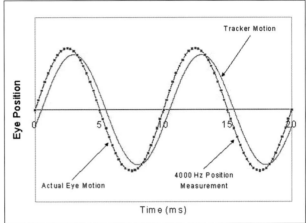

Figure 12-7. Active eye tracking characteristics of the LADARVision device. The system measures the location of the eye at the treatment plane 4000 times every second, as indicated by the light blue dots in the figure, or 40 times for each 100 Hz sinusoidal oscillation indicated by the dark blue curve in this example. The device then repositions internal mirrors to compensate for the detected motion, with a closed-loop bandwidth of 100 Hz. The red curve slightly lagging the true eye motion indicates the closed-loop compensation.

customized surgical procedure with the exception of the dimensions of the optical zone and blend zone. The optical zone is defined as the region over which the full refractive correction is applied while the blend zone is an annulus outside of this zone in which the ablation depth smoothly decreases to zero. Definition of these is performed in the LADARVision system prior to surgery and can be varied so as to optimize the optical zone size and ablation depth on a per-patient basis. In all CustomCornea clinical trials performed so far, the optical zone diameter has been 6.5 mm and a blend annulus of 1.25 mm has been used, resulting in a total ablation diameter of 9 mm.

A first-order algorithm for determining the ablation profile is shown in Figure 12-6. The desired wavefront is a perfect plane wave, as would be seen with an ideal emmetrope. The optical path difference (OPD) between the measured wavefront and this ideal is calculated at each transverse location in the corneal plane. Ablative treatment replaces corneal tissue in the wavefront path with air, which has a lower refractive index. Selective ablation at one site will "speed up" the wavefront in that region relative to surrounding areas that receive less treatment. The ablation profile is found by multiplying the OPD by minus one, then dividing by the difference in refractive indices between cornea and air.

It should be noted that additional factors (eg, corneal curvature, corneal biomechanics, etc) must be taken into account in optimizing the refractive correction. Details of these effects are proprietary. The approach shown in Figure 12-6 represents a good starting point in determining the correction needed. It is not the complete method we use in our treatments.

Active Eye Tracking

The LADARVision eye tracker detects and compensates for motion of the iris/pupil boundary. The tracker has a 4000 Hz sampling frequency and a closed loop bandwidth of 100 Hz. What these specifications mean in practical terms is shown in Figure 12-7. The dark blue trace indicates sinusoidal motion (ie, back and forth movement through some reasonable distance) of the eye 100 times each second. The lighter blue dots indicate position measurements by the LADARVision eye tracker. The device makes 40 such measurements during each eye motion cycle. The red trace indicates the active compensation of

The tracker has a 4000 Hz sampling frequency and a closed loop bandwidth of 100 Hz.

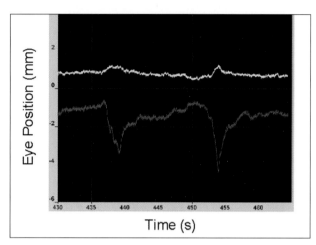

Figure 12-8. Actual eye motion during a CustomCornea surgery. The horizontal axis indicates time in seconds. Excimer laser treatment started at about the 430-second mark. The vertical axis plots eye position in millimeters, with the yellow trace showing vertical eye motion and the red trace showing horizontal movement. Twice during the treatment the eye made large-amplitude rapid excursions predominantly to the side.

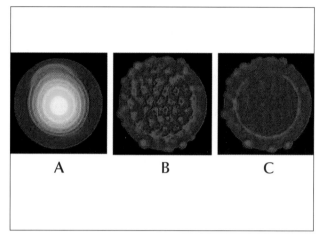

Figure 12-9. Simulated treatment of the eye with the motion profile shown in Figure 12-8. A: the target CustomCornea ablation profile with a 6.5 mm diameter optical zone and a surrounding 1.25 mm-wide blend zone. B: the ablative outcome in the absence of an active eye tracker (see text). Ideally, the post-treatment profile would be uniformly black. The color fluctuations in panel B indicate treated surface height errors of greater than 5 microns. C: shows the simulation outcome when the eye is stabilized with the LADARVision active eye tracker.

the eye motion by mirrors within the LADARVision system. The system tracks the eye motion with a slight following error. For eye oscillations up to ~100 Hz this error is small.

Figure 12-8 shows actual eye motion during one of our CustomCornea LASIK surgeries. The horizontal axis in the plot indicates time in seconds during the procedure (the excimer laser was activated at approximately the 430-second mark). The vertical axis indicates eye position in millimeters, with vertical (superior/inferior) motion shown by the yellow trace and side-to-side motion shown in red. During this ~3 diopter (D) myopic correction, the eye underwent two large amplitude motions predominantly to one side.

Figure 12-9A shows the desired ablation profile for this surgery. The field of view is a 10 x 10 mm square. The pseudocolor display shows the depth of the ablation over the 6.5-mm diameter optical zone and surrounding 1.25-mm blend zone. Deepest ablation (~45 µm) is indicated by the whitish color in the center of the figure, while the dark red color depicts minimal ablation. Figure 12-9B and C indicate computer-simulated treatment of this eye. In both cases the desired outcome is a uniform black surface, indicating that the starting error of Figure 12-9A has been

accurately removed. In Figure 12-9B a 1 Hz eye tracker has been included in the computer simulation to approximate a physician moving the eye manually to correct for eye motion. The treated surface contains height errors in excess of 5 microns. In Figure 12-9C the active eye tracker of the LADARVision system is included in the simulation. This obviously results in a much more uniform treated surface with residual height errors that are generally submicron in height (as indicated by the fairly uniform dark red color). Providing accurate ablative correction is simply not possible without a high performance eye tracker stabilizing the treatment surface.

> Providing accurate ablative correction is simply not possible without a high performance eye tracker stabilizing the treatment surface.

Narrow-Beam Corneal Shaping

The excimer laser in the LADARVision system produces a gaussian beam at the treatment plane that has a full-width half-maximum (FWHM) diameter of < 0.9 mm and a pulse energy of < 3 mJ. Each laser fir-

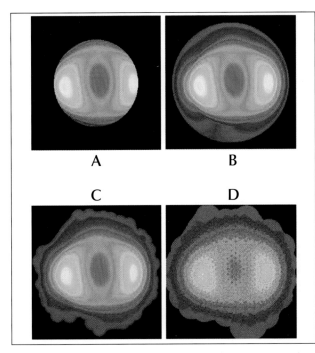

Figure 12-10. Simulated treatment of a patient with a complex preoperative wavefront. A: the desired ablation profile over a 6.5-mm optical zone. B: the ablation profile with the surrounding 1.25 mm blend zone added. C: the simulation outcome when the excimer laser is assumed to have the beam characteristics of the LADARVision system. D: the simulated ablation using a 2-mm diameter "top-hat" excimer beam. Panel C much more closely approximates the desired profile of panel B.

closely approximates the target profile of B. In contrast, D shows computer simulation of the desired profile using a 2-mm excimer beam with a "top-hat" fluence profile and a 10 mJ pulse energy. This last result only crudely approximates the intended treatment. The larger diameter beam simply is not capable of ablating this complex profile with high fidelity.

PATIENT OUTCOMES TO DATE

At the time of this writing, 20 patients have received CustomCornea LASIK surgery in one eye and conventional LADARVision treatment in the contralateral "control" eye. (In addition, a handful of patients have received CustomCornea PRK treatment, but it is too early in the postoperative course to perform meaningful analyses on these cases.) These procedures have been conducted as part of a US Food and Drug Administration (FDA) feasibility phase trial of the CustomCornea technology. The very first cases showed little difference in outcome between the two eyes. Over the course of the FDA CustomCornea trial, we have refined the CustomCornea algorithm and generally seen consistent improvement in the wavefront-based treatment outcomes.

> Over the course of the FDA CustomCornea trial, we have refined the CustomCornea algorithm and generally seen consistent improvement in the wavefront-based treatment outcomes.

ing removes ~450 picoliters of corneal tissue so that several hundred to a few thousand pulses are used in typical refractive corrections.

One of the patients enrolled in our CustomCornea clinical trial was retreated for refinement of an original refractive laser surgery. The retreatment was based on preoperative wavefront data. The desired ablation profile over the 6.5-mm optical zone is shown in Figure 12-10A. Deepest ablation (~25 microns) is again indicated by the whitish color peripherally on either side of the optical zone. This obviously complex surface is made more so by the addition of the customized blend zone, shown in Figure 12-9B, which uniformly tapers the ablation to zero depth at 9-mm diameter. Panel C shows computer-simulated ablation of the desired profile using the nominal LADARVision excimer laser beam. The simulation outcome within the optical zone very

One of our more promising cases is shown in Figure 12-11. Preoperatively, this patient had a measured spherical refractive error of –2.25 D, with an additional –1.25 D of astigmatism. Preoperative wavefronts are shown in panels A and B of Figure 12-11. Panel A indicates the total wavefront over a 5-mm diameter circle, while panel B shows the same wavefront with the spherocylindrical portion removed. Red indicates the highest point in the wavefront, while blue indicates the lowest. Preoperatively, the wavefront was dominated by the spherocylindrical error. However, measurable higher-order aberrations are also clearly present in panel B. Panel C shows the total wavefront measured at the 1-month postoperative visit, while panel D shows the higher-order postoperative wavefront. CustomCornea surgery has produced a much flatter wavefront, as indicated by the fairly uniform color as compared to panel A. In addition, the surgery has reduced the higher-order aberrations, as can be seen by comparing panel D with B. Clinically, this patient had a preoperative best-corrected visual acuity in this eye of 20/20, as measured with a backlit Early Treatment Diabetic Retinoscopy Study (EDTRS) chart under mesopic illumination. Postoperatively under the same examination conditions, the patient had an uncorrected visual acuity of 20/12.5 in this eye.

This result indicates the potential of the CustomCornea technology. In the near future we hope to report many outcomes such as this.

REFERENCES

1. Krueger RR. In perspective: eye tracking and Autonomous LADARVision ladar radar. *J Refract Surg.* 1999;15:145-149.

2. Liang J, Williams DR. Aberrations and retinal image quality of the normal human eye. *J Opt Soc Am.* 1997;14:2873-2883.

3. He JC, Marcos S, Webb RH, Burns SA. Measurement of the wavefront aberration of the eye by a fast psychophysical procedure. *J Opt Soc Am.* 1998;15:2449-2456.

4. Mrochen MM, Kraemmerer M, Seiler T. Wavefront-guided laser in situ keratomileusis: early results in three eyes. *J Refract Surg.* 2000;16:116-121.

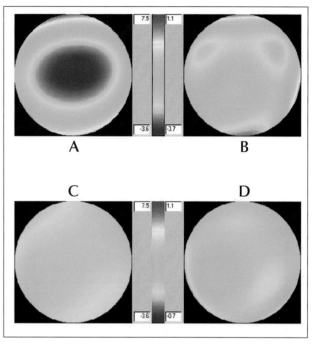

Figure 12-11. Actual wavefront data for one patient enrolled in the CustomCornea LASIK trial. A: the preoperative wavefront over a 5 mm circular region, with the color scale as indicated to the right of the picture. B: the wavefront with the spherocylindrical errors removed using the color scale shown to the left of the plot. By phoropter exam, this patient had a preoperative spherical refractive error of –2.25 D, with an additional astigmatic error of –1.25 D at an axis of 11 degrees. C and D: corresponding postoperative wavefront data 1 month after surgery. Visual acuity in this eye was 20/12.5 at the 1-month exam.

Chapter Thirteen

Customized Ablation Using the VisX WaveScan

Josef F. Bille, PhD
Joana Buechler Costa, Dipl Phys
Frank Mueller, Dipl Phys

Introduction

Wavefront technology was originally developed for astronomical applications. It was used to measure wavefront distortions that occurred when light traveling through the atmosphere entered an optical telescope. By applying adaptive optical closed-loop controls, the speckle patterns of the star images could be resolved toward diffraction-limited performance. Most of the technology was developed in association with research related to antimissile defense systems in the late 1970s.

Starting in 1978, the principle of wavefront measurement and compensation was adapted at the University of Heidelberg, Germany for ophthalmic applications. The technique is based on Hartmann-Shack wavefront sensing, measuring the optical path of light rays through the eye to detect all aberrations at all points in the optical system of the human eye. Adaptive optical systems were developed that measure and compensate wave aberrations of the human eye with closed-loop control.[1-4]

Recently, the application of wavefront sensing for preoperative evaluation of refractive surgical procedures has been proposed. Adaptive optical closed-loop systems can be used to subjectively measure and compensate the higher-order optical aberrations of the human eye to guide the surgeon in the selection of parameters of the procedure.

Measurement of the Optical Aberrations of the Human Eye

In Figure 13-1, the principle in operation of a Hartmann-Shack wavefront sensor is demonstrated. On the lefthand side, the processing of an ideal plane wave is depicted. The incident plane wave results in a square grid of spots in the focal plane of the microlens array. On the righthand side, the imaging of a distorted wave is shown. The distorted wavefront causes lateral displacements of the spots on the CCD array. From the spot pattern, the shape of the incident wavefront can be reconstructed based on appropriate curve fitting algorithms.

In Figure 13-2, the results of wavefront measurements on two human eyes are shown. The dependence of the root mean square (RMS) wavefront error (RMS in microns) on the diameter of the pupil is plotted. The data show that optical aberrations of the human eye increase considerably with larger pupil sizes. Figure 13-3 shows the reproducibility of Hartmann-Shack wavefront measurements after a few minutes and after 1 week. One shade of gray corresponds to a $\lambda/10$ wavefront deviation, the pupil size is approximately 3 mm.

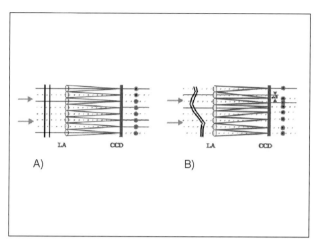

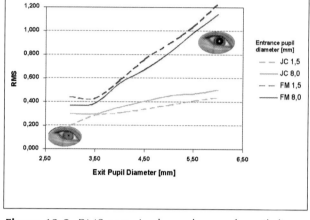

Figure 13-1. Principle of operation of a Hartmann-Shack wavefront sensor. A: plane wave; B: distorted wave.

Figure 13-2. RMS error in dependence of pupil diameter.

CLINICAL RESULTS OF REFRACTIVE WAVEFRONT MEASUREMENTS

The clinical validity of wavefront measurements was tested on human volunteer and refractive surgical patient eyes. In Figure 13-4, the computer display of the WaveScan instrument (VisX, Inc) is shown demonstrating the wavefront results of a human volunteer eye. In the lower left part of the display, the acuity map over a 5-mm pupil is depicted. In the lower center of the display, the higher orders of the optical aberrations beyond sphere and astigmatism are plotted demonstrating considerable wavefront deviations in the outer segments of the pupil, even in the case of a 20/15 human eye. In Figure 13-5, the computer display of the WaveScan instrument is shown depicting the measurement data of a patient eye that underwent a photorefractive keratectomy (PRK) surgical procedure. The image of the high-order optical aberration in the lower part of the display indicates the presence of a small coma aberration.

PRINCIPLE OF ADAPTIVE OPTICAL CLOSED-LOOP CONTROL

In Figure 13-6, the principle of adaptive optical closed-loop control is schematically demonstrated. The wavefront of light that is distorted due to optical aberrations of the optical system (eg, the human eye) is measured by a wavefront sensor. The reconstruct-

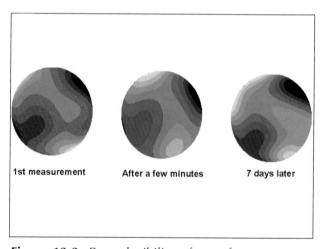

Figure 13-3. Reproducibility of wavefront measurements of the human eye taken at different times.

ed wavefront is dithered on a wavefront controller (ie, an active mirror) in order to compensate for the associated optical aberrations. Finally, an ideally aberration-free optical image through an aberrating medium can be achieved.

In Figure 13-7, a number of active mirrors and wavefront sensors developed and used in the Kirchhoff Institute of Physics, University of Heidelberg, during the past 20 years are depicted. The first-generation foil mirror was successfully

Recently, a multisegment microchip mirror was introduced. This mirror has approximately 100,000 facets, each able to slightly shift the phase of a local component of the wavefront in order to compensate for the detected wavefront error.

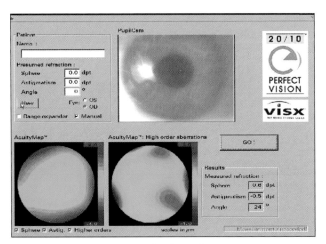

Figure 13-4. Computer display of acuity map images of a normal eye.

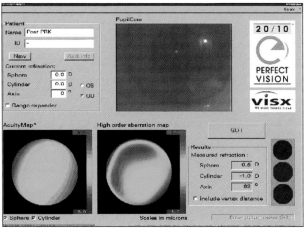

Figure 13-5. Computer display of acuity map images of a post PRK eye.

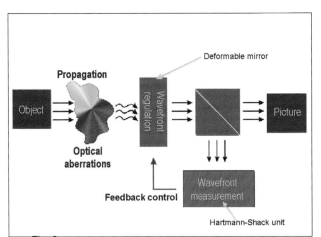

Figure 13-6. Schematics of a closed-loop adaptive optical system.

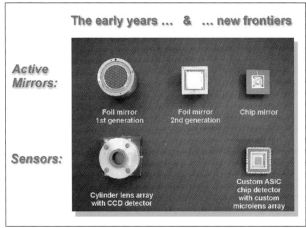

Figure 13-7. Diagram of different active mirrors and wavefront sensors.

applied for the real-time compensation of aberrations of the human eye for high-resolution imaging of the retina.1 In this paper, closed-loop operational results of the second-generation foil mirror7 are reported. Recently, a multisegment microchip mirror was introduced. This mirror has approximately 100,000 facets, each able to slightly shift the phase of a local component of the wavefront in order to compensate for the detected wavefront error and create a perfectly concentrated spot on the retina. In the lower part of Figure 13-7, two different Hartmann-Shack wavefront sensors are shown. On the lefthand side is a diagram of a cylinder lens array with CCD-detector, which was first used to measure the aberration of the human eye in real-time.3 On the right-hand side is a custom ASIC chip detector, which is used in combination with a custom microlens array.

The ASIC chip is divided into a matrix of clusters consisting of photodetectors and signal processing circuitry. By analog signal processing in winner-takes-all circuitry, the highest photocurrent is detected and its position calculated. The obtained data are evaluated in real-time for reconstruction of the wavefront of light.

SIMULATION OF THE PERFORMANCE OF A CLOSED-LOOP ADAPTIVE OPTICAL SYSTEM

Figure 13-8 shows two examples of low-order optical aberrations compensated by a continuous membrane mirror.7 The membrane mirror consists of

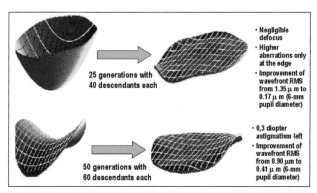

Figure 13-8. Compensation of low-order aberrations by a membrane mirror using genetic algorithms.[8]

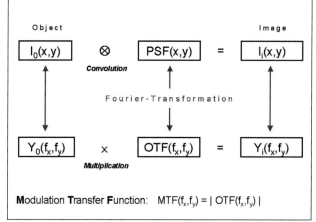

Figure 13-9. Summary of Fourier transform calculations.

a silicon nitride membrane coated with aluminum. It is deformed by electrostatic forces of 37 underlying electrodes arranged in a hexagonal grid. The device is compact (15-mm aperture) but needs voltages of up to 250 V.

Since the real-time compensation with a closed loop requires that the eye not move or change its state of accommodation to obtain an ideal result, another approach was chosen. An attempt was made to obtain a wavefront from the mirror that corresponded to that of a given set of aberrations but with a different sign. A genetic algorithm was used to determine the voltages that yielded the best compensation.[8]

In the upper part of Figure 13-8, the compensation of defocus is shown. A considerable improvement can be observed, but there are some leftover residual aberrations. The compensation of astigmatism (shown in the lower part of the figure) yields poorer results: though the wavefront RMS drops to less than half, the archived residual RMS of 0.41 microns is much too high to obtain near diffraction-limited imaging.

SIMULATION OF COMPENSATION OF HUMAN OPTICAL ABERRATIONS

The simulation of compensation of the optical aberrations of the eye uses methods of Fourier optics.[5,6] Fourier optics use the fact that a real image can be described as a perfect image of the object convoluted with the point spread function (PSF), which in turn represents the real image of a single (infinite-

ly small) point in object space. The upper part of Figure 13-9 demonstrates this correlation. As a convolution in object space corresponds to a simple multiplication in Fourier space, it is convenient to look at the problem in Fourier space. The lower part of Figure 13-9 depicts this representation: the Fourier transform of the object multiplied by the Fourier transform of the PSF results in the Fourier transform of the image. The Fourier transform of the PSF is called the optical transfer function (OTF). Since Fourier space is frequency space, the absolute value of the OTF represents the "amplification" of the associated spatial frequencies of the image. Because of this simple interpretation, the absolute value of the OTF is often used in analysis of optical systems and is called modulation transfer function (MTF).

Some calculations are necessary to obtain the MTF from acquired wavefront information (eg, from a Hartmann-Shack sensor). The first step is the calculation of the PSF. The pupil function P that represents the wavefront is Fourier transformed and the absolute value of the result is squared (equation 1):

$$PSF\ (x,y) = 1\ FT\ (P\ [x,y])\ 1^2$$

Having calculated the PSF, it is easy to compute the Strehl ratio, which is the ratio of the maximum intensity (and therefore the maximum PSF value) of an ideal focus spot to the maximum intensity of the real focus spot.

The inverse Fourier transformation of the PSF then yields the optical transfer function and hence the MTF (equations 2 and 3):

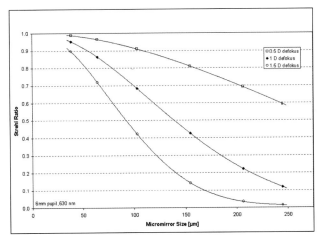

Figure 13-10. Strehl ratio in dependence of micromirror size for different defoci.

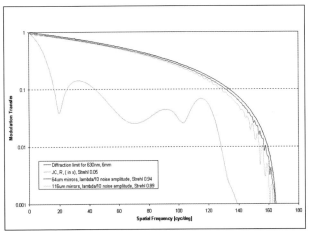

Figure 13-11. Preoperative simulation of refractive outcome using closed loop adaptive optical control.

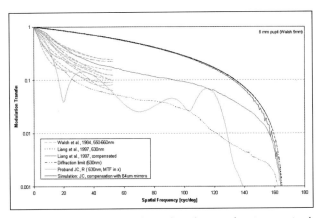

Figure 13-12. MTFs with and without adaptive optical compensation of different surgeons.

$$OTF\ (f_x,\ f_y) = FT^{-1}\ (PSF\ [x,y])$$

$$MTF\ (f_x,\ f_y) = 1\ OTF\ (f_x,\ f_y)$$

For simulations of adaptive optics, the wavefront modulation of the adaptive optical element is applied to the pupil function corresponding to the original wavefront and the above-described calculations are performed. Errors introduced by supporting structures of the micromirrors were neglected, and the original wavefront was assumed to be completely known. The results then represent the absolute limits of performance of the examined segmented micromirror.

In Figure 13-10, the results of simulation calculations regarding the obtainable Strehl ratio versus micromirror size for three different amounts of defocus are presented. It can be seen that in all situations for micromirror sizes < 50 μm, a Strehl ratio of more than 90% can be achieved.

PREOPERATIVE SIMULATION OF SURGICAL OUTCOMES USING ADAPTIVE OPTICS CLOSED-LOOP CONTROL

In Figure 13-11, measurements and simulations of the preoperative evaluation of aberration-free refractive surgical procedures are summarized. The simulation results are based on the application of multi-micromirror-integrated active mirror matrices. In all situations the MTF is plotted versus the spatial frequency (cycles per degree). Specifically, the MTFs for an ideal 6-mm pupil for a normal human eye and simulating active mirrors closed-loop compensation for mirrors with 64-micron micromirror size and 116-micron micromirror size, respectively, are demonstrated. These data suggest that the application of multisegment microchip mirror systems can be reliably applied to simulate the diffraction-limited performance of the human eye. This enables the surgeon to preoperatively and subjectively test the influence of higher-order optical aberrations on the visual performance in a clinical setting.

In Figure 13-12, the results of simulation calculations for adaptive optical closed-loop operations based on multi-micromirror technology are compared to previous results by other authors. The MTFs are plotted versus spatial frequency. The measure-

These data suggest that the application of multisegment microchip mirror systems can be reliably applied to simulate the diffraction-limited performance of the human eye. This enables the surgeon to preoperatively and subjectively test the influence of higher-order optical aberrations on the visual performance in a clinical setting.

ment data are based on results of Charman,[9] Liang, et al,[10] and our group. It is obvious that segmented micromirror systems have the potential of a nearly perfect compensation of optical aberrations of the human eye.

CONCLUSION

It has been demonstrated that based on new developments in microtechnology the measurement and evaluation of optical aberrations of the human eye can be accomplished. With adaptive optical closed-loop control systems, the measured aberrations can be compensated for so that better than normal vision (ie, "perfect vision") can be achieved. The limits of adaptive optical compensation systems due to the finite size of micromirror elements of multimirror microchip mirrors have been studied. It was found that microchip mirrors with sufficient numbers of elements are superior to standard deformable mirrors with a low number of controllable elements, especially mirrors with a contiguous, large surface.

REFERENCES

1. Dreher AW, Bille JF, Weinreb RN. Active optical depth resolution improvement of the laser tomographic scanner. *Applied Optics.* 1989;28(4):804-808.
2. Claflin ES, Bareket N. Configuring an electrostatic membrane mirror by least square fitting with analytically derived influence functions. *J Opt Soc Am A.* 1986;3(11):1833-1839.
3. Liang J, Grimm W, Goelz S, Bille JF. Objective measurement of the wave aberrations of the human eye using a Hartmann-Shack wavefront sensor. *J Opt Soc Am A.* 1994;11(7):1949-1957.
4. Bille J, Freischlad K, Jahn G, Merkle F. Image restoration by adaptive optical phase conjugation. Proceedings of the 6th International Conference of Pattern Recognition. Munich, Germany; 1982.
5. Goodman JW. *Introduction to Fourier Optics.* 2nd ed. New York, NY: McGraw-Hill; 1996.
6. Born M, Wolf E. *Principles of Optics—Electromagnetic Theory of Propagation, Interference and Diffraction of Light.* 6th ed. Oxford, England: Pergamon Press; 1984.
7. Vdovin GV. Adaptive mirror micromachined in silicon. Thesis. Delft, Netherlands: University of Delft.
8. Wühl S. Aktive korrektur optischer aberrationen mittels genetischer algorithmen. Thesis. Heidelberg, Germany: University of Heidelberg.
9. Charman WN. Wavefront aberration of the eye: a review. *Optom Vis Sci.* 1991;68(8):574-583.
10. Liang J, Williams DR. Supernormal vision and high-resolution retinal imaging through adaptive optics. *J Opt Soc Am A.* 1997;14(11):2884-2892.

Wavefront-Guided Custom Ablation

CLINICAL SCIENCE SECTION

Retinal Imaging Aberrometry

Ronald R. Krueger, MD

The main differentiating feature of retinal imaging aberrometry is that the wavefront error pattern is defined by subtle deviations in the ideal position of individual laser rays projected into the eye and imaged on the retina—hence the words "retinal imaging." This form of wavefront sensing is uniquely characterized and described by the principles of Tscherning.

To best understand these principles in more detail, let us begin by reviewing the history of this form of wavefront sensing. Its earliest application was in the late 1800s when Tscherning first described it in defining the monochromatic aberrations of the human eye.[1] The leaders of ophthalmic optics, including Gullstrand, however, did not support Tscherning's description, and it was not favorably accepted. It was not until the 1970s that

> It was not until the 1970s that Howland and Howland used Tscherning's aberroscope design together with a cross cylinder lens to project a grid pattern of laser light onto the retina that subjectively monitored the monochromatic aberrations of the eye.[2]

Howland and Howland used Tscherning's aberroscope design together with a cross cylinder lens to project a grid pattern of laser light onto the retina that subjectively monitored the monochromatic aberrations of the eye.[2] Most recently, Seiler modified this concept to project a 1-mm grid pattern onto the retina that could also be objectively imaged and photographed with a small para-axial aperture optical system.[3] At the same time, Molebny and coworkers from the Ukraine devised a retinal ray tracing modification of the Tscherning technique whereby individual rays were sequentially projected and imaged on the retina. The sequential tracing of the position of these retinal spots as a whole defined the wavefront aberration pattern.[4]

These simple principles of "retinal imaging" aberrometry are shown in Figure II, which demonstrates the ingoing direction of rays of light and how each of the rays are deviated by the optics of the eye. The extent of their deviation is then seen within the grid pattern projected onto the retina, and that image is then captured to define the wavefront aberration pattern.

The commercial systems described in the chapters that follow include the modified Tscherning aberrometer, which is commercially available by both Wavelight Technologies and Schwind Inc (Chapter Fourteen), as well as the retinal ray tracing method commercially available by Tracey Technologies Inc (Chapter Fifteen).

In addition, double pass aberrometry techniques have been previously described and used to define the point spread function on the retina but have not yet been developed into commercial systems for clinical ophthalmic use.[5]

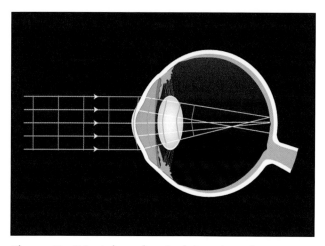

Figure II. Principles of retinal imaging aberrometry (Tscherning). Rays of light enter the eye and are deviated to form an aberrated retinal image, which is photographed to define the wavefront aberration pattern (photo courtesy of D. Huang).

References

1. Tscherning M. Die monochromatischen aberrationen des menschlichen auges. *Z Psychol Physiol Sinn.* 1894;6:456-71.

2. Howland HC, Howland B. A subjective method for the measurement of monochromatic aberrations of the eye. *J Opt Soc Am A.* 1977;67:1508-18.

3. Meirdel P, Wiegard W, Krinke HE, Kaemmerer M, Seiler T. Measuring device for determining monochromatic aberrations of the human eye. *Ophthalmology.* 1997;6:441-5.

4. Molebny VV, Pallikaris IG, Naoumidis LP, Chyzh IH, Molebny SV, Sokurenko VM. Retinal ray tracing technique for eye-refraction mapping. Proceedings of the SPIE. 1997;2971:175-83.

5. Artal P, Santamaria J, Bescos J. Retrieval of wave aberration of human eyes from actual point-spread-function data. *J Opt Soc Am A.* 1988;A5:1201-6.

Chapter Fourteen

Wavefront-Guided LASIK Using a Tscherning Wavefront Analyzer

Michael Mrochen, PhD
Maik Kaemmerer, PhD
Peter Mierdel, PhD
Theo Seiler, MD, PhD

INTRODUCTION

The optical quality of the human eye suffers from ocular monochromatic aberrations that have long been recognized as early as the mid 19th century.[1,2] Shape factors of the refractive surfaces, such as the cornea and lens, and their decentrations result in wavefront errors that degrade the retinal image quality and may, therefore, reduce the visual acuity for large pupils. The wavefront aberration function[3,4] is a fundamental description of the eye's optical characteristics from which traditional measures of the image quality, such as the subjective refraction, may be calculated. The recently achieved clinical introduction of wavefront-guided laser surgery or high-resolution imaging of the fundus requires a direct measurement of the wavefront aberrations.[5,6] Currently available methods to determine wavefront aberrations of the human eye fall into two broad categories—subjective or objective—but they are all based on a common principle: the direction of rays passing through selected points in the pupil area are monitored, and the aberrations are quantified by the deviation of these selected rays from the trace of rays in an aberration-free system.

Since scanning spot excimer lasers are available to remodel the corneal surface for correction of refractive errors such as myopia, hyperopia, and astigmatism, monochromatic aberrations may also be individually treated.[7] As a first step, the wavefront error of the individual eye has to be measured preoperatively. The wavefront error may then be expressed numerically in terms of a surface irregularity at the level of the outer corneal surface, which can be remodeled by means of the excimer laser with submicron precision. Following this strategy, the aim of wavefront-guided laser-assisted in situ keratomileusis (LASIK) is to improve or at least not deteriorate mesoptic vision and best-corrected visual acuity (BCVA).

THE WAVEFRONT ANALYZER BASED ON THE PRINCIPLES OF TSCHERNING

In 1894, Tscherning introduced a new way to subjectively analyze the ocular optical aberrations of human eyes.[8] Therefore, he used an optical lens of approximately +4.0 diopters (D) with a grid at the lens surface that consisted of equidistant lines. During the investigations, the subjects were advised to fixate on a star and sketch their own optical aberrations. Here, the light of a star can be assumed to be parallel with a plane wavefront due to the enormous distance between the star and the subject's eye. Today, the use of modern technology such as lasers, CCD cameras, and personal computers allows the conversion of Tscherning's initial subjective method into an objective method to measure the optical aberrations of a human eye. A scheme of the Tscherning

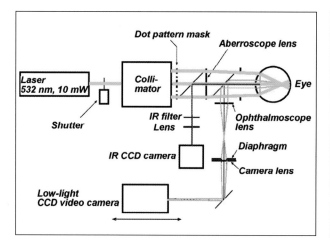

Figure 14-1. Technical setup of the wavefront analyzer based on the principles of Tscherning's aberrometry.

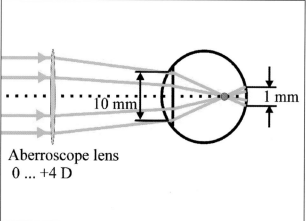

Figure 14-2. Ingoing optics of the wavefront analyzer used for projecting a spot pattern onto the cornea that is refracted on the retina by the optical conditions of the subject's eye. The diameter of the spot pattern at the cornea is 10 mm and the diameter of the retinal image can be kept constant at 1 mm by means of different aberroscope lenses.

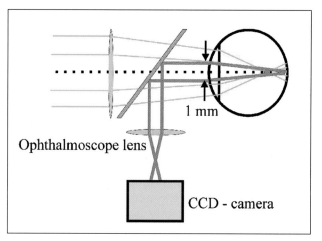

Figure 14-3. Outgoing optics of the wavefront analyzer based on the principle of indirect ophthalmoscopy. The retinal image is grabbed by a highly sensitive CCD camera through an artificial pupil (diameter 1 mm) in the exit pupil plane.

wavefront analyzer, developed at the Department of Ophthalmology of the Technical University of Dresden, Germany, is shown in Figure 14-1.[7]

Basically, the wavefront analyzer based on Tscherning's principle consists of two different optical pathways named the in- and outgoing optics. The "ingoing" optics (Figure 14-2) are used to project a grid or, as used in this system, a spot pattern onto the cornea. The optical behaviors of the subject's eye refracts the initial equidistant spot pattern, forming a somewhat distorted image pattern on the retinal level. The formed retinal image of the spot pattern can now be photographed by means of a highly sensitive CCD camera using the principle of indirect ophthalmoscopy (Figure 14-3). The optical pathway used for photographing the retinal image through an aperture of 1 mm in the exit pupil plane is termed "outgoing" optics. Considering the ingoing and outgoing optics, the wavefront analyzer represents a double-pass optical system. However, the small aperture used for the outgoing optics allows one to assume that the optical pathway of the outgoing optics is diffraction-limited and, as a consequence, the wavefront analyzer can be assumed to be a single-pass system.

In our system,[7,9] a frequency-doubled Nd:YAG laser emitting light at a wavelength of 532 nm was used. The dot pattern mask creates 168 single (13 x 13) light rays from the Nd:YAG laser beam. The center of the mask design was empty to avoid light reflections at different optical surfaces of the human eye, which might deteriorate the quality of the captured retinal image. The diameter of the spot pattern at the cornea is 10 mm, and the diameter of the reti-

Considering the ingoing and outgoing optics, the wavefront analyzer represents a double-pass optical system. However, the small aperture used for the outgoing optics allows one to assume that the optical pathway of the outgoing optics is diffraction-limited and, as a consequence, the wavefront analyzer can be assumed to be a single-pass system.

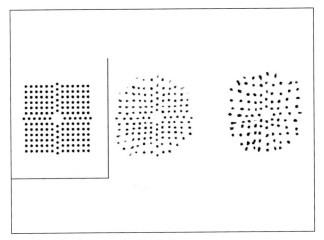

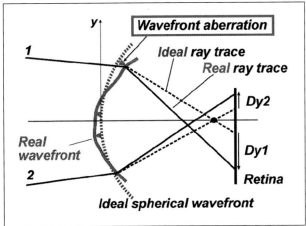

Figure 14-4. Examples of spot patterns. Ideal retinal image of a spot pattern for an emmetropic eye without optical aberrations (left). This spot pattern is equal to the mask design. Examples of measured retinal spot patterns (middle and right) demonstrate a distorted image due to optical aberrations.

Figure 14-5. Reconstruction of the wavefront aberrations from the ideal and measured spot positions. The shift in the positions of the ideal retinal spots (Dy1 and Dy2) resulting from light rays 1 and 2 are representing the difference of the ideal spherical wavefront and the real wavefront at a given position within the entrance pupil. Mathematical models allow the reconstruction of the wavefront aberrations based on the shifts of each single retinal spot with very high accuracy.

nal image can be kept constant at 1 mm by means of different aberroscope lenses (Figure 14-4). Here, the number of dots projected onto the retina depends only on the subject's pupil size and the mask design. The total illumination time is 60 milliseconds (ms) with a laser power far below the international safety requirements; the overall capture time for one image is 40 ms.

The retinal image is "grabbed" by means of a highly sensitive CCD camera that is linked to a personal computer. The optical aberrations of the investigated eye can now be calculated by analyzing the retinal image. Basically, each real spot position taken from the retinal image is compared to its corresponding ideal spot position. From the resulting deviations, the wavefront aberrations are mathematically reconstructed at the corneal apex (Figure 14-5). In this approach, the size of the ideal spot pattern is calculated by the use of Gullstrand's eye model. This assumption, however, does not influence the measurement of the higher-order optical aberrations but might lead to an error of < 0.25 D for the determination of the defocus (spherical refraction). The accuracy of the device was tested by measuring several dif-

> Basically, each real spot position taken from the retinal image is compared to its corresponding ideal spot position. From the resulting deviations, the wavefront aberrations are mathematically reconstructed at the corneal apex.

ferent telescopes that are assumed to be aberration-free.

One of the important factors in wavefront sensing is the correct centration of the subject's eye. The strong impact of decentrations on ocular aberrations forces better solutions on the centration problem in wavefront measurements and refractive surgery. Presently, it is common to aim on the center of the entrance pupil while the patient fixates a target coaxial with the wavefront system or the excimer laser beam.[10] The straight line connecting the center of the entrance pupil and the fixation target is termed "line of sight" in the physiologic optics literature.[11] There is another point visible on the cornea, which is easily defined by the surgeon—the first Purkinje image (P) of the fixation target (Figure 14-6). Assuming the fixation target is coaxial with the surgeon's view (which is correct in our excimer laser delivery system), the Purkinje image is located somewhat paracentral with reference to the entrance pupil's center (E'). This distance can be 1 mm or more in hyperopic eyes and eyes with high myopia, but in most cases is < 0.5 mm.[11] The problem is, however, more complicated because according to geometrical optics, the true visual axis that connects the fovea with the target goes through the nodal point N, and this line crosses the cornea in N' (see Figure 14-6), located between the points E' and P. This would be the ideal point of

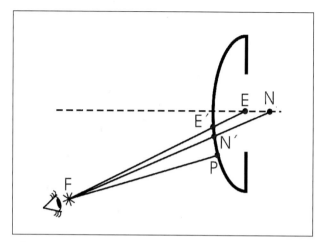

Figure 14-6. Centering points at the cornea. F: fixation target; E: center of the entrance pupil; E': center of the pupil at the cornea; P: Purkinje image; N₁: nodal point; N': ideal point of centration of the ablation zone (the geometries of the diagram are exaggerated).

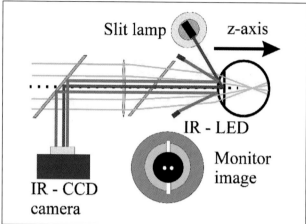

Figure 14-7. Scheme of the centration system used in the wavefront analyzer. The monitor image demonstrates the corneal reflexes of the IR diodes used to determine the center of the pupil, as well as the slit lamp image from the iris used for alignment of the z axis.

centration of the ablation zone. Until now, except in the rare cases, the topic of centration was not an issue because the distance E'-P was small compared to the pupil diameter and the diameter of the ablation zone. Therefore, it was considered negligible. Based on the data presented, however, decentrations as small as 0.2 mm must be considered clinically important, hence we may have to develop more precise methods to find the point N' on the cornea.

The wavefront analyzer uses an infrared video system to perform the alignment of the measuring system onto the line of sight of the subject's eyes. Thus, the line of sight is determined as the reference axis for the purpose of measuring and calculating the optical aberrations. The centration of the dilated pupil is done by means of infrared LEDs and a CCD camera that records the reflection of the LED light from the cornea. In addition to this, the accurate alignment of the z axis is done by centering the iris reflex of a modified slit lamp onto the pupil center. An overview of the centration system used for the wavefront analyzer is given in Figure 14-7.

Another important point when introducing new technology into ophthalmology is the reproducibility of the measurements in patients' eyes. From 300 eyes (five measurements in each eye; pupil size > 7 mm)

> The wavefront analyzer uses an infrared video system to perform the alignment of the measuring system onto the line of sight of the subject's eyes.

Table 14-1		
Reproducibility of the Wavefront Analyzer		
	RANGE	±*SD*
Sphere	+2 to -12 D	0.08 D
Cylinder	up to -4 D	0.08 D
Axis	0 to 180 degrees	2 degrees
RMS	up to 10 μm	0.04 μm
RMSH	up to 2 μm	0.02 μm
(Pupil Size 7 mm)		

measured with the Tscherning aberrometer, the absolute reproducibility for the sphere and cylinder was found to be ± 0.08 D. The reproducibility for the root mean square (RMS) wavefront error and the RMS of the higher-order optical aberrations are shown in Table 14-1. The standard deviation for the RMS was found to be in the order of 40 nm. In the case of a large pupil (> 7 mm), the Zernike polynomials up to the eighth order (45 Zernike coefficients) can be calculated with high accuracy.

The image quality of the retinal light spots depends on the optical transparency of intraocular mediums passed by the ingoing and outgoing optical pathways. Some opacities of the cornea, ocular lens,

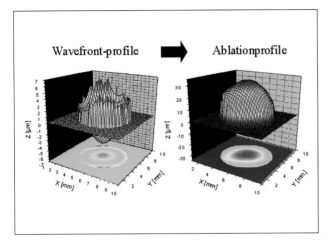

Figure 14-8. Conversion of the wavefront aberration map (left) into an ablation profile that is used for corneal laser surgery.

or vitreous body can considerably diminish the intensity of rays passing these turbid media and, as a consequence, spots may not be detected by the image processing program.

TECHNICAL ASPECTS OF THE LASER LINK-UP

For wavefront-guided treatment, the aberrations were measured by means of a wavefront analyzer (described in Chapter Ten). The patients' entrance pupils were dilated to diameters of at least 7 mm, and the patients fixated on a target in the center of the laser spot grid. From the deviations of the measured retinal spot pattern from their reference grid points, the gradient of the wavefront deviation in the corneal apex plane at the corresponding corneal position was calculated. Using corresponding mathematical models, the wavefront aberrations are approximated by means of Zernike polynominals including third, fourth, fifth, and sixth-order aberrations.[3] The wavefront aberration map is then converted numerically into a corresponding ablation profile, including a transition zone of at least 0.5 mm (Figure 14-8).[12] Finally, the resulting ablation profile must be approximated by a series of spot ablations including appropriate overlaps. These calculated positions of each single excimer laser spot on the cornea are then transferred to the computer-assisted input of the laser.

Preoperative planning of the treatment also includes determining the attempted optical zone.

After measuring the central corneal thickness by means of optical or ultrasonic pachymetry, the maximum ablation depth was approximated by the following equation (with a maximum diameter of 7.0 mm for the optical zone):

max ablation depth = corneal thickness – flap thickness – min residual stromal thickness

Diameter of optical zone = square root (3 x max ablation depth/spherical refraction)

Here, the flap thickness was 130 ± 30 μm for the used microkeratome (Supratome, Schwind, Kleinostheim, Germany); and for the minimum residual stromal thickness, a value of 300 μm was assumed to be appropriate. The following examples (considering a 480 μm and a 540 μm corneal thickness) might explain the selection of the optical zone for a -6 D myopic correction based on the wavefront measurements. In the case of the thinner cornea, the maximum ablation depth is 70 μm and for the thicker cornea, 110 μm. Therefore, the corresponding optical zones are 5.9 and 7.4 mm in diameter and chosen to be 5.9 and 7.0 mm.

Prior to the treatment, each ablation profile was tested under standard conditions (with eye tracking and simulated eye movement) on polymethylmethacrylate (PMMA) plates and by measuring the surface profile with a surface profiling system after the ablation. Also, the correct alignment of the eye tracking system was checked by using an artificial pupil printed onto an overhead folio. The standard system check for the excimer laser included the measurement of the pulse energy and the beam profile, which had to be gaussian with a correlation coefficient r = 0.95 or better. The spot diameter on the cornea was 1.0 mm and the repetition rate was 200 Hz.

CLINICAL RESULTS

Thirty eyes of 28 patients that were scheduled for LASIK to correct myopia and astigmatism were included in a prospective study. The LASIK surgery, including early postoperative healing, was uneventful in all eyes. The manifest refraction (spherical equivalent) changed from –3.9 ± 2.8 D preoperatively to +0.1 ± 0.5 D at 1 month after surgery. The cylinder was reduced from 1.0 ± 0.7 D to 0.2 ± 0.4 D.

At the 1-month follow-up examination, the increase factor of the monochromatic fourth, fifth,

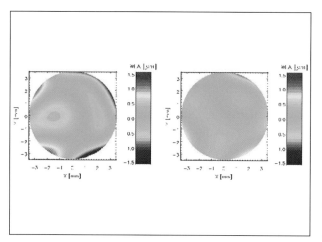

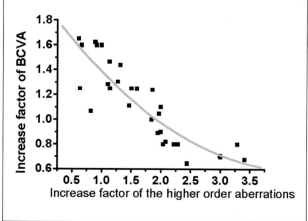

Figure 14-9. Preoperative and 1-month postoperative wavefront maps of one eye of the study group. The maps do not include tilt, defocus (spherical error), and astigmatism, but only coma-like and spherical-like optical aberrations to facilitate comparison. The demonstrated optical zone corresponds to the used ablation optical zone of 7 mm in diameter.

Figure 14-10. Increase of best-corrected visual acuity in dependence on the increased factor of higher-order optical aberrations' ratio of post-RMS to pre-RMS. A decrease in the higher-order aberrations leads to an increase in best-corrected visual acuity.

> All patients (20%) with a postoperatively supernormal vision of 20/10 showed a reduction in RMS wavefront error.

and sixth-order aberrations (post RMS/pre RMS) ranged from 0.6 to 3.2 with an average of 1.6. Figure 14-9 displays the pre- and 1-month postoperative wavefront deviation of one of the eyes treated. All patients (20%) with a postoperatively supernormal vision of 20/10 showed a reduction in RMS wavefront error.

The increase in visual acuity was statistically significantly correlated with the reduction in RMS wavefront error ($R^2 = 0.79$; $p < 0.001$), as shown in Figure 14-10. This key finding (that visual acuity can be increased by an operative improvement of the optical quality of the retinal image) supports the basic idea of wavefront-guided LASIK.

At this point, however, it is not clear whether a supernormal visual acuity of approximately 20/10 represents the real upper limit of visual acuity or whether we did not obtain better acuities because the correction of the wavefront errors was far from complete. Even in eyes with an increase in visual acuity, we achieved only a reduction of the wavefront errors of maximally -40%. On the other hand, this reduction of aberrations was significantly correlated with the increase in visual acuity, indicating that in many eyes visual acuity is limited by optical aberrations con-

sisting of cornea and lens. By compensating the aberrations by means of adaptive optics, Liang and coworkers could even resolve fine gratings (55 c/deg) that were invisible under normal viewing conditions.[5] The mean increase in wavefront error by 60% is a disappointing result on first glance; however, it is very promising when compared with the more than five-fold increase after standard excimer laser surgery.[13,14]

Corneal healing after surgery may stabilize the operatively changed shape of the outer cornea but may also level out the newly formed structure. Although stromal remodeling is considered minimal after LASIK, hyperplasia of the corneal epithelium may occur, which is also responsible for some regression of the refractive effect during the first 3 to 6 months after LASIK. Longer follow-up is necessary to estimate the influence of regression on visual acuity. Also, we expect that different wavefront errors will specifically be affected by regression (eg, spherical aberration and n-fold may be influenced more than coma-like aberrations). Such effects can be overcome by the strategy of tuning factors in the ablation algorithm that are different for different aberrations. However, such tuning factors should be determined only after 6 months, when regression is most probably over.

Currently, the technique of wavefront-guided LASIK is proposed as an additional feature during refractive laser surgery for correction of ametropia.

Although the procedure may be considered safe in this series because no visual loss occurred, this has to be substantiated in prospective trials that include a larger number of patients. Once it has proven to be a safe and more effective procedure, wavefront-guided LASIK may also apply to emmetropic eyes aiming toward an improved visual acuity only, especially under night conditions.

REFERENCES

1. Volkmann AW. Sehen. In: R Wagner, ed. *Handwörterbuch der Physiologie III*. Braunschweig, Germany: Vieweg und Sohn; 1846:289-93.

2. von Helmholz H. Handbuch der physiologischen *Optik*. Verlag von Leopold Voss; 1909.

3. Born M, Wolf E. *Principles of Optics*. 5th ed. Oxford, England: Pergamon Press; 1975.

4. Mahajan VN. *Aberration Theory Made Simple*. Bellingham, Wash: SPIE Optical Engineering Press; 1991.

5. Liang J, Williams DR, Miller DR. Supernormal vision and high-resolution retinal imaging through adaptive optics. *J Opt Soc Am A*. 1997;14:2884-92.

6. Mrochen M, Kaemmerer M, Seiler T. Wavefront-guided laser in situ keratomileusis: early results in three eyes. *J Refract Surg*. 2000;16:116-121.

7. Mierdel P, Krinke HE, Wiegand W, Kaemmerer M, Seiler T. Messplatz zur bestimmung der monochromatischen aberration des menschlichen auges. *Ophthalmologe*. 1997;96:441-5.

8. Tscherning M. Die monochromatischen aberrationen des menschlichen auges. *Z Psychol Physiol Sinne*. 1894;6:456–471.

9. Mierdel P, Kaemmerer M, Mrochen M, Krinke HE, SeilerT. An automated aberrometer for clinical use. *SPIE Proceedings 2000*. In press.

10. Uozato H, Guyton DL, Waring III GO. Centering corneal surgical procedures. In: GO Waring III, ed. *Refractive Keratotomy for Myopia and Astigmatism*. St. Louis, Mo: Mosby-Year Book; 1993:491–505.

11. Le Grand Y, El Hage SG. *Physiological Optics*. New York, NY: Springer-Verlag; 1980:72-74.

12. Klein SA. Optimal corneal ablation for eyes with arbitrary Hartmann-Shack aberrations. *J Opt Soc Am A*. 1998;2580-2588.

13. Martinez C, Applegate R, Klyce S, McDonald M, Medina I, Howland CK. Effects of pupillary dilation on corneal optical aberrations after photorefractive keratectomy. *Arch Ophthalmol*. 1998;116:1053-62.

14. Seiler T, Kaemmerer M, Mierdel P, Krinke HE. Ocular optical aberrations after photorefractive keratectomy for myopia and myopic astigmatism. *Arch Ophthalmol*. 2000;118:17-21.

Chapter Fifteen

Tracey Retinal Ray Tracing Technology

Vasyl V. Molebny, DSc
Ioannis G. Pallikaris, MD
Sophia I. Panagopoulou, PhD
Jean Brandau, MBA
Joe S. Wakil, MD

"Perfect vision" is an elusive goal that is obtained most often by chance and not by calculation. The input of desired refractive correction is by itself one of the largest errors in the refractive surgery procedure. The high degree of subjectivity involved in assessing a patient's refraction leaves the yearning for a truly reliable, objective measurement of refraction and total visual quality. Without an exact understanding of a patient's refraction, we can never expect to achieve perfect visual results.

Fundamentally, refraction is the core of refractive surgery and the reason it is called refractive surgery in the first place. Refraction is the "gold standard"—the ultimate measure of our clinical results. Simply put, our goal is to successfully change the refractive status of our patients. With the advances of modern refractive surgery, it has become increasingly important to understand the dynamics of vision. New diagnostic instrumentation, such as corneal topography, has increased refractive surgeons' appreciation of the detail and variability of the cornea's shape and, hence, its refractive power. However, with the cornea providing roughly 70% of the refractive power of the eye, it is a critical element but not the entire picture.

As in the case of corneal topography, the keratometer became obsolete after a device was created that makes no assumption of spherocylindrical optics and describes in point-by-point detail the cornea's surface both within and outside of the opti-

cal zone. With full appreciation of both optical and shape characteristics of the cornea, corneal topography provides a complete picture of corneal optical performance.

The time has come for us to look at the entire refraction of the eye with the same level of objective measure and detail. In the same measure, to view a refractive map of the entrance pupil that colors the refractive power of the entire eye on a point-by-point basis (as opposed to the basic refractive numeric summary of sphere and cylinder) will have at least as much impact in understanding vision as the corneal topography maps of the mid 1980s.

Measuring refraction on a spatially resolved basis requires the ability to look at the wavefront aberrations of the eye on a point-by-point basis. The problem with the human eye is that we cannot just remove the patient's retina and replace it with a CCD chip to measure how the eye focuses light passing through it. Instead, we must analyze light that is directed into the eye and focused onto the retina, creating a secondary light source as it is reflected from the retinal surface and projected out through the exit pupil. There are several principles, such as Tscherning aberroscopy, Hartmann-Shack wavefront sensing, and thin-beam ray tracing, that may be utilized to measure the complete aberrations of the human visual system. At Tracey Technologies, LLC (Bellaire, Tex), we have chosen the fundamental principle of thin-beam ray tracing to generate this infor-

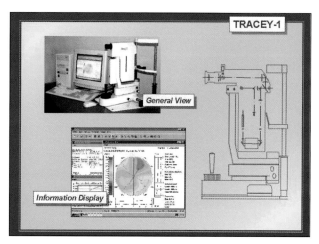

Figure 15-1. Tracey-1 device and diagnostic refractive profile map.

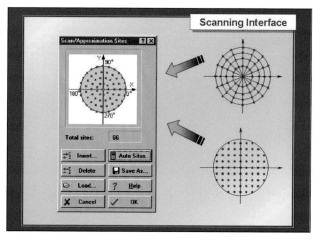

Figure 15-2. Selectable scanning patterns of rapid fire "bullets" of light passed through the entrance pupil.

mation in a unique design to provide a new diagnostic platform in which to study the human eye.[1,2] Tracey's proprietary technology (multiple patents pending) was developed in Eastern Europe and is fully owned by Tracey Technologies, LLC. The company also owns technology that will enable it to develop second- and third-generation diagnostics that build on the Tracey 1 platform to expand the available diagnostics beyond refraction to the assessment of total visual function (Figure 15-1).

The Tracey ray-tracing refractometer uses the fundamental thin-beam principle of optical ray tracing to measure the total refractive power of the eye on a point-by-point basis. The simplicity of measuring one point in the entrance pupil at a time is unique to this device as compared to other competing technologies. Both of the competing technologies, the Tscherning aberroscope and Hartmann-Shack lenslet array system, measure all the data points passing through the entrance pupil at once, making these technologies easily susceptible to the criss-crossing of data points in a highly aberrated eye. The Tracey system is designed to rapidly fire a sequence of very small parallel light beams into the eye, much like bullets out of an old-fashioned Gattling gun. These "bullets" of light pass through the entrance pupil in an infinite selection of software-selectable patterns. These selectable patterns (Figure 15-2) enable Tracey

The Tracey system is designed to rapidly fire a sequence of very small parallel light beams into the eye, much like bullets out of an old-fashioned Gattling gun.

to actually concentrate on particular areas of the entrance pupil, not only the entire aperture (eg, concentrating points around the exterior of the entrance pupil for assessment of aberrations caused by a LASIK flap or centrally on a keratoconus patient). This flexibility to easily program any myriad of patterns and number of desired data points through the entrance pupil is unique to Tracey.

Second, by design, the fovea is represented by the conjugate focal point of the system from the patient's fixation. Semiconductor photodetectors detect the location where each bullet of light strikes the retina and provide raw data of the (x,y) error distance from the fovea or conjugate focal point. These raw data are direct measures of the transverse aberration for each particular point in the entrance pupil and can very easily provide refractive correction needed with only simple computational processing, as opposed to systems that require advanced image processing algorithms. The speed of this system is tremendous, measuring 64 points five times each (320 individual measurements) in just over 10 milliseconds (ms). The ability to make iterative measurements for each data point greatly improves the system reproducibility because individual data point readings are averaged any selectable number of times (eg, five times over a very small area of the aperture). Variability is dramatically reduced compared with a system using a CCD camera that typically takes at least 33 ms to capture a single data measuring image.

The retinal spot diagram is analogous to the point spread function (PSF) of the eye and from its concentration of points, or the spread of points (Figure 15-3); one can correlate this to contrast sensitivity of the

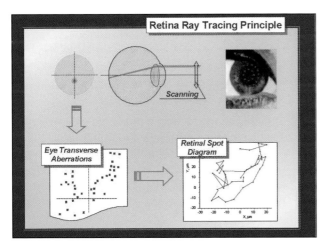

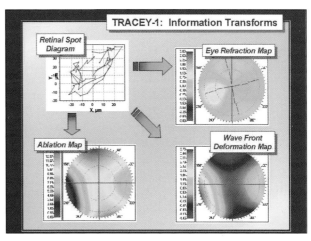

Figure 15-3. Retinal spot diagram demonstrating the concentration of spread of points striking the retina (similar to the PSF).

Figure 15-4. Tracey-1 transformation maps including the eye refraction map, wavefront deformation map, and ablation map.

patient. The tighter the retinal spot diagram, the greater concentration of photons striking any one spot on the retina. This will maximize contrast sensitivity. On the contrary, the more spread the diagram, the lower density of photons will strike any one spot on the retina, leading to poor contrast sensitivity. The ability to present the color map of the entrance pupil whereby each point is color coded by the refractive correction required at such point is of extreme benefit to the practitioner as he or she examines a patient's visual function and creates a plan for optimizing that patient's vision.

With new photodetector system designs, Tracey can easily measure a large dynamic range of refractive aberrations while maintaining high resolution. This should provide for a significant advantage when measuring a physiologic system, such as the eye, which can easily have a tremendous dynamic range of refractive errors as is typically seen in keratoconus or the edge of a LASIK flap. Additionally, since each point is sequentially measured, there is never any confusion of which entrance pupil location registers with the retinal spot detected. As the Tracey system is practically a direct measure of the PSF of the eye with its retinal spot detection, it can then easily provide for full calculation of wavefront deformation maps, the modulation transfer function (MTF) of the eye, and eventually the calculation of a

> Additionally, since each point is sequentially measured, there is never any confusion of which entrance pupil location registers with the retinal spot detected.

customized corneal ablation map utilizing the patient's corneal topography data (Figure 15-4).

As for the competitive principles to Tracey, Tscherning aberroscopy generally requires a two-dimensional image of a rectilinear grid projected into the eye, which is then imaged as a distorted grid on the retina.[3] This two-dimensional image on the retina contains distortions directly related to the nonhomogenous optics of the eye. When this image is viewed through a direct ophthalmoscope (small aperture optics), a digital image is captured via a CCD camera. This captured image is then subjected to a great amount of digital image processing to evaluate the distortions of the grid image on the retina and to calculate the aberrations responsible for the pattern change. This technique is limited by the resolution of the aberroscope grid pattern in resolving points within the entrance pupil and subject to high variability by requiring captured images to be averaged over large fractions of a second.

The Hartmann-Shack lenslet array measures the slope changes of the distorted wavefront as it exits the eye.[4] This technology utilizes a bundle of light entering the eye and reflecting from the retina as a secondary light source. It is assumed that this secondary light source is ideal and nondistorted, which is not the case and complicates this technique. As the reflected light travels retrograde through the eye, it is subject to the eye's aberrations and projects out through the exit pupil, striking a lenslet array. This is a grid of tiny lenses each of which focuses a small part of the wavefront onto a CCD imaging chip. The location of each lenslet's focusing point on the CCD is an indication of the slope of that specific part of the wavefront. The number of lenslets in the array limits the spatial resolution of this system, and the sensitivity of this system is limited by the focal length of the lenses used in the lenslet array. There is a trade-off between the greater number of lenses and the greater light-gathering power, or aperture, of each lens. The focal length of the lenslet array must also be selected and fixed. In other words, the design, much like the aberroscope, is limited to the selection of the lenslet array. Once selected, it fixes the resolution and sensitivity of the unit. There is no programmable flexibility. Also, since the CCD imaging system must digitize the image of each lens in the array and then process its location before calculating the aberration, there is a great deal of computation involved. These systems tend to have a limited dynamic range in measuring higher-order aberrations. With post-refractive surgery patients or corneal pathologies, this may become a significant limitation. This device, like the aberroscope, takes a single full aperture measurement at a time, requiring significant computation, and is also susceptible to greater variability from shot-to-shot.

CLINICAL VALUE OF TRACEY

The Tracey system for objectively measuring the refractive status of the eye provides new information for assessing the quality of vision of our patients.[5] This ability to measure the dynamics of vision and provide quantitative information can be summarized by the following three principle improvements over traditional objective refraction technology:

- Objective measurement that directly correlates to contrast sensitivity.
- Spatial resolution of refractive aberrations in both day and night pupillary conditions.
- Quantification of accommodative volume and speed between near and far fixation. With this new objective, clinical refraction data, and a real understanding of visual quality, ophthalmologists will be able to better plan their refraction corrections to achieve "perfect vision" by calculation rather than chance.

REFERENCES

1. Molebny VV, Pallikaris IG, Naoumidis LP, Chyzh IH, Molebny SV, Sokurenko VM. Retinal ray tracing technique for eye refraction mapping. *Proc SPIE.* 1997;2971:175-183.

2. Molebny VV, Panagopoulou SI, Molebny SV, Wakil YS, Pallikaris IG. Principles of ray tracing aberrometry. *J Refract Surg.* 2000;16:S572-5.

3. Mrochen M, Kaemmerer M, Mierdel P, Krinke HE, Seiler T. Principles of Tscherning aberrometry. *J Refract Surg.* 2000;16:S570-1.

4. Thibos LN. Principles of Hartmann-Shack aberrometry. *J Refract Surg.* 2000;16:S563-5.

5. Pallikaris IG, Panagopoulou SI, Molebny VV. Clinical experience with the Tracey technology wavefront device. *J Refract Surg.* 2000;16:S588-91.

Wavefront-Guided Custom Ablation

CLINICAL SCIENCE SECTION

Ingoing Adjustable Refractometry

Ronald R. Krueger, MD

The main differentiating feature of ingoing adjustable refractometry is that the wavefront error pattern is defined by a compensatory adjustment of ingoing rays of light relative to the fovea, hence the words "ingoing adjustable." This form of wavefront sensing is most similar to that of clinical refraction and retinoscopy and is uniquely characterized and described by the principles of Scheiner. Historically, its earliest application was by Smirnov in 1961 as a form of subjectively adjustable refractometry.[1] Peripheral beams of incoming light were subjectively redirected toward a central target to cancel the ocular aberrations from that peripheral point. Recently, Webb and coauthors modified this as a subjective form of wavefront refractometry of the human eye.[2] This method of

> The method of spatially resolved refractometry utilizes approximately 37 testing spots, which are manually directed by the patient to overlap a central target in defining the wavefront aberration pattern.

spatially resolved refractometry utilizes approximately 37 testing spots, which are manually directed by the patient to overlap a central target in defining the wavefront aberration pattern. Objective variants of this method are based on a form of slit retinoscopy (skioloscopy), which is rapidly scanned across a specific axis and orientation. The fundus reflection is then captured to define the wavefront aberration pattern. The retinoscopic technique is sequential at various axes of orientation and allows for a more rapid capture of information.

These principles of ingoing adjustable refractometry are shown in Figure III, which demonstrates ingoing rays of light all focusing on the retina because the course of their entry has been adjusted to bring all the rays of light into sharp focus, similar to subjective refraction and retinoscopy.

The commercial systems described in the chapters that follow include the spatially resolved refractometer, which is being clinically implemented by the Emory Vision Correction Group (Chapter Sixteen) and the Nidek OPD Scan slit skioloscopy device (Chapter Seventeen).

References

1. Smirnov HS. Measurement of the wave aberration in the human eye. *Biophys.* 1961;6:52-66.
2. Webb R, Penny CM, Thompson K. Measurement of ocular local wavefront distortion with a spatially resolved refractometer. *Applied Optics.* 1992;31:3678-86.

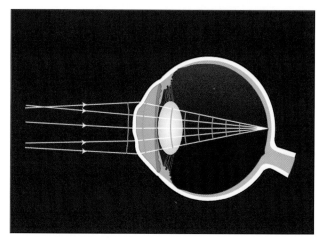

Figure III. Principles of ingoing adjustable refractometry (Scheiner). Rays of light enter the eye and are adjusted into focus on the retina, thereby changing the course of their entry to define the wavefront aberration pattern (photo courtesy of D. Huang).

Chapter Sixteen

Measurement of Image Quality with the Spatially Resolved Refractometer

Stephen A. Burns, PhD
Susana Marcos, PhD

INTRODUCTION

With the prospect of improved techniques for the precise control of the refracting elements of the eye, there has been a renewed interest in characterizing the wavefront aberrations of the eye. In the past, the true clinical utility in measuring the optical quality of the eye was mainly restricted to the measurements of spherical and cylindrical errors in refraction since these two optical quantities were all that could be corrected. While wavefront measurements were useful for evaluating clinical success or reasons for a failure in patient satisfaction, they were not widely used outside of the research laboratory. The development of plans for detailed, point-by-point correction of the optics of the eye has re-awakened interest in the measurement of aberrations more complex than sphere and cylinder. This chapter describes the technique we use to evaluate wavefront aberrations of the eye.

The ability of the eye to form an image on the retina depends on the quality of the optics of the eye. If the optics are poor, a low-quality image is formed on the retina and the image is blurred. If the optics are relatively good, a sharp image is formed on the retina. The simplest forms of image blur arise from the errors in the refractive state of the eye. Defocus and astigmatism can be corrected by the appropriate use of lenses combining spherical and astigmatic corrections. However, even if the sphere and astigmatism are perfectly corrected, the retinal images are still blurred more than predicted by diffraction from the edges of the pupil, especially when the pupil is large. This blur arises from higher orders of imperfections in the optical properties of the eye. Different regions of the pupil direct light to different places on the retina, even when the eye is optimally corrected with glasses or contact lenses. The total image-forming ability of the eye (ignoring scatter) can be described mathematically by the eye's pupil function. This pupil function has two components: an intensity apodization function and a phase function, which is proportional to the wavefront aberration of the eye. The ray aberrations of the eye represent the angular deviation of a ray of light from ideal as it passes through the optics of the eye (alternatively, the wavefront aberrations represent the phase distortions at the pupil plane with respect to an ideal spherical wavefront). An ideal optical system would have a flat wavefront aberration (ie, all values would be equal). The most familiar form for the apodization function is the pupil size. The image on the retina depends on the size of the pupil. For small pupils, refractive errors are not very important because the wavefront aberration of normal eyes does not vary rapidly across the pupil, but diffraction from the edges of the pupil are important. At the end of this chapter we describe how the cone photoreceptors also contribute to the apodization of the eye, but for the majority of the chapter we will be discussing the wavefront aberrations.

In principle, the local slopes of the wavefront

aberration of the eye can be measured by passing the image of a light source through each point in the pupil and determining where that ray strikes the retina with respect to a reference. In a simplified form, this is the technique described by Scheiner to measure the refractive error of the eye. We use a more complicated form of a Scheiner optometer—the spatially resolved refractometer (SRR)[1-3]—to measure the deviation of a ray of light for 37 different entry locations within the eye's pupil. This chapter describes an implementation of the spatially resolved refractometer and gives sample results.

METHODS

Measuring Ray Deviations

To measure the wavefront aberrations of the eye, we use a psychophysical ray-tracing approach. This is the same approach used in Scheiner's disc, and the concept is shown in Figure 16-1. Basically, if a subject has perfect optics and was emmetropic, no matter where in the pupil light from a distant object (eg, a star) entered the eye, it would be focused into a very small region of the retina, and the observer would view a diffraction-limited point. However, eyes are not perfect, and as a result, light entering the pupil at different positions is directed to slightly different locations on the retina. With Scheiner's disc, if light is allowed into the pupil from two small apertures, one at the top of the pupil and the other in the center of the pupil (rays A and B in Figure 16-1), the myopic subject sees two spots on the retina (points A' and B'). The hyperopic subject would also see two points, but the relative positions would be reversed. The emmetropic subject, however, would see only one spot. Thus, the amount and direction of the displacement of the retinal location from the ideal is a measure of the ray deviation for that point in the pupil. The ray deviation, in turn, is proportional to the slope of the wavefront aberration function for that pupil location. By turning the ray entering the periphery of the pupil on and off and simply asking the subject if the spot is above, below, or coincident with the spot formed by the central ray, we can determine if the subject is hyperopic, myopic, or emmetropic. If we now add a lens and make the same test, we can determine if we have under- or overrefracted the subject. This observational test (do we get one spot or two), while not practical for a complete refraction, suggests how we can make pre-

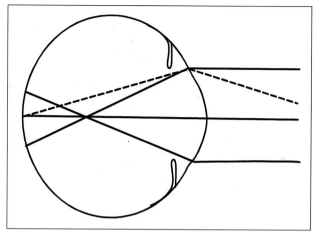

Figure 16-1. Demonstration of the principle of the SRR. Here we show the path of rays of light entering the eye from a distant object for an eye whose only aberration is spherical defocus (a myopic eye). The rays from the three pupil entry positions (solid lines) all cross in front of the retina. If the ray entering the eye at the top of the pupil is tilted (eg, it is coming from a nearby object), it can be made to strike the retina at the same location as the centrally entering ray. The amount of tilt needed to align the rays is the slope of the wavefront at that location.

cise measurements of the ray deviation. We simply change the angle at which the light ray strikes the cornea until the subject sees both points in the same location (angle α in Figure 16-1). If this measurement is performed for a whole series of entry positions within the pupil while keeping the reference position at the center of the pupil, we can determine the ray deviations across the whole pupil. We can then use standard mathematical techniques[4,5] to turn these slope measurements into an estimate of the wavefront.

The principles of the apparatus have been described in detail.[1] In our current implementation, the gimballed mirror has been replaced with an oscilloscope screen, as described in Marcos, et al.[6] The apparatus works by collecting light emitted from an illuminated point on an oscilloscope. The light is passed through a wheel mounted on a stepper motor. This wheel is optically conjugate to the eye's pupil, and the wheel has a series of 1-mm diameter precision drilled holes. By rotating the stepper motor to a series of preset positions, the holes are scanned across the pupil in 1-mm steps. Thus, the subject sees the illuminated point on the oscilloscope through each point in the pupil. If the eye had no aberrations, then every point on the pupil would project to the

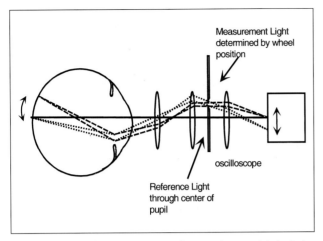

Measurement Light
determined by wheel
position

oscilloscope

Reference Light
through center of
pupil

Figure 16-2. The SRR varies the angle at which light enters the eye by moving a point in the image space. In this example, a spot is generated on the face of an oscilloscope. The location at which light enters the pupil is controlled by placing an aperture (a hole drilled in a metal wheel, which can be rotated by a motor) optically conjugate to the pupil of the eye. To change the angle at which light enters the eye, we can simply move the point on the face of the oscilloscope until the subject sees the point aligned to a reference target seen through the center of the pupil. To measure the next pupil position, the wheel can be rotated to bring a new hole into the pupil—the spot is then aligned again.

> The angle required to null the aberrations at each pupil position represents the slope of the wavefront at that location. The task for the subject is simply to use a joystick to align a spot to a cross. Make a response, then do it again.

same point on the retina. The eye does have aberrations, however, so the position of the oscilloscope point on the retina changes for each pupil entry position. By moving the image of the oscilloscope point with a joystick, the retinal location is moved (Figure 16-2). If it is moved so it aligns visually with a reference mark (the image of a cross provided by another optical channel), then the aberrations for that location in the pupil can be cancelled. The angle required to null the aberrations at each pupil position represents the slope of the wavefront at that location. The task for the subject is simply to use a joystick to align a spot to a cross. Make a response, then do it again. This is an extremely simple task for most subjects, and most people can make the alignment with very high precision. For the experimenter, the task is to keep the pupil centered on a video screen (pupil

position is monitored using an infrared-sensitive CCD). The computer presents the stimuli in random order, one at a time, through each pupil location. A single run takes about 4 minutes, and we generally collect three separate runs for a total measurement time of 12 to 15 minutes.

Determining the Wavefront From the Slope Measurements

We then use a standard fitting procedure[4,5] to fit the slope measurements to a set of Zernike polynomials.[7,8] The resulting Zernike expansion is an estimate of the wavefront height. The advantages of the Zernike polynomials for this purpose have been discussed elsewhere.[3,7-11] The advantage of the different Zernike terms is that they are quite simple in form and, in a number of cases, relate directly to well-known optical factors. For instance, the lower-order terms correspond to tilt, astigmatism, and sphere. Higher-order terms are related to coma and spherical aberration, as well as a number of optical errors that do not have a familiar name. The primary practical advantage of wavefront reconstruction is that it lets us also calculate the quality of the image that the eye forms.

Defining Retinal Image Quality

The goal of measuring wavefront aberrations is to accurately assess the quality of the image formed on the retina. The goal of refractive correction is to improve the quality of the image formed on the retina. Unfortunately, there is no generally agreed upon definition of retinal image quality. Clinical studies often use visual acuity as an endpoint. However, visual acuity is not an ideal estimate since many everyday visual tasks are dependent on the image quality at lower spatial frequencies and less dependent on fine detail. In addition, while there are fundamental neural limits that restrict the amount of improvement in acuity that can be expected with wavefront-guided corrections, for some observers, larger improvements in the contrast sensitivity at midfrequencies may be possible.[12] In optically "good" imaging systems, a commonly used metric is the root mean square (RMS) wavefront error, which is the average distance from the reference sphere and represents the smoothness of the wavefront (a diffraction-limited optical system has an RMS error of zero). However, RMS wavefront error has some major problems in optical systems that are highly aberrated, such as the eye. As an alternative, we pre-

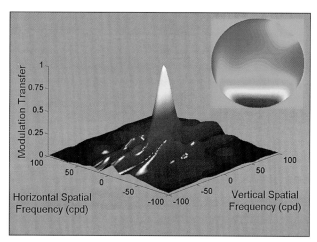

Figure 16-3. An example of the wavefront map for a 7.6-mm pupil (inset, upper right) and the resulting MTF for that eye. Note that in this particular eye, the optics are relatively good across the horizontal extent of the pupil (there are few variations in wave height) but poor vertically. This translates into good contrast sensitivity for vertical spatial frequencies but poor for horizontal ones.

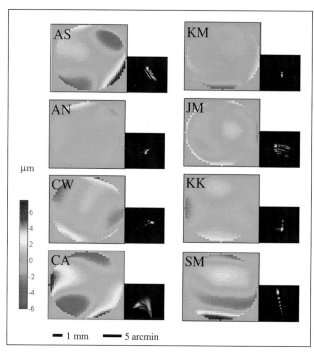

Figure 16-4. Wavefront aberrations for eight subjects. Defocus has been cancelled in all cases. The grayscale images represent the images of a distant point source that would be formed on the retina (the PSF), computed from the wavefront aberration assuming a 6-mm pupil size and considering the cone's directionality apodization function (which was independently measured for each subject). Note that greater retinal blur is associated with larger amounts of aberration. The color bar shows the scale in microns for the wavefront error. Scale bars indicate pupil scale (in millimeters) for the wavefront aberration and retinal scale (in arc/minute) for the PSF, respectively.

fer a metric that provides information on the light distribution that is available at the retinal level. The first of these is the point spread function (PSF), which can be thought of as the retinal image of a distant point (such as a star). Probably even better, since it is more easily quantified and related to clinical tests such as contrast sensitivity, is the modulation transfer function (MTF) of the eye, which is simply the proportion of the contrast at each frequency and orientation that is transmitted by the optics. Since the MTF is the magnitude of the Fourier transform of the PSF, the two are directly related. To obtain a single number, the MTF can be summed across frequencies and orientations to give the MTF volume. For comparison to specific subjective tests, such as contrast sensitivity tests, the MTF at that frequency can be computed. Figure 16-3 shows an example of a wavefront (inset, upper right) and the resulting two-dimensional MTF for that eye. Note that this particular eye has very good image quality in one axis but is poor along the other axis. This is not an uncommon feature of human eyes.

RESULTS

Basic Wavefront and Point Spread Function Measurements

The optical quality of the eye varies considerably across individuals. Figure 16-4 shows reconstructed wavefront maps and the resulting PSFs on the retina for eight relatively young subjects (ages 23 to 35). In these wavefronts we show the results if the subjects had a perfect refractive correction for a small pupil. It is clear that the aberration pattern, as well as its magnitude, changes greatly across subjects.

Reproducibility of the Spatially Resolved Refractometer

Overall reproducibility has been reported by He, et al.[1] We find that subjects can reliably measure ray aberrations with a standard error of the mean of 0.27 milliradians, which is equal to the ray deviation produced by 0.09 diopters (D) of blur at the edge of a 6-mm pupil. This is about the minimum resolvable blur for the human eye, providing a good match between the measurements and the visual capacity

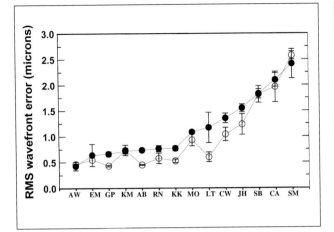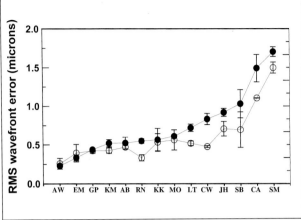

Figure 16-5. A comparison of the RMS wavefront error for the natural (solid symbols) and dilated (open symbols) pupil in 15 subjects. All calculations are for a 7.6 mm pupil. Left: The RMS wavefront error is calculated excluding only spherical defocus. Right: RMS is calculated excluding spherical and astigmatic defocus.

of the subjects. Testing on healthy laboratory subjects, we found that the results are reproducible over a time period of 2 years. Finally, it was possible to test subjects ranging from 11 years[13,14] to over 60 years old.[15]

Changes in Wavefront with Static Accommodation

We have used the SRR to measure the change in the wavefront with static accommodation.[16] We find that there are systematic changes that occur in the wavefront quality of the eye with accommodation. In general, subjects tend to have the lowest RMS wavefront error when they are accommodating about 1 to 2 D in from their far point.

Changes in the Wavefront with Mydriatics

We have also made a series of measurements of the wavefront aberrations of the eye under various pharmacological states. Figure 16-5 shows the effect of dilation with 5% tropicamide compared to the natural pupil (where mydriasis was achieved by using low light conditions) for 15 subjects. We show both the changes in the RMS error for all the aberrations except spherical error (see Figure 16-5, left) and the change in aberrations for discounting spherical and astigmatic errors (see Figure 16-5, right). Note that in general the optical quality of the eye is better in the natural as opposed to the pharmacologically dilated pupil.

The Effect of Wavelength

The SRR is also useful for examining the effect of wavelength on the wavefront aberrations of the eye.

In general the optical quality of the eye is better in the natural as opposed to the pharmacologically dilated pupil.

The largest aberrations for most eyes are the changes in focus that occur across wavelengths with polychromatic (white) light. Chromatic aberrations arise from the difference in the index of refraction of the eye's tissue across wavelengths. These changes in refractive index cause changes in both the refractive power of the eye with wavelength and changes in the magnification of images with wavelength. The refractive power of the eye varies by about 2 D across the visible spectrum.[6,17-19] The change in spherical refractive power is commonly called the longitudinal chromatic aberration (LCA). In addition to this difference in refractive power, there is also a difference in where the images at different wavelengths fall on the retina. This occurs because ocular optics comprise a compound lens system and because the fovea is not on the optical axis of the eye (magnification changes that occur with wavelength), producing wavelength-dependent displacements. These displacements with changes in wavelength are generally called transverse chromatic aberrations (TCAs). TCA varies from subject to subject.[6] In addition, the actual perceived TCA varies considerably whether one accounts for the influence of the cones (the Stiles-Crawford effect, or SCE20) or not.[6] In general, the changes in higher-order aberrations with changes in wavelength are relatively small. Figure 16-6 shows the calculated MTFs (radial profiles) of the effect of "perfect" aberration correction for one of our sub-

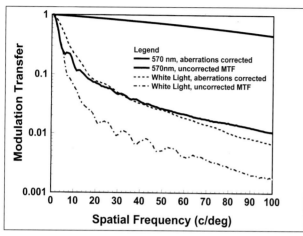

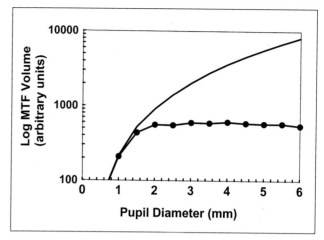

Figure 16-6. The calculated effect of "perfect" customized corneal ablation on the monochromatic and white light MTF (data from Marcos S, Burns SA, Moreno-Barriusop E, Navarro R. A new approach to the study of ocular chromatic aberrations. *Vision Res.* 1999;39(26):4309-4323). The full wavefront aberrations were measured at six wavelengths. In addition, the TCA at each point in the pupil was measured. We then calculated the MTF for white (lower dashed curve) and 570 nm (lower solid curve) light. We next calculated the MTF if all monochromatic aberrations were corrected for both white (upper dashed curve) and 570 nm (upper solid curve) light. Clearly, while such surgery improves the MTF, the effect in white light is much smaller than that in monochromatic light.

> If one considers only the monochromatic aberrations, a very significant improvement in the MTF is theoretically possible. However, for the white light the possible improvement is reduced, though still significant.

ject's eyes that was corrected at 570 nm but viewed broadband white light. For this calculation the aberrations were measured at six wavelengths from 460 nm to 650 nm, and the data for other wavelengths were estimated from these. TCA was measured using a two-wavelength technique.[6] If one considers only the monochromatic aberrations, a very significant improvement in the MTF is theoretically possible (top curve). However, for the white light the possible improvement is reduced, though still significant. What is not shown here is that for subjects with large amounts of TCA, the resulting MTF is highly asymmetric since TCA tends to decrease contrast in one dimension while leaving it relatively unaffected in the other dimension.

Figure 16-7. The change in MTF volume with pupil diameter for a diffraction-limited eye (solid line) and a real eye (circles). For small pupil diameters, the eye is close to diffraction limited. However, for larger pupil diameters the eye is severely limited by aberrations.

The Role of Photoreceptors and Image Apodization

It is well known that the image quality of an optical system depends on the size of the pupil used. For instance, it is common in ophthalmology to check the visual acuity of a subject when viewing an acuity target through a small artificial pupil (or pinhole). This small pupil serves to limit the importance of the aberrations (Figure 16-7) by limiting the area over which light enters the eye to a relatively uniform region of the wavefront (this limitation is called apodization). When the spatial variation in the wavefront is small relative to the pupil size, the optical system is essentially diffraction limited. In a real eye, it is not only the pupil that acts to apodize the wavefront aberrations, but also the cone photoreceptors themselves. It has been known for over 30 years that the visual system has different sensitivities to light coming from different points in the pupil. The effect, known as the SCE,[20] occurs because the cones themselves act as waveguides[21-23] and are oriented toward specific portions of the pupil. This differential sensitivity of the cones to light from different points in the pupil can have an important influence on the aberrations of the eye.[24,25] Recently, we have shown that when the actual wavefront aberrations and the cones are directionality measured[26] in the same subjects, the cones can improve the retinal image quality.[27]

Figure 16-8 shows sample results for one subject. Here we have shown the change in the MTF volume as a function of defocus, because the combination of

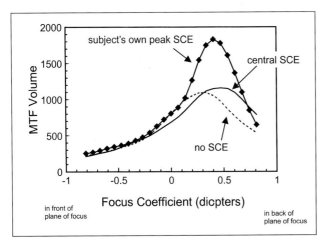

Figure 16-8. The change in volume of the two-dimensional MTF with the addition of the cone directionality. The dashed line shows the whole pupil (6 mm) MTF volume for various positions around the small pupil focus. The addition of a central SCE improves the imaging for hyperopic defocus (solid line). Placing the Stiles-Crawford peak at this subject's own optimal location greatly increases the image quality (solid lines plus symbols).

the aberrations and the apodization in a real eye causes the best MTF to occur at a different focus than the paraxial defocus, which is predicted by the Zernike fits. It should be noted that this subject has an unusually large improvement of the MTF by cone apodization. In our larger sample, the effect tends to be smaller.

DISCUSSION

The SRR can be a valuable tool for investigating the image-forming ability of the eye. In our laboratory we have been able to test individuals ranging in age from 20 to over 60 years of age. Other researchers have successfully applied the device to both pediatric[13,14] and clinical populations. The current system implemented in our laboratory does have some limitations, mainly in that it has three separate optical channels that require careful alignment. However, we are currently constructing a more compact system.[27]

Using the SRR we have identified a number of factors that can limit the ability of wavefront-guided refractive surgery to improve vision. We have shown that in young observers, accommodation is an important factor. Wavefront aberrations are at a minimum at the resting point of accommodation,[13] and

this needs to be factored into surgical decisions. We have also shown that chromatic aberrations are very important, and in some observers TCA can be both large and change dynamically with pupil size.[6] A correction of monochromatic aberrations will not provide perfect optics if the chromatic aberrations are not also compensated. Finally, the pharmacological state of the pupil is important. While we showed results for the effects of mild mydriatics, we have observed in two subjects that cyclopentelate can also alter the wavefront aberrations. While these pharmacological effects are not particularly large, they are not always in the same direction and require better understanding of the causes before we can properly talk about eliminating wavefront aberrations. Finally, we have found that there are potentially large interactions between the region in the pupil toward which the photoreceptors are oriented and the wavefront quality of the eye. There is considerable individual variation in photoreceptor alignment in the normal population,[26-28] as a result this factor could be important in understanding the result of surgery. A simple example is that for some subjects, the maximum visual sensitivity is found for light entering the eye up to 3 mm from the center of the dilated pupil. For these subjects, a large pupil and a surgical transition zone that overlays the region of maximum sensitivity could be quite bothersome.

CONCLUSION

The spatially resolved refractometer is a reliable, reproducible technique for measuring the wavefront aberrations of the human eye. Working with Navarro, et al[29] we found that the SRR gives essentially identical estimates of the wavefront aberrations to measurements in the same eye using either a Hartmann-Shack wavefront sensor or a laser ray-tracing technique.[30] It has both strengths and weaknesses related to other techniques in use for measuring the wavefront aberrations of the eye. Because it uses the subject's own visual system to determine the wavefront, it is truly a single pass measurement. There are no assumptions about the reflecting layers in the eye and their spatial relation to the photoreceptors. While this is not an important assumption in normal eyes,[31] it may be important in older or diseased eyes. However, at the same time it is slower than the optical measurements, although the time involved is not a problem for most subjects. We can currently obtain a full measurement in 3 to 4 min-

> The SRR is a sequential technique, which means the patient's pupil could be sampled adaptively, with increased density of pupil sampling in bad regions (much as do modern automatic perimetry programs).

utes, and there is room to improve this. The SRR is a sequential technique, which means the patient's pupil could be sampled adaptively, with increased density of pupil sampling in bad regions (much as do modern automatic perimetry programs). However, techniques such as the Hartmann-Shack wavefront sensor can be used in less than a second. The Hartmann-Shack has the disadvantage that it can be quite difficult to apply in some eyes with large aberrations,[32,33] lens changes, and it requires a strong reflection from the retina.

Acknowledgments

Supported by NEI RO1-EY04395, Human Frontier Science Program LT-542/97, and Department of Energy Center of Excellence Grant DE-FG-02-91ER61229.

References

1. He JC, Marcos S, Webb RH, Burns SA. Measurement of the wavefront aberration of the eye by a fast psychophysical procedure. *J Opt Soc Am A*. 1998;15(9):2449-2456.

2. Penney CM, Webb RH, Tieman JT, Thompson KP. Spatially resolved objective refractometer. US Patent; 1993.

3. Webb RH, Penney CM, Thompson KP. Measurement of ocular wavefront distortion with a spatially resolved refractometer. *Applied Optics*. 1992;31:3678-3686.

4. Cubalachini R. Modal wavefront estimation from wavefront slope measurements. *J Opt Soc Am A*. 1979;69:972-977.

5. Southwell WH. Wavefront estimation from phase derivative measurements. *J Opt Soc Am A*. 1980;70:998-1006.

6. Marcos S, Burns SA, Moreno-Barriusop E, Navarro R. A new approach to the study of ocular chromatic aberrations. *Vision Res*. 1999;39(26):4309-4323.

7. Mahajan VN. Zernike circle polynomials and optical aberrations of systems with circular pupils. Engineering and laboratory notes. *Optics and Photonics News*. 1994;21-24.

8. Malacara D. *Optical Shop Testing*. New York, NY: Wiley; 1992.

9. Born M, Wolf E. *Principles of Optics*. Oxford, England: Pergamon Press; 1983.

10. Schwiegerling J, Grievenkamp JE, Miller JM. Representation of videokeratoscopic height data with Zernike polynomials. *J Opt Soc Am A*. 1995;12:2105-2113.

11. Wang JY, Silva DE. Wavefront interpretation with Zernike polynomials. *Applied Optics*. 1980;19:1510-1517.

12. Lopez-Gil N, Howland HC. Influence of coma and spherical aberration on contrast sensitivity of the human eye. *Invest Ophthalmol Vis Sci*. 1999;40(4):1941.

13. He JC, Gwiazda J, Held R, Thorn F, Ong E, Marran L. Wavefront aberrations in the eyes of myopic and emmetropic school children and young adults. Presented at the VIII International Conference on Myopia. Boston, Mass; 2000.

14. He JC, Ong E, Gwiazda J, Held R, Thorn F. Wavefront aberrations in the cornea and the whole eye. *Invest Ophthalmol Vis Sci*. 2000;41:S104.

15. McLellan JS, Marcos S, Burns SA. The change in wavefront aberration of the eye with age. *Invest Ophthalmol Vis Sci*. 1999;40(4):189B149.

16. He JC, Burns SA, Marcos S. Monochromatic aberrations in the accommodated human eye. *Vision Res*. 2000;40(1):41-48.

17. Bedford RE, Wyszecki GW. Axial chromatic aberration of the human eye. *J Opt Soc Am A*. 1957;47:564-565.

18. Morrell A, Whitefoot HD, Charman WN. Ocular chromatic aberration and age. *Ophthalmic Physiol Opt*. 1991;11(4):385-390.

19. Thibos LN, Bradley A, Zhang XX. Effect of ocular chromatic aberration on monocular visual performance. *Optom Vis Sci*. 1991;68(8):599-607.

20. Stiles WS, Crawford BH. The luminous efficiency of rays entering the eye pupil at different points. *Proceedings of the Royal Society (London) B*. 1933;112:428-450.

21. Enoch JM. Visualization of waveguide models in retinal receptors. *Am J Ophthalmol*. 1961;51:1107-1118.

22. Snitzer E. Cylindrical dielectric waveguide modes. *J Opt Soc Am A*. 1961;51:491-498.

23. Toraldo de Francia G. Retina cones as dielectric antennas. *J Opt Soc Am A*. 1949;39:324.

24. Metcalf H. Stiles-Crawford apodization. *J Opt Soc Am A*. 1965;35:72-74.

25. Mino M, Okano Y. Improvement in the OTF of a defocused optical system through the use of shaded apertures. *Applied Optics*. 1971;10:2219-2225.

26. Burns SA, Wu S, Delori FC, Elsner AE. Direct measurement of human cone photoreceptor alignment. *J Opt Soc Am A*. 1995;12(10):2329-2338.

27. Burns S, Marcos S. *Evaluating the Role of Cone Directionality in Image Formation.* Washington, DC: Optical Society of America; 2000.

28. Webb RH, Burns SA, Penney M. *Coaxial Spatially Resolved Refractometer.* Boston, Mass: Schepens Eye Research Institute; 1999.

29. Applegate RA, Lakshminarayanan V. Parametric representation of Stiles-Crawford functions: normal variation of peak location and directionality. *J Opt Soc Am A.* 1993;10:1611-1623.

30. Navarro R, Moreno-Barriuso E, Marcos S, Burns S. Comparing laser ray tracing, Hartmann-Shack wavefront sensor, and spatially resolved refractometer to measure ocular aberrations. *Invest Ophthalmol Vis Sci.* In press.

31. Navarro R, Losada MA. Aberrations and relative efficiency of light pencils in the living human eye. *Optom Vis Sci.* 1997;74(7):540-547.

32. Williams DR, Brainard DH, McMahon MJ, Navarro R. Double-pass and interferometric measures of the optical quality of the eye. *J Opt Soc Am A.* 1994;11:3123-3135.

33. Moreno-Barriuso E, Navarro R. Laser ray tracing versus Hartmann-Shack sensor for measuring optical aberrations in the human eye. *J Opt Soc Am A.* In press.

Chapter Seventeen

Customized Ablation Using the Nidek Laser

Scott M. MacRae, MD
Masano Fujieda, MA

PRINCIPLE OF THE SCANNING SLIT REFRACTOMETER

Overview

This chapter presents the approach of using a scanning slit refractometer (the OPD Scan, Nidek) in conjunction with a corneal topography system to guide customized corneal ablation. Optical path difference (OPD) refers to the differences in optical path lengths. This is discussed in more detail in Chapter Nineteen. This diagnostic system is coupled with the Nidek EC-5000 system, which combines scanning slit and a scanning small area ablation (1.0 mm) to perform a customized ablation.

INTRODUCTION

Customized corneal ablation can be done using a variety of diagnostic techniques including the Hartmann-Shack wavefront sensing aberroscope, the spatially resolved refractometer (SRR), and a variety of other diagnostic instruments.[1-4] Nidek Co, Ltd has developed a diagnostic instrument based on retinoscopic principles. This is a specialized autorefraction system coupled with a corneal topography system. The resulting diagnostic information can then be used in conjunction with the new Nidek EC-5000, which has a larger area scanning slit as well as small area ablation capabilities to perform excimer laser customized ablation.

METHODS

The OPD Scan measuring principle uses retinoscopic information obtained in the following fashion. There is a projecting system and a receiving system. Both the projecting system and the receiving system rotate around an optical axis synchronously to measure the refraction at each 1-degree meridian.

The projecting system consists of an infrared LED that emits light, which goes through a chopper wheel, then a projecting lens and several mirrors (Figure 17-1). The chopper wheel, with its slit apertures, is located between the light source (LED) and the projecting lens. It rotates constantly at high speed to scan the retina. The chopper wheel has slit apertures that create slit-shaped light bundles. The projecting system rotates 180 degrees in 0.4 seconds across both hemimeridians so that 360 meridians are covered. The slit light rays go into the retina and are reflected back out the eye and through a receiving lens, an aperture stop, and finally a group of pho-

> The slit light rays go into the retina and are reflected back out the eye and through a receiving lens, an aperture stop, and finally a group of photodetectors that receive the light signal.

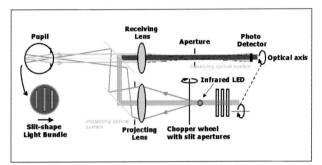

Figure 17-1. OPD Scan projecting and receiving system. Infrared light is generated and passes through a chopper wheel, which creates slits of light that pass through a projecting lens and mirrors. The light slits then go into the eye and reflect off the retina through a receiving lens, an aperture, and onto photoreceptors. The projecting and receiving system rotates synchronously around an optical axis.

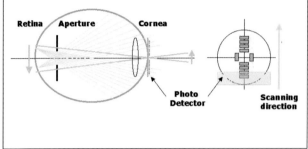

Figure 17-2. OPD Scan photodetectors. The LED (see Figure 17-1) and photodetectors are conjugate with the cornea. There are four photodetector pairs (above and below the optical axis) that measure light at 2 to 5.5 mm in diameter at the corneal plane. There is also a pair of photodetectors located horizontally, which locates the center of the four photodetector pairs. This determines the center of the optical axis.

todetectors that receive the light signal. The LED and photodetectors are conjugate with the cornea. The aperture stop is conjugate with the retina when the eye is emmetropic. In myopia, the aperture stop is in front of the retina; in hyperopia, the aperture stop is behind the retina.

There are four photodetectors above and four photodetectors below the optical axis. There are also two photodetectors, one on each side, which detect the center of the photodetector pairs. This center point determines the optical axis of the eye (Figure 17-2) when the optical axis of this device and the examined eye are aligned correctly. The photodetectors measure light at the corneal plane at diameters of 2.0, 3.2, 4.4, and 5.5 mm.

Figures 17-3 through 17-11 demonstrate the system in myopia, emmetropia, and hyperopia.

In the myopic eye, the aperture stop is located in front of the retina. The incoming slit-shaped light bundle bounces off the retina and the reflecting slit moves in an opposite direction compared to the incoming slit. This causes the lower photodetector cells to be stimulated earlier than the upper photodetectors, indicating myopia (see Figures 17-3 to 17-6).

In the emmetropic eye, the aperture stop is located directly on the retina. Under these conditions the incoming slit-shaped light bundle goes into the retina and comes out synchronously so that all of the photodetectors are excited simultaneously (see Figure 17-7).

In hyperopia, the aperture stop is located behind the retina. The scanning slit light is reflected off the

retina and the reflecting slit moves in the same direction as the incoming slit light. Thus, the upper photo detectors are stimulated earlier than the lower photo detectors by the returning light, as noted in Figures 17-8 to 17-11.

The time difference generated at any point on the cornea is based on the optical path distance between the retina and the aperture. The time difference between the center and each photodetector in the four pairs is converted into the refractive power.

The placido rings are used to measure corneal topography and integrate these data into the assessment.

RESULTS

Figure 17-12 demonstrates the output data for the OPD Scan for a patient with mild myopia and slight cylinder. The data output includes an axial topography map (upper left). This axial topography map can then be converted to a refractive power map (lower left). In addition, the slit light bundle autorefraction system generates a refractive power map, shown in the upper right. The refractive power map from the topography and autorefraction can be combined as well, as shown in the lower right portion of Figure

> The refractive power map from the topography and autorefraction can be combined... The corneal topography data can be helpful in eyes that have a corneal opacity that may interfere with data acquisition using the autorefractor.

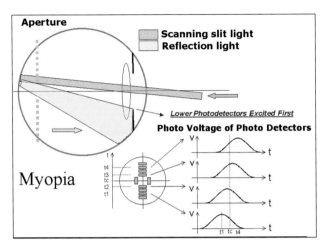

Figure 17-3. OPD Scan scanning light slit in myopia. The slit light goes in (blue) and reflects off the retina (yellow) and stimulates the lower photodetectors before the others.

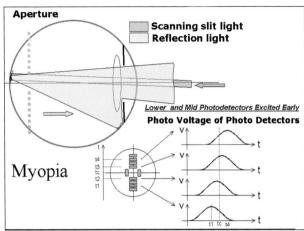

Figure 17-4. OPD Scan in myopia. The lower and mid photodetectors are excited early.

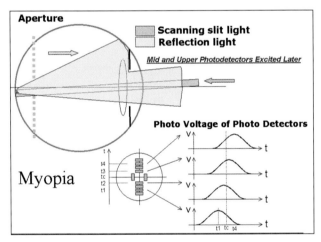

Figure 17-5. OPD Scan in myopia. The mid and upper photodetectors are excited later.

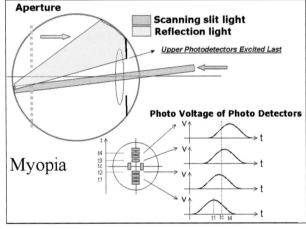

Figure 17-6. OPD Scan in myopia. The upper photodetectors are excited last.

17-12, which is a normal myope with moderate astigmatism. Figure 17-13 demonstrates the same series of maps on a postoperative PRK eye that had -4.25 diopters (D) of myopia preoperatively.

DISCUSSION

The Scanning Slit Diagnostic Approach— OPD Scan

There are some key points to this system:
1. It measures the time difference between the center of the cornea and each of the photodetectors.
2. The time difference is proportional to the refractive power.
3. The refractive power range is wide (0 to ± 20 D spherical, 0 to ± 12 D).
   - Sphere 0 to ± 20 D
   - Cylinder 0 to ± 12 D
4. This retinoscopic autorefractive system does not assume the eye is symmetric (previous autorefractors assumed the eye's symmetry).

The number of diameters measured for each half of the cornea can be increased. The addition of another photodetector at the 6.0 to 6.5 mm diameter is also being considered. It will also be very interesting to

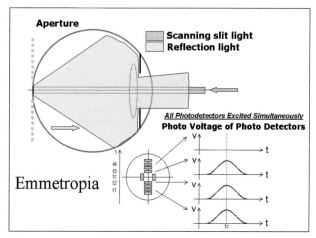

Figure 17-7. OPD Scan scanning light slit in emmetropia. All photodetectors are excited simultaneously.

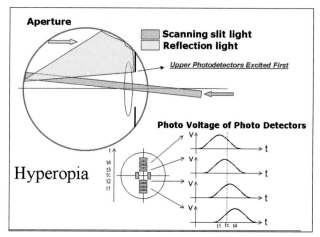

Figure 17-8. OPD Scan scanning light slit in hyperopia. The slit light excites the upper photodetectors before the others.

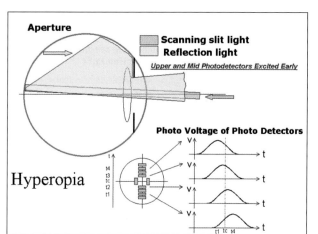

Figure 17-9. OPD Scan in hyperopia. The slit light exits the upper and mid photodetectors early.

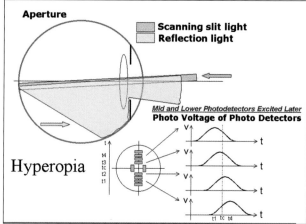

Figure 17-10. OPD Scan in hyperopia. The slit light exits the mid and lower photodetectors later.

integrate the corneal topography data with the autorefraction data and see how these two systems interact pre- and postoperatively. The corneal topography data can provide feedback on how the cornea has been reshaped after the laser treatment. The corneal topography data can also be helpful in eyes that have a corneal opacity that may interfere with data acquisition using the autorefractor.

THE NIDEK EC-5000 SCANNING SLIT AND SMALL AREA ABLATION

The system can be combined with the Nidek EC-5000 in a unique fashion. The Nidek EC-5000 has a scanning slit delivery system that can treat over 7.5

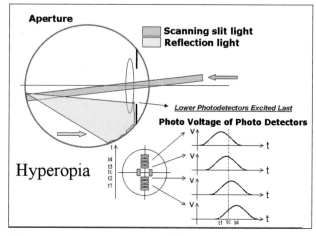

Figure 17-11. OPD Scan in hyperopia. The slit light exits the lower photodetectors last.

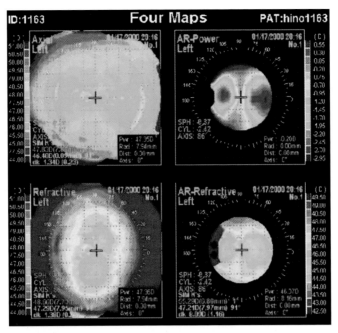

Figure 17-12. Corneal topography with OPD Scan with myopic astigmatism. The upper left figure demonstrates an axial topography map. The lower left figure is a refractive power map based on the axial topography. The upper right figure demonstrates the slit light autorefraction system that also generates a refractive power map. In the lower right figure, the refractive power map from the topography and autorefraction are combined into a refractive power map.

mm of the cornea in myopia and up to 10 mm of the cornea in hyperopia. It uses 10 to 40 Hz. The larger area ablation can be combined with a new small area (1.0 mm) ablation over a 10-mm diameter of the cornea. This combination of the scanning slit system with the segmental small area ablation (1.0 mm) allows for more efficient treatment and shorter treatment times.

The segmental spot uses a 1.0-mm small area ablation that can be implemented at the end of the traditional sphere and cylinder treatment, which uses the scanning slit. The segmental small area ablation treatment can be used to treat subtle irregularities for a customized ablation based on the OPD Scan diagnostic system.

Figure 17-14 demonstrates the segmental small area ablation. There are six apertures that can deliver more than one small area ablation treatment at a time for greater efficiency. Figure 17-15 demonstrates the combination of the scanning slit in the segmental ablation program. Shown in this figure is the regular spherical treatment, aspheric treatment, and segmen-

> The segmental small area ablation (1.0 mm) can treat subtle aberrations after the traditional sphere and cylinder treatment, which uses the scanning slit.

tal small area ablation programs. The segmental small area ablation (1.0 mm) can treat subtle aberrations that are detected by the OPD Scan.

SUMMARY

The Nidek customized ablation system utilizes retinoscopic principles in the OPD Scan system to give wavefront data. This information is combined with corneal topography for the pre- and postoperative evaluation. The new Nidek EC-5000 laser delivery system combines the traditional scanning slit with a newer segmental small area (1.0 mm) of ablation to maximize laser efficiency. Further evaluation of this system will be of great interest to the refractive surgical community. Such combination strategies may be more common in the future.

Figure 17-13. Demonstration of the same display sequence as in Figure 17-12 in a patient who was treated with a -4.25 D spherical PRK.

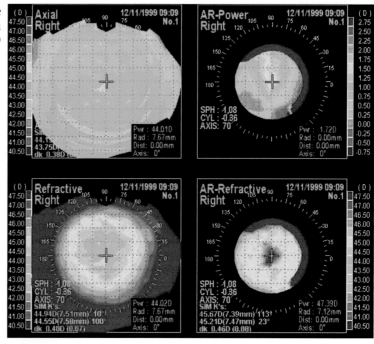

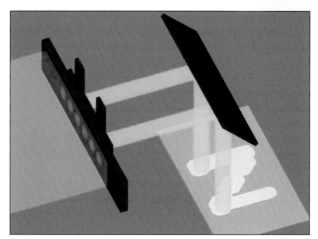

Figure 17-14. Nidek EC-5000 segmental small area ablation. Six apertures deliver small area ablation (1.0 mm) over a 10 mm diameter area. Several apertures can be opened simultaneously for greater efficiency, as shown.

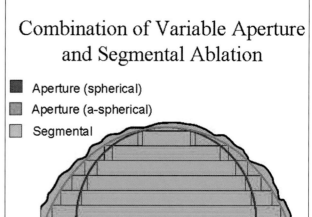

Figure 17-15. Nidek EC-5000 combines the variable aperture of the current scanning slit system with the segmental small area (1.0 mm) ablation. It can treat with spherical (red outline, upper left) and newer aspheric (green, upper right) ablation using the current scanning slit system. The aspheric program is used to reduce spherical aberration. The segmental small area ablation (gold area removed) removed a customized treatment area of more subtle irregularities detected by the OPD Scan.

REFERENCES

1. MacRae SM. Supernormal vision, hypervision and customized corneal ablation. *J Cataract Refract Surg.* 2000;26:154-157.

2. Liang J, Williams DR, Miller DT. Supernormal vision and high-resolution retinal imaging through adaptive optics. *J Opt Soc Am A.* 1997;14:2884-2892.

3. Liang J, Grimm B, Geolz S, Bille JF. Objective measurement of wave aberrations of the human eye with the use of a Hartmann-Shack wavefront sensor. *J Opt Oct Am A.* 1994;11:1949-1957.

4. Howland HC, Howland B. A subjective method for the measurement of monochromatic aberrations of the eye. *J Opt Soc Am A.* 1977;67:1508-1518.

Corneal Topography-Guided Ablations

Basic Science Section

Chapter Eighteen

What Corneal Topography Can Tell You About Corneal Shape

Tim N. Turner, PhD

Corneal topography measures surface shape, not optical power. The fundamental measures of surface size and shape are curvature, slope (or inclination), height, and relative elevation. They are related but distinctly different measures. Height measures position in space. Elevation measures position relative to some close-fitting reference surface. Slope and inclination measure the orientation of tangent and normal lines (Figure 18-1). Curvature measures bending (the sharper the bend, the greater the curvature) and is inversely proportional to radius of curvature. All are local, meaning their values are determined by a small neighborhood or surface patch surrounding the point of interest. Height and elevation are uniquely valued (every surface point has but one value), while slope and curvature have an infinite number of values at each surface point, one for each direction of measurement. Directed curvatures and slopes are those measured in definite directions.

HISTORICAL PERSPECTIVE

Because of its historical connection with keratometry, maps of corneal surface curvature have been expressed in dioptric units of optical power. This unfortunate tradition has confused geometric shape and optical power. To cut through this haze, the recently adopted American National Standards Institute (ANSI) *Standards in Corneal Topography*[1] (see Appendix Two) has defined the "keratometric

diopter (D)" to be a unit of curvature, not optical power. It applies only to the anterior surface of the cornea,[1] inverse millimeter of curvature equaling 337.5 keratometric D (eg, an 8 mm radius sphere has a curvature of one-eighth inverse millimeter or 337.5/8 keratometric diopters).

This does not mean that corneal topography can not yield optical information. Nevertheless, optical power maps and point spread functions (PSFs) derived from topography are necessarily optical simulations based on refractive index models supplementing surface shape and are calculated via ray tracing.

Although all corneal topography instruments measure shape, different technologies directly measure different geometric properties of the cornea. Reflective devices (all placido ring instruments) directly measure radial surface slope from reflected images. From these data, surface curvature and height are deduced. Projective devices (eg, Orbscan, Par, and Euclid) directly measure surface height by triangulating projected light beams. As all corneal topography instruments, excepting Orbscan (Bausch & Lomb Orbtek, Salt Lake City, Utah), measure only the anterior tear film, inferred corneal shape must assume tear film uniformity. When the tear film is broken or pooled, this assumption breaks down, making the data invalid (Figure 18-2).

A projective slit-scan system (such as Orbscan) is unique in that it measures several ocular surfaces

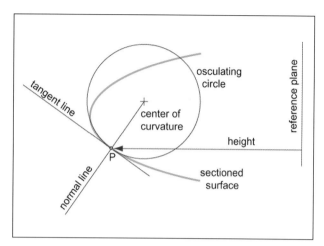

Figure 18-1. Height, slope, and curvature. This meridional section through a prolate surface (like the anterior cornea) illustrates the geometric constructs required to determine the height, slope, and curvature of the surface at a point P. The normal line is the local perpendicular to the surface. It passes through the local center of curvature, defined by the osculating circle that just "kisses" or best fits the sectioned surface at P. Height is just the three-space position of P. It is measured in millimeters. Slope and inclination both refer to the orientation of the tangent line through P. Slope is the dimensionless ratio of rise over run, while inclination is the equivalent angle. Curvature equals the reciprocal radius of the osculating circle. Its natural units are inverse millimeters.

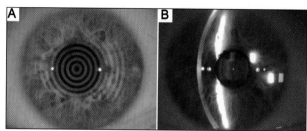

Figure 18-2. Raw data images. A: single placido ring image used in reflective systems. This image, which covers the cornea, is generated by the anterior tear film surface. B: one of many Orbscan slit-beam images. The light beam penetrates the cornea and lens, locating edges on both corneal surfaces, the anterior lens, and anterior iris. Forty slit-scan images taken in succession are required to cover the cornea.

(interfaces between light scattering tissues and non-scattering humors) within the anterior segment. Internal surfaces are ray trace triangulated, which requires the use of refractive index models but removes any optical distortion induced by looking through the cornea.

Since instrument accuracy is limited by the weakest link in a system, it can vary dramatically between instrument makes and models. Nevertheless, useful generalizations can be made about instrument classes. Reflected data are inherently the most precise but are also very sensitive to tear film irregularity and corneal pathology. In the absence of surface irregularities, reflective devices typically measure curvature accurately. Projective devices often have difficulty with curvature because of the mathematical differentiation required to translate height into curvature. However, projective devices are much more robust and able to measure height over greater corneal area and with uniform accuracy. Corneal pathologies like keratoconus, which may confuse reflective placido devices, are easily characterized by projective systems.

It is important to realize that all instruments have some background level of random measurement noise, that this noise level may vary with map type (eg, curvature versus elevation), and that any instrument will at one time or another take a bad exam. To get a feel for the noise level of a particular instrument and map, take three exams of the same eye and compare them. Unrepeatable variations are noise, not genuine irregularity. Another useful test is to compare right and left eyes of the same patient. Genuine irregularities often possess mirror symmetry.

Early corneal topography instruments displayed anterior corneal shape in the form of one or two color-contour maps: axial curvature and meridional curvature. These are new ANSI standard names (Table 18-1 gives translations to older terminology). Meridional curvature is measured locally in meridional directions. Axial curvature is the radial average of meridional curvature from the map center to the point of interest. Axial curvature maps are always broader and smoother than their meridional counterparts, precisely because they are averaged or smoothed meridional maps. Their utility has more to do with looks and tradition than with science.

> Axial curvature maps are always broader and smoother than their meridional counterparts, precisely because they are averaged or smoothed meridional maps.

CURVATURE MAPPING

Curvature (erroneously called power) (Figure 18-3), although at one time was the only corneal topography descriptor in use, is now being superceded by

Table 18-1	
Corneal Topography Map Names	
ANSI Name[1]	*Obsolete Traditional Name*
Axial curvature	Axial or sagittal power, color map
Meridional curvature	Tangential or instantaneous power
Mean curvature	Mean power
Toricity	Astigmatic power

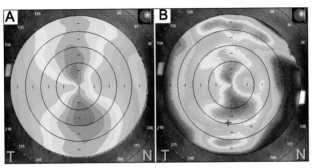

Figure 18-3. Curvature of regular astigmatism. A: axial curvature map, which is the radially averaged version of the meridional curvature map. B: the irregular contours are repeatable and real. When viewed with high-resolution topography (Orbscan II), even normal corneas have fine-scale irregularity. Note that relatively large curvatures (sharp or steep) are colored with red hues, while smaller curvatures (flat) are colored with blue hues.

surface height. Initially, curvature was important because it is proportional to the paraxial power of a surface. To be precise, we must specify a particular point of the surface because, like curvature, paraxial power is local in nature depending only on geometric and physical properties within a narrow thread-like region surrounding a prescribed optical axis. In contrast, the light forming the retinal image is not confined to a narrow paraxial thread but is a relatively broad beam, limited only by the pupil. To accurately calculate the retinal image and its optical aberrations, paraxial optics have been superceded by the more accurate theory of ray trace optics, which require surface height and slope data but not curvature.

If curvature no longer has optical importance (except for crude back-of-the-envelope estimates), does it have any other significance? Surprisingly, the answer is probably not. Modern ablation patterns do not specify change in curvature but do specify

height. As compared to curvature, a height correction is easy to calculate. A surface viewed in a curvature space is typically incomplete (some data required to completely characterize the surface are missing) and may be artifact ridden (eg, the bow tie is an artifact of displaying curvature measured only along intersecting meridians). While interpretation of curvature is hard, height is intuitive.

HEIGHT MAPPING

The problem with corneal height is that it cannot be directly displayed. The disparity of scales between local features of interest (microns high) and the global radius of curvature (millimeters in radius) does not permit global shape and local features to be viewed simultaneously. The problem is similar to viewing terrestrial mountains from space. When your field of view is large enough to encompass the whole earth, its mountains become imperceptible.

Terrestrial topography maps solve this problem by displaying local elevation relative to the mean sea level. Dry land above sea level is positively elevated, while sea floors below are negatively elevated. The same approach is taken in corneal topography, except that the cornea has no anatomic "mean sea level." Instead, the corneal topography instrument provides a symmetrical and close-fitting reference surface. Although a number of different shapes are used, the sphere is the simplest and provides the most generally useful reference surface. Local surface features lying above or outside the reference sphere have positive elevation and are colored with spectral hues on the red side of green. Features lying below or within the reference sphere are negatively elevated and are colored with hues on the blue side of green. Green ribbons separating red highs from blue lows mark areas where the reference sphere intersects (or is very near) the cornea. This color scheme, which applies to both corneal surfaces, fol-

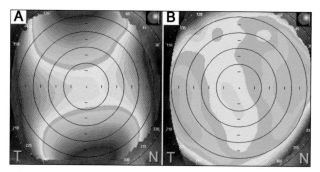

Figure 18-4. Normal astigmatic eyes. A: elevation map of the same with-the-rule astigmatic eye as in Figure 18-3. B: elevation map of an against-the-rule astigmatic eye. The steep meridian—the one having the sharpest curvature—always runs from "sea-to-sea" in elevation.

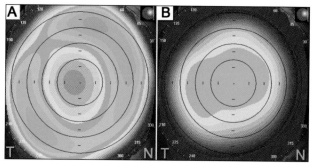

Figure 18-5. Normal spherical eye. A: elevation map with a 10-mm fit zone. B: elevation map of the same eye with a 3-mm fit zone. Elevation is surface height measured relative to a reference surface, which is constrained to fit the cornea as close as possible but only within a prescribed fit zone. Thus, changing the fit zone changes the map.

> The first thing one notices about elevation is that steepest and flattest meridians appear reversed. To properly interpret an elevation map, you must remember that it is not curvature (or power) but surface height measured relative to some reference surface, often called the best-fit sphere.

lows the pattern set long ago by terrestrial topography (Figure 18-4).

The first thing one notices about elevation is that steepest and flattest meridians appear reversed. To properly interpret an elevation map, you must remember that it is not curvature (or power) but surface height measured relative to some reference surface, often called the best-fit sphere. The steepest meridian has the sharpest curvature, which causes the corneal surface to drop below the best-fit sphere and be colored blue. The flattest meridian rises above the best-fit sphere and is colored red. Thus, the steep axis, which follows red in curvature, runs from "sea-to-sea" in elevation (ie, from blue to blue).

The second thing to notice about elevation is that a normal "spherical" eye (ie, one devoid of astigmatism) does not have a spherical cornea. The normal cornea is prolate, meaning it is sharper centrally than peripherally—similar to the pointy end of an egg. Such a shape has a distinctive elevation map: the central region rises above the best-fit sphere (red "hill"), the midperipheral zone falls below the sphere (annular blue "sea"), and the far peripheral zone again rises above (red peripheral "highlands"). The more prolate the cornea, the higher the central area will rise above the best-fit sphere.

This distinctive form (Figure 18-5A) only occurs

when the reference surface best fits the cornea over the entire map. If the area of best fit is reduced to a central disc, the resulting map (see Figure 18-5B) is centrally green (it follows the sphere) and is very high peripherally. Therefore, changing the fit zone changes the whole complexion of an elevation map.

This arbitrariness is a consequence of the cornea having no anatomic mean sea level. It also means that contours separating yellow from green or green from blue are no more significant than any other contours separating different shades of blue or yellow. Do not fall into the color trap, thinking one color is more significant than any other. Likewise, do not worry that different fit zones yield different elevation maps. Relative elevation is used only for human comprehension. Ablation patterns are calculated from absolute surface height. Nevertheless, to fairly compare eyes or exams, the same fit zone must be used.

The utility of a user-selectable fit zone is evident when comparing pre- and postoperative corneas corrected by refractive surgery. The goal of a myopic correction is to centrally flatten the cornea, which is done by centrally ablating tissue and reducing height. You can use an elevation difference (Figure 18-6) map to check the centration and depth of the ablation, but to do this, the two independently measured surfaces must be "properly" aligned one to the other. As tissue was only removed centrally, one might expect the periphery to remain unaltered. By selecting a large annular fit zone, the surfaces can be brought together peripherally. Now the central difference is a measure of the ablation depth.

Of course, the assumption that the cornea is only

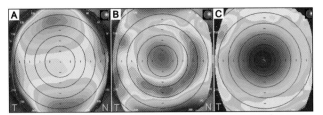

Figure 18-6. Pre- and post-LASIK elevation. A: Preoperative anterior elevation shows some with-the-rule astigmatism. B: Postoperative anterior elevation shows central flattening with some asymmetry. C: Post-minus preoperative elevation difference shows the ablation to be centered and symmetric. As the two exams were aligned peripherally (7- to 10-mm annular fit zone), the elevation difference (-137 microns) gives an estimate of the ablation depth.

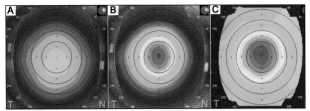

Figure 18-7. Pre- and post-LASIK corneal thickness. Ablation depth is more accurately measured via pachymetry difference. A: preoperative corneal thickness of the eye in Figure 18-6A. B: postoperative corneal thickness of the eye in Figure 18-6B. C: post minus preoperative pachymetry difference gives a central ablation depth of 169 microns. Notice the cornea also thickened peripherally (at least superiority), which is a secondary biomechanical effect that enhances the primary central ablative effect.

altered locally is fiction. Typically, central ablation also induces peripheral thickening (see Chapter Nine). These changes are best viewed by looking at a difference map of corneal thickness (Figure 18-7).

POSTERIOR CORNEAL SURFACE

The posterior corneal surface, although not as important optically as the anterior, is structurally more fluid and is therefore a sensitive indicator of abnormality. This occurs because corneal swelling allows posterior fibers to buckle inward, while anterior fibers remain under tension and retain their form. Because of this nature, the normal posterior surface is always more irregular than the anterior. Often, transience rather than just the magnitude of posterior irregularity is the best indicator of corneal instability whether due to disease, healing, or ectasia.

SURGICAL ECTASIA AND KERATOCONUS

One of the insidious complications of laser-assisted in situ keratomileusis (LASIK) surgery is ectasia: stromal thinning and weakening sometimes leading to anterior protrusion, which may be stable or progressive. As anterior protrusion results in loss of effect following a myopic correction, it is important to know the cause of regression. If the cause is ectasia, surgical enhancement will only worsen the result. Following the rule that stromal pathology always affects the posterior surface first, ectasia is most easily recognized in a series of posterior elevation maps (Figure 18-8).

One of the main uses of corneal topography has been to recognize subclinical keratoconus. Numerous indices and classifiers have been employed with success, except for the alarming number of false positives. When looking only at the anterior surface, nonpathological anomalies (sometimes introduced by contact lens wear) are sometimes impossible to differentiate from those incident to disease. Keratoconus (being a disease of the stroma) will first affect the structurally more sensitive posterior surface. In fact, one finds that every anterior cone always overlays a more significant and more easily identifiable posterior cone. When anterior and posterior elevations are perused together with corneal thickness maps, keratoconus detection is unequivocal (Figure 18-9).

Where is the apex of the keratoconus cone? Maps of elevation and corneal thickness all show the cone to be nearly symmetrical in shape. Apices at the centers of symmetry in each case (anterior protrusion, posterior excavation, and corneal thinning) all lie close to one another—the only exception being when anterior protrusion is still negligible. Thus, maps of elevation and thickness yield an unequivocal apex location. What is interesting is that this apex does not align with the area of maximum curvature on either the axial or meridional curvature map. The answer to this puzzle will help us understand why these axis-based curvatures tend to distort reality.

> Keratoconus (being a disease of the stroma) will first affect the structurally more sensitive posterior surface. In fact, one finds that every anterior cone always overlays a more significant and more easily identifiable posterior cone.

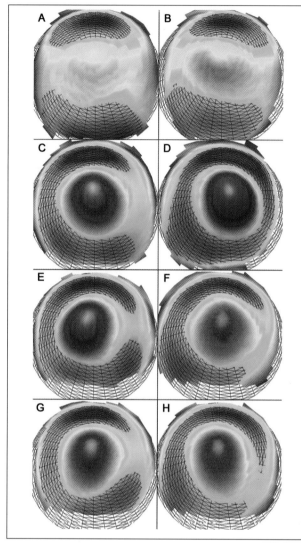

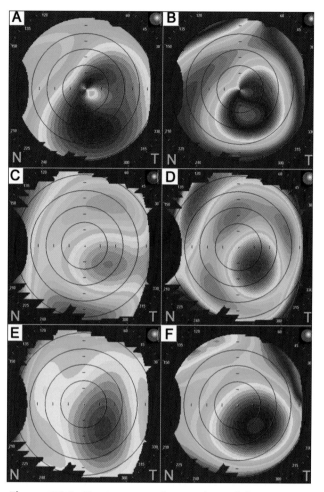

Figure 18-8. Post-LASIK ectasia. A: postoperative time series of both eyes of a bilateral LASIK patient (OD on the left, OS on the right). Although anterior elevation shows little change, these three-dimensional views of posterior elevation (A and B at 8 weeks postoperatively, C and D at 16 weeks, E and F at 32 weeks, and G and H at 90 weeks) show significant bilateral ectasia, which eventually reversed. The increase and eventual subsidence of posterior ectasia correlated to similar trends of decreasing and eventual improvement in best spectacle-corrected visual acuity.

Figure 18-9. Keratoconus. A: anterior axial curvature. B: anterior meridional curvature. C: anterior elevation. D: posterior elevation. E: corneal thickness. F: anterior mean curvature. The following topographic signs are characteristic of this disease. The posterior cone (D) is always significantly larger than the anterior cone (C). The cone is often geometrically symmetrical about coincident apices in elevation (C, D), the thickness minimum (E), and the mean curvature maximum (F). As the apex is a local maximum in mean curvature, the anterior cone is prolate (sharper toward the apex). The apex lies not at a meridional curvature maximum, but between the arms of the bent bow tie (B). Traditional axis-based curvature maps (A, B) give a distorted view of the corneal surface.

To measure surface curvature in a particular direction, the surface must be theoretically sliced by a plane. True curvature only results when the plane is perpendicular to the surface at the point of measurement. Such a plane is called a normal plane, and the resulting curvature is called normal curvature. Oblique curvature results when the surface is sliced by non-normal oblique planes. Oblique curvature, depending on the angle of obliquity, can have any value, from its true or normal value up to infinity. For example, consider a sphere with radius R and normal curvature 1/R. Its oblique curvature ranges from 1/R to infinity as the sphere is sliced first through the middle, then off center, and finally tangentially (Figure 18-10).

Both axial and meridional curvatures are oblique

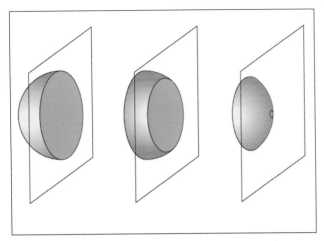

Figure 18-10. Slicing a sphere. When a sphere is sliced, its section is always a circle. The radius of the circular section depends on how the sphere was sliced. Normal sections (left) sliced through the center give the largest radius (smallest curvature). Oblique sections (middle) always give smaller radii (larger curvatures). Tangential oblique sections (right) approach zero radius or infinite curvature. Only normal sections yield the true curvature of the sphere.

except for the clinically uninteresting case in which the cornea is perfectly axisymmetric. For an offset bump, the apex is actually a "saddle point" of meridional curvature. That is, it has a maximum along the apical meridian but a minimum when compared circumferentially to adjacent meridians slicing the foot of the bump. The true keratoconic apex is located at the same radial distance of the meridional maximum but along a meridian between the enclosing arms of the "bent bow tie." Because axial curvature is radially averaged, its maximum is always more peripherally located than the meridional maximum (see Figure 18-9 and compare oblique curvatures A and B with four other nondistorting maps: anterior and posterior elevation, thickness, and mean curvature).

A keratoconic bump can be clearly seen on a mean curvature map. For the mathematically astute, mean curvature is the local mean of the two principal curvatures, which in turn are the minimum and maximum values bounding the range of normal curvatures existing at every smooth surface point. Geometrically, it can be understood as the continuous distribution of curvature having an infinite array the spheres, each best-fitting the surface locally. In other words, mean curvature measures the local sphericity of a surface. Similarly, the local difference of the principal curvature, or toric curvature, measures local toricity. Both show keratoconus and other anomalies as they exist, undistorted by any axial artifact. We also know a keratoconic cone is truly prolate or cone shaped, because its apex corresponds to a local maximum in mean curvature.

REFERENCE

1. ANSI Z80.23-1999. American National Standard for Ophthalmic Instruments-Corneal Topography Systems-Standard Terminology, Requirements. New York, NY: American National Standards Institute.

Chapter Nineteen

Corneal Topography in Customized Ablation

Charles Campbell, PhD

In a certain sense, all refractive corrections of the eye are customized because each eye has a unique refractive error. It is that unique error that must be corrected. But the term "customized ablation" has come to take on a special meaning to differentiate those procedures that correct more complicated refractive errors from those more common procedures that only correct simple spherocylindrical error. The first corneal refractive surgical procedures attempted to correct only mean spherical error and as a result, the ablation patterns exhibited a great degree of spatial symmetry and were fairly insensitive to minor positional errors. When correction for astigmatism was added, rotational symmetry was broken and the relationship of the cylinder axis of the ablation to that of the eye became critical. However, from an optical point of view, minor positional errors in the placement of the ablation pattern on the cornea were not too important.

We find the same thing to be true in the more familiar case of spectacle lenses in which we know that the correction for astigmatism in single vision lenses remains good even as the eye turns to look through different portions of the lens, in effect simulating a decentered ablation pattern. The situation is quite different once we attempt to correct localized refractive errors and so attempt a customized ablation. If such an ablation is not precisely aligned both in position and rotational orientation, the refractive result will quite likely be worse than before the pro-

cedure, whereas if alignment is correct, vision will be improved. So, when a customized ablation is to be used, it is quite important that the measurements of localized error, both magnitude and location, are precisely made. The alignment requirements will be discussed later.

It is the shape of the cornea that is altered during any type of ablative procedure, so it is only reasonable that we would wish to measure that shape prior to any surgery and use this information to attain our goal—improvement of vision through the removal of refractive error. Corneal topography is a means to measure that shape, and in this chapter we will investigate what role corneal topography can have in obtaining this information. Before we can discuss how the information gained through corneal topography can be used to guide customized ablation procedures, it is best to first establish what is measured by corneal topography, how it is presented, and what it means to the refractive state of the eye.

THE OPTICAL ROLE OF THE CORNEA

The cornea is one of the principal refractive elements of the eye. It has a highly curved surface and exists at the interface between the outside world—usually air—and the tissue of the eye itself. We can think of the action of any optical refractive surface element to be governed primarily by two parameters: the curvature of the surface and the change of index of refraction across that surface. The term *optical refractive surface element* is used to define an optical element in which refraction occurs only at the surface, thus differentiating it from an optical element in which the index of refraction changes in some continuous fashion in the bulk of the material, thereby causing refraction to occur throughout the element. This is an important consideration for the eye because the optical action of the cornea may be thought to occur solely on its surfaces, whereas the refractive action crystalline lens not only comes from its surfaces but also from an index of refraction gradient throughout the bulk of the lens.

For an optical refractive surface element, the refractive power is directly proportional to the product of the change of index of refraction across the surface and the magnitude of the curvature of the surface. With these thoughts in mind, it is easy to see why the cornea is the major refractive element of the eye. It has a very highly curved surface with a radius of curvature in the vicinity of 8 mm and the refractive index at its anterior surface changes from 1.00 in air to 1.336 in the anterior tear film. The crystalline lens has a curvature very similar in magnitude to that of the cornea on its surfaces, but the index change is very much less, changing at the surfaces from 1.336 in the aqueous humor to 1.386 at the edge of the cortex of the lens. This change of 0.050 is 15% of that at the anterior tear film interface, so the refractive action of the lens surface is much less than that of the cornea. It is the product of the refractive index change and the curvature that determines the refractive power of any optical element. It also suggests that any local curvature changes in lens surfaces will have proportionally less overall effect on the refractive state of the eye than changes of the same magnitude in the curvature of the cornea.

It would seem then that the curvature of the cornea and changes to that curvature are the most important parameters to consider when changing the refractive state of the eye via corneal refractive surgery. However, for the purposes of deciding how to control the action of a laser ablation system, curvature is not the most convenient parameter to use. Before explaining why this is the case, let us first consider what the corneal topographer measures at a fundamental level.

MEASUREMENTS THAT CAN BE MADE BY A CORNEAL TOPOGRAPHER: CURVATURE VERSUS HEIGHT

If we were talking about the topography of the surface of the earth or the topography of some three-dimensional object, we would most likely be thinking of describing topography in terms of the height or elevation of the surface at designated locations above some fixed plane or reference surface. We would be describing the topography in terms of the three-dimensional coordinates of the surface. But, for mostly historical reasons, this is not what is generally meant when one speaks of corneal topography. Corneal measurements were first taken with instruments called ophthalmometers or keratometers. These instruments measured the curvature of small areas of the cornea by measuring the magnification of luminous targets, known as mires, by the highly curved corneal surface. The values thus found were curvature values, and it was in terms of curvature that ophthalmic professionals came to characterize the corneal surface. It was therefore reasonable, when corneal topographers first became available, to present their topographical data in terms of curvature at various locations on the cornea. However, this created a problem in presentation because the curvature at a given location (x,y) on a surface cannot be expressed as a single value as can surface elevation (z). Curvature needs three values (eg, sphere, cylinder, and axis) to express it at a given location. So normal topographical maps using contour lines or colors to represent the elevation variables in terms of two positions are inadequate to fully represent curvature. The compromise that was settled upon for corneal topographical curvature maps was to pick one component of the curvature and represent it in a color-coded contour map. The chosen component was the one in the direction of the meridians of a polar coordinate system drawn on the corneal surface and centered on the corneal vertex.

> Curvature requires three values—sphere, cylinder, and axis—to express it at a given location. So normal topographical maps using contour lines or colors to represent the elevation variables in terms of two positions are inadequate to fully represent curvature.

Methods of Measuring Curvature

Keratometric Analysis Method

How is this curvature information to be obtained by the corneal topographer? It is possible to analyze a multiple ring corneal topographer image (placido ring system) in the same way one analyzes a keratometer ring image. Each of the multiple rings is considered to be a keratometer ring by itself. Using the *keratometer analysis method*, curvature values are found for each ring.

Arc Step Method

It turns out that there is a better way to analyze the image of a placido ring system created by the corneal surface. This method considers the deflection of rays from the source rings by the surface and uses the laws of reflection and ray tracing techniques to find the slope of the surface at measured locations. This slope information is then used to calculate values related to the local curvature of the surface at a great number of points on the corneal surface. If the method used to find these slope values is the iterative method known as the *arc step method*, the elevation of the surface is also found at each measured location along with the surface slope.

It must be noted that surface slope information is only found along the meridians. Nothing is found as to the surface slope in other directions, hence information on surface curvature is incomplete. This is because curvature can only be found along meridians when present-day corneal topographer analysis methods are employed. Such partial displays of curvature have proved extremely useful to clinicians to get an overall subjective idea of the refractive state of the cornea, but they are not particularly useful for optical analysis of the cornea via ray tracing and other analytical methods.

For ray tracing, one needs to know the surface normal at various locations. The surface normal is a line passing through a point on the surface perpendicular to a plane tangent to the surface at that point. To know the surface normal, one needs to know not only the surface slope along a meridian but also the slope at right angles to the meridian. It seems that corneal topography, as currently performed, is not adequate for detailed analysis of refractive error. However, if the elevation information, which is obtained in addition to slope information in certain analysis methods, is considered, the situation changes and there is a way to analyze the optical action of the cornea in great detail.

Treatment of the Optical Action of a Refractive Element in Terms of its Thickness (Optical Path Length)

The optical action of a refractive element has thus far been considered to be governed by the change in index of refraction at its surfaces and by the surface curvatures. There is a very different way to treat optical action that is just as valid and useful as the more common approach. Instead of considering the refraction of light rays by a surface, one considers the change in *optical path length* (OPL) for different rays as they pass through an optical element and impose the restraint that each ray, as it progresses from an initial wavefront to a refracted wavefront, has the same OPL. The OPL for a segment of a ray is defined as the physical distance along the ray segment multiplied by the index of refraction found in that segment (equation 1):

OPL = physical distance x index of refraction

> The OPL for a segment of a ray is defined as the physical distance along the ray segment multiplied by the index of refraction found in that segment.

To see how this creates optical action, consider a simple positive lens. Such lenses are thicker in the middle than at the edge. This means that the OPL of a ray passing through the middle of the lens has a longer OPL than does a ray passing through the edge. Now let this positive lens have a plano front surface and a convex back surface and suppose that a plane wavefront enters the flat front surface so that all rays enter the lens at once. Because the OPL for edge rays is less than for central rays, they exit the lens sooner and travel some distance beyond the lens before the central rays exit. This causes the refracted wavefront to take a convex curvature, producing the focusing action of the lens. This is illustrated in Figure 19-1.

This is a very simple example, but the approach is general and it allows the optical behavior to be expressed in terms of change in lens thickness or other optical elements as the position on the element changes. In addition, this method allows aberrations to be treated by considering them to be differences in OPL between the actual wavefront and some ideal wavefront at various positions on the wavefront. We can therefore use distance measures in the form of elevation changes of a surface to analyze its optical performance instead of using curvature information or surface slope information. In many ways this is a better approach because it allows the use of very powerful optical analysis theorems to predict the quality of images without having to resort to ray tracing. Ray tracing is difficult to perform precisely in eyes because of uncertainly regarding the optical characteristics of an individual crystalline lens. There is no convenient way to precisely measure the surface profile or the index of refraction within this gradient index lens in the living eye. Even if precise ray tracing could be done, interpretation of ray intercepts with the fovea is not as easy as interpretation of point spread functions (PSFs) and spatial frequency spectrums, which can be directly related to contrast sensitivity and visual acuity (computed directly from wavefront error information).

For the purposes of controlling a laser ablation system, the thickness approach to characterizing a lens is the only practical one. Refractive correction is accomplished when using a PRK or LASIK procedure by removing a tissue lens with the laser system. This tissue lens is referred to as the *treatment lenticle*. The power of this treatment lenticle is the power of the refractive error. As the laser selectively removes tissue to remove the treatment lenticle, it needs to know how much tissue to remove at different locations. When the treatment lenticle is characterized by thickness, the information needed by the laser is immediately available. In fact, for simple refractive errors there is no need for information on the topography of the cornea. A treatment lenticle with the correct thickness gradient to produce the desired correction is removed and the optical result is the desired one regardless of the shape of the corneal surface.

> Refractive correction is accomplished when using a PRK or LASIK procedure by removing a tissue lens with the laser system. This tissue lens is referred to as the *treatment lenticle.*

Customized Ablation

We have defined customized ablation as a corneal refractive surgical procedure that corrects more complicated refractive errors than simple spherocylindri-

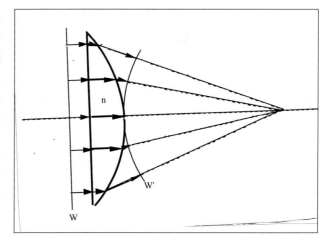

Figure 19-1. Optical path length. A plane wavefront enters the flat front surface of a plano convex lens so that all rays enter the lens at once. The optical path length for the peripheral rays is less than for the central rays. They exit the lens sooner and travel some distance beyond the lens before the central rays exit. This causes the refracted wavefront to take a convex curvature, producing the focusing action of the lens.

cal ones. We may wish to do this for a variety of reasons: an earlier procedure may have induced corneal irregularity that we wish to remove. We may wish to remove higher-order aberrations of the eye in addition to spherocylindrical error, thereby increasing the resolution of the eye. No matter what the reason for customization, it will be necessary to measure the aberrations of the eye carefully so that they are well characterized not only in magnitude but also in location with respect to the pupil of the eye. This information must then be converted to instructions for the laser ablation system on the amount of tissue to be removed at specified locations.

Wavefront Error

The most convenient form of aberration information is *wavefront error.* The wavefront error is the OPL difference at each location between the desired wavefront and the actual wavefront. Since OPL is the product of the index of refraction and the physical path length, a method that measures an actual surface and compares it to a desired surface is in essence the wavefront error. In the case of the cornea, the index of refraction to use is the stroma (1.376).

We can now see how information from a corneal topographer can be used if the system can measure the three-dimensional position of the surface. What the corneal topographer does not measure is the shape of the desired corneal surface. This must be supplied in some fashion. There are a number of reasonable approaches.

One approach uses a combination of the desired spherocylindrical correction and considerations on aberration-free surfaces. Usually there is a spherocylindrical refractive error to be removed, and the ablation profile to accomplish this can be found without any reference to the cornea surface (as was noted above). The elevation values associated with the spherocylindrical correction can then be directly subtracted from the measured corneal elevation values to give the surface that will exist after the basic correction. It is known that surfaces that minimize aberration are very smooth in the sense that their curvature changes slowly as a function of position. In the eye there two refractive elements that can contribute to aberration—the lens and the cornea. The lens is a very regular optical structure and is very unlikely to contribute to higher-order aberration caused by rapid changes in curvature or index. The cornea, on the other hand, can exhibit fluctuations in curvature on a very local basis. If these local fluctuations can be removed, the higher aberrations will also be reduced. This can be done by fitting the surface found by subtracting the spherocylindrical ablation pattern from the measured surface to a smooth function such as general ellipsoid. The elevation difference between this surface and the best-fit smooth surface gives the extra amount of ablation needed to remove corneal irregularities and the resulting higher aberrations from the eye.

A variation on this approach is to constrain the fitted general ellipsoid to have a given eccentricity. One of the higher aberrations—spherical aberration—can be reduced if the eccentricity of the corneal surface is properly chosen. For instance, as it is known that a corneal eccentricity of 0.55 (p-value of 0.7) gives an optimal reduction of spherical aberration for an average eye, this would a reasonable value to use. However, for such an approach to be fully successful, the fitted ellipsoid should be properly centered on the pupil.

ALIGNMENT PRECISION NEEDED FOR CUSTOMIZED ABLATIONS

There is no way that a hard and fast rule can be given for necessary alignment precision because of the wide variation in the size and severity of localized refractive errors found in practice. It is helpful,

though, to think of the situation in this way. Suppose that there is a local corneal irregularity that degrades vision by some amount. We may think of the correction for this irregularity as the addition of second corneal irregularity, which is equal but opposite to the original so that the two cancel out one another. Let us suppose that we misalign the correction so that it does not fall on the original. It then adds a refractive error similar in magnitude to the original error without causing the original to go away. We have thereby essentially doubled the problem for the visual system. On the other hand, if our misalignment is only partial, then some cancellation of error will occur and the net result may be an improvement. This is a very simple approach to what in practice will be a fairly complicated optical situation, but it certainly gives us good direction in our thinking on this matter. It must also be noted that errors of alignment can be rotational as well as translational, a concept well known from our experience in correcting astigmatism. Perhaps the most important idea, as we consider the alignment precision needed for customized ablation, is that the size of the local irregularity is not only important from the point of view of its effect on vision but also on the precision with which we must apply a correction ablation to remove its effect. A second important idea is that the magnitude of the irregularity is also important. To see this, consider the familiar case of correction for simple astigmatism and the need to correctly orient cylinder axis. The residual refractive error when the axis is misaligned is proportional to the product of the axis error (the rotational positional error) and the original magnitude of the cylinder error.

REQUIREMENTS FOR CORNEAL TOPOGRAPHERS WHEN USED TO GUIDE CUSTOMIZED ABLATION

A corneal topographer must be able to measure the elevation of the corneal surface for it to be useful for planning customized ablation. Systems that only measure curvature may be useful for subjective evaluation of the corneal surface, but they are not adequate tools for planning customized ablation. For those corneal topographers that can make elevation information available, only those with sufficient precision of measurement are truly useful. To guide us on setting limits for this necessary precision we have the characteristics of laser ablation systems and the magnitude of expected aberrations. It is best to express aberrations in terms of OPL—the appropriate unit is the wavelength of light. Therefore, errors are best expressed in microns, as the midrange wavelength value for the visible spectrum is 0.55 microns. Laser ablation systems typically remove 0.25 microns of tissue per pulse. As this is stromal tissue with an index of refraction of 1.376, the optical path length removed per pulse is 0.62 waves (divide equation 1 by the wavelength).

$$OPL = \frac{\text{physical distance x index of refraction}}{\text{wavelength}}$$

$$OPL = \frac{0.25 \times 1.376}{0.55} = 0.62 \text{ waves}$$

Since we are interested in the change wavefront error caused by the ablation, what is important is the change in OPL from the case of light traveling through stromal tissue to that of light traveling through air when the stromal tissue is removed. The change in OPL—d(OPL)—is the physical distance multiplied by the change in index of refraction. A single ablation pulse changes the OPL, in waves, by 0.17 waves.

$$d(OPL) = \frac{\text{physical distance x (index of refraction in tissue - index of refraction in air)}}{\text{wavelength}}$$

$$d(OPL) = \frac{0.25 \times (1.376 - 1.000)}{0.55} = 0.17 \text{ waves}$$

Certainly, there is no need to measure surface details to an accuracy greater than the minimum amount of tissue that can be removed.

To get an idea of the elevation resolution needed to use custom ablation, let us first consider the variation in thickness for a tissue lens that represents a change in refractive power of 0.25 D. A change in refractive power of this magnitude can be expressed in terms of wavefront error if a pupil diameter is assumed using the simple approximation for sag of a sphere (equation 2):

$$sag = \frac{D^2P}{8}$$

where D is the diameter of the aperture (in millimeters) and P is the power (in diopters); the sag is expressed in microns. The wavefront error, W, from the center to the edge of the aperture given in waves is the sag divided by the wavelength of light (equation 3):

$$W = \frac{sag}{\text{wavelength}} = \frac{D^2P}{8 \text{ wavelengths}}$$

If a 3-mm pupil is chosen and the wavelength is 0.55 µm, W is 0.51 waves. It should be noted in passing that this is twice the Rayleigh criterion for wavefront error perceptibly changing image quality. This fact provides a physical reason for the observation that 0.25 D blur is just noticeable under normal visual conditions. We should also note that often the wavefront error is not expressed as the difference from the aperture center to the edge but in terms of the root mean square (RMS) wavefront error. To convert W to RMS error for simple surface forms such as spheres, ellipsoids, and toric surfaces, a good approximation is found by multiplying W by the factor 0.3 (equation 4):

$$RMS \text{ error} \cong 0.3 \times W$$

The RMS error corresponding to the Rayleigh quarter wave criterion is 0.75 waves.

$$0.75 = 0.3 \times 0.25$$

To find out what such an error means in terms of the variation in thickness of a corneal tissue lens, we may use a simple formula widely used to calculate ablation depths (equation 5):

$$d = D^2P/8(n-1)$$

where d is the variation in lens thickness (in microns), D is the diameter (in millimeters), P is the power (in diopters), and n is the index of refraction of the tissue. We find that the thickness variation from tissue lens center to edge is 0.49 µm. As this thickness is equivalent to the ablation effect of just two nominal pulses, it first shows us that customized ablation will require an ablation system to operate at the limit of its capability in any case. It is of interest to note that the change in measured RMS wavefront error for recent LASIK studies shows changes in

The elevation resolution needed to use customized ablation to within 0.25 D results in a thickness variation from the tissue lens center to the edge of 0.49 µm.

higher-order aberrations and increases in wavefront error of around 0.15 waves. Removal of this error is certainly at the limit of a system that removes 0.17 waves per pulse.

It is clear that a corneal topography system needs to be able to measure surface elevation differences to better than 1.0-μm resolution to be useful in guiding customized ablation. This not to say that corneal topography systems with less resolution are not useful to assess larger corneal surface features and are valuable in monitoring change both following corneal procedure and for other purposes. Wavefront errors beyond those of normal refractive errors are of a size that will not be detected unless a measurement system has this resolution. Current placido disc-based corneal topography systems using arc step reconstruction algorithms are able to resolve corneal surface elevation variations to about 0.7 microns. These systems give the best resolution available today.

> This means that the highest resolution corneal topography systems available are just able to detect the presence of surface variations that will contribute to higher-order wavefront errors, as 0.7 microns of tissue removal converts to 0.48 waves of wavefront change.

For those more familiar with the performance of corneal topography systems expressed in axial curvature values (keratometric diopters), the following example illustrates the relationship between variation in surface elevation and variation in axial curvature in a local area of the corneal surface. Let us take a circular area of the cornea that is 1.5 mm in diameter with an axial curvature value 1 D greater than the surrounding area. Using equation 5 and the nominal index of refraction value taken to express keratometric diopters of 1.3375, we find the variation in elevation, d, to be 0.833 microns. As we know that the better corneal topography systems can detect curvature changes of this size over this area, we see that they have resolution in the range that is useful for customized ablation. This simple test can, of course, be used to judge the suitability of any corneal topography system used as a guide for customized ablation.

COMPARISON OF CORNEAL TOPOGRAPHY TO WAVEFRONT SENSING AS A GUIDE TO CUSTOMIZED ABLATION

When corneal topography is used as a guide for customized ablation, the desired surface is not known and some reference surface is needed to find the wavefront error so that a correcting ablation profile can be generated. Wavefront error sensing devices, such a Shack-Hartmann wavefront sensor, can be configured to directly measure the wavefront error of the entire eye on the area of the pupil. For this area, they supply the information needed to create an ablation profile directly, and in so doing also account for aberration induced by the lens in addition to that created by the cornea. They would therefore seem to be superior to a corneal topographer as a guide to planning a customized ablation. However, certain characteristics of these devices must first be considered before completely accepting this view.

Wavefront sensing devices can only sample in the pupil area, so it is important that the pupil be fully dilated so that areas only used in low light conditions are sampled. It is also best if accommodation is paralyzed during the measurement to remove the accommodation uncertainty in the crystalline lens. In essence, wavefront sensors are automatic refractors with a very high sample density, so all the known precautions associated with obtaining good refractive information with automatic refractors applies directly to them. Corneal topographers, on the other hand, sample over a much larger area of the cornea and are unaffected by accommodation, pupil size, or other refractive effects.

Wavefront sensing devices measure the entire refractive state of the eye and cannot tell if measured aberrations are caused by the cornea or by a combination of effects of the cornea and crystalline lens. Unlike corneal topographers, they give no direct information on the state of the corneal surface.

Wavefront sensing devices sample in a different way from corneal topographers. In general, the sample density is somewhat less and the sample pattern is different. Wavefront sensors divide the pupil in small areas, usually in a rectangular grid, and measure the average deflection of light exiting from each area. This deflection information is then processed to yield wavefront error. The most common corneal topographers sample the cornea with concentric rings and may be thought to measure the surface either only at boundaries between light and dark or averaged over the area illuminated by a ring. In addition, sampling is typically lower in the center of the corneal topographer image for these devices.

On the other hand, it seems that if wisely used, wavefront sensing devices serve better as guides for customized ablation than do corneal topographers. However, corneal topographers should not be dismissed because they give direct information on the shape of the cornea, which is unavailable from a wavefront sensor. They should be routinely used as a "second opinion" when planning a customized ablation.

In addition, there are cases in which a wavefront sensor will not work well because wavefront sensing devices must be able to send and receive light from the retinal surface without significant interference from the ocular tissue. In corneal trauma, the cornea may be compromised to the extent that it is not possible for the incoming beam of the wavefront sensing device to form a reasonably well-focused spot on the retina. When this happens, the detected spots of light may be so badly deformed that good measurement of higher-order aberrations is not possible. The corneal topographer has no such limitation. It can measure the corneal surface shape even in the presence of serious irregularity, and this information is quite sufficient to plan an ablation pattern to correct this defect. Since the crystalline lenses is assumed to be a regular optical element, even though its exact details are not known, its effect can safely be assumed in calculations; the true cause of the degradation of vision—the corneal irregularity—can be corrected using only corneal information. This suggests that the correlation between wavefront error measured with a wavefront sensor and wavefront error measured with a corneal topographer needs to be established so that when it is not possible to obtain wavefront error information from a wavefront sensing device, corneal topographical information can be reliably substituted.

OTHER USES FOR CORNEAL TOPOGRAPHY TO ASSIST WITH CORNEAL ABLATION PROCEDURES

There are other uses of corneal topographical information to guide in performing customized ablations of the cornea in addition to using the information to decide the amount of tissue to remove.

Corneal topography displays can be used to simulate an ablation that graphically illustrates what can be expected with different ablation patterns. Displays showing the difference in corneal shape from the expected are useful to allow the surgeon to alter procedure and get desired results.

A simulated ablation feature first allows an ablation pattern to be specified. This specification includes such variables as the desired ablation zone size, the refractive error to be removed, the specification of transition zones between the corrected central optical zone and the unablated peripheral cornea, and the centration of the pattern with respect to the pupil center. Alternatively, the ablation pattern may be supplied by the laser ablation system. In either case, the ablation pattern is removed from the corneal shape as measured by the corneal topographer and software program, to produce a new corneal shape. This new shape is then displayed on the topographer. The practitioner who is familiar with corneal topography map presentations and their meaning can now judge if the proposed ablation pattern will produce the desired effect.

A second effective way to use corneal topography information to assist with laser refractive surgery procedures is to use difference maps to graphically show the difference between two corneal surfaces. The first use of such a technique was to monitor changes in the corneal shape before and after surgery and then to monitor subsequent changes over time as corneal healing progressed. Another use of the differencing method is to combine it with simulated ablation. The presurgery corneal shape is used to create a simulated shape by using the ablation pattern that was used in surgery. This simulated shape is then compared via a difference map with the actual postsurgery corneal shape. In this way, actual results can be compared with expected results in a visual way. Since actual results are often slightly different from expected results, studies of this kind can serve as a guide to alter ablation patterns and achieve the desired results.

Chapter Twenty

Corneal Aberrations and Refractive Surgery

Raymond A. Applegate, OD, PhD
Howard C. Howland, PhD
Stephen D. Klyce, PhD

INTRODUCTION

The corneal-air interface represents the largest refractive index change in the eye. As can be seen in equation 1, using para-axial optics, the power of the corneal first surface (48.83 diopters [D]) represents over 80% of the total power (58.64 D) of the Gullstrand schematic eye #1 (equation 1):

$$F = \frac{n' - n}{r} = \frac{1.376 - 1}{0.0077} = 48.83 \text{ D}$$

where n' is the index of the cornea, n is the index of air, and r is the radius of curvature of the corneal first surface in meters.

> Traditional clinical teaching is that the "power of the cornea" averages 43 D in the human adult. This arises from the fact that the back surface power of the cornea (approximately –6 D) is added to the expression given in equation 1. This convention is not used in this chapter, as substantial errors can arise when the curvature of only the corneal first surface is changed as it is with excimer laser surface-ablating refractive surgical procedures.

All other optical interfaces in the eye have radii of curvatures that are similar (within a factor of 2) to the corneal first surface radius. However, the other optical interfaces are formed by two optical media, both

having a high water content. This makes the change in refractive index across the interface small (the largest being 0.05) compared to the index change at the corneal first surface (0.376). Consequently, the powers of all other optical interfaces within the eye are small compared to the corneal first surface.

Because of the large index change and relatively steep curvature, small alterations in the corneal shape have large effects on corneal first surface refractive power, making corneal refractive surgery effective. For the same reasons, unwanted changes or technically compromised refractive surgeries can induce large changes in the eye's aberration structure.

> Small alterations in the corneal shape have large effects on corneal first surface refractive power, making corneal refractive surgery effective.

In this chapter we will present:
1. Methods for using corneal topography to define the surface and/or aberration structure of the corneal first surface.
2. Methods for specifying the corneal first surface aberration structure.
3. Corneal first surface aberration of the normal eye as a function of age.
4. Corneal first surface aberration structure induced by radial keratotomy (RK), photorefractive kerate-

ctomy (PRK), and laser-assisted in situ keratomileusis (LASIK).

5. Corneal first surface aberration as a function of attempted correction.

6. Corneal first surface aberration and visual performance.

7. Corneal topography-driven refractive surgery.

8. The future: combining corneal topography and total eye wavefront measurements for "super vision."

Corneal Topography and Corneal First Surface and/or Aberration Structure

Corneal topographers provide maps of the corneal first surface. Although traditionally displayed as dioptric maps, elevation maps are just as easily generated and have the advantage of fundamentally defining the optical surface, allowing corneal first surface aberration to be calculated.[1-18] Just like elevations on the earth's surface, elevations of the corneal surface are measured with respect to a reference. The selection of the reference surface can either hide or reveal surface structure of interest.

> Just like elevations on the earth's surface, elevations of the corneal surface are measured with respect to a reference.

This point is illustrated in Figure 20-1, which shows corneal first surface elevations of an RK eye. In the left panel, surface elevations are plotted with respect to a best-fitting sphere. In the right panel, the same surface elevations are plotted with respect to a reference surface constructed by combining the best-fitting sphere with a fourth-order Taylor polynomial fit to the residual elevations displayed in the left panel. This reference surface more closely follows the actual corneal first surface topography and allows one to easily visualize residual surface characteristics. Notice that RK incisions are now clearly revealed, whereas in the left panel only hints of the incisions are evident. Had corneal elevations been referenced to a plane, all subtleties of the corneal surface would have been lost.

The ideal corneal elevation reference would render the eye diffraction limited when combined with

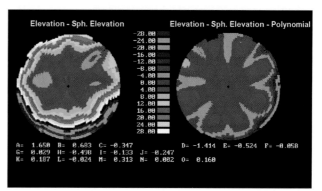

Figure 20-1. Corneal elevations of an RK patient with respect to a best-fitting sphere (left panel) and corneal elevations (right) with respect to the best-fitting sphere combined with a fourth-order Taylor polynomial fit to the residual elevations displayed in the left panel. A through O are the coefficients of the fourth-order Taylor polynomial least squares fit to elevations displayed in the left panel (reprinted with permission from Applegate RA, Howland HC, Sharp RP, Cottingham AJ, Yee RW. Corneal aberrations and visual performance after radial keratotomy. *J Refract Surg.* 1998;14:397-407).

> Unfortunately, corneal topography by itself does not define the structure of the ideal corneal first surface.

all other optical elements. Unfortunately, corneal topography by itself does not define the structure of the ideal corneal first surface.

Like elevations, aberrations are specified with respect to a reference. For the corneal first surface, the ideal reference would be the wavefront (or surface) that, when combined with the rest of the eye's optics (eg, corneal back surface, crystalline lens), would render an aberration-free foveal image of the object point of interest. This ideal wavefront is simply the wavefront formed by refraction through the ideal corneal surface from the object point of interest (generally, a foveally fixated object point at optical infinity). Unfortunately, like corneal first surface elevations, corneal topography by itself provides little insight as to the nature of the ideal reference wavefront. Consequently, the choice of the reference wavefront for specifying corneal aberrations from corneal topography is somewhat arbitrary.

In the work of Applegate and Howland, two different reference surfaces have been used to calculate corneal first surface aberration structure: a best-fitting sphere to the central presurgical cornea and the presurgical cornea. Experience has taught that the

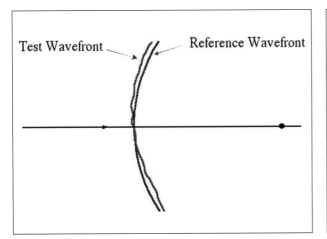

Figure 20-2. The difference between the test wavefront and the reference wavefront as a function of location in the exit pupil defines the aberration structure of the test wavefront.

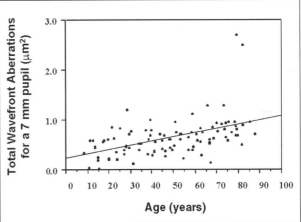

Figure 20-3. Total corneal first surface wavefront aberrations due to the higher-order terms (piston, prism, defocus, and astigmatism removed) show a statistically significant increase with age ($p < 0.001$) (adapted from Oshika T, Klyce SD, Applegate RA, Howland HC. Changes in corneal wavefront aberrations with aging. *Invest Ophthalmol Vis Sci.* 1999;40:1351-1355).

aberrations over a 7-mm pupil induced by refractive surgeries studied prior to the year 2000 are so large that the choice of reference surface made no significant difference in the analysis.[10] However, as surgeries improve, it will become increasingly important to use the ideal reference to optimize surgical outcomes in an effort to create super vision (discussed later in this chapter).

SPECIFICATION OF ABERRATIONS

The difference between the test wavefront and the reference wavefront (Figure 20-2) as a function of exit pupil location defines the aberration structure. As a matter of convention, wavefront error is set to zero at the center of the exit pupil. Typically, the differences are plotted as a contour map or, for a more quantitative representation, fitted with a polynomial. For corneal first surface optics (as opposed to the eye's optics), the exit pupil is placed at the corneal first surface. In the work reported here, the center of the exit pupil is centered on the eye's natural pupil as measured by the corneal topographer.

The variance of the wavefront from the reference is termed the *wavefront variance* and is a single number we use to characterize the quality of the optical system. If the differences between the actual wavefront and reference wavefront are fitted with a Zernike polynomial that is appropriately normalized

(see Appendix One), the magnitude of the wavefront variance is equal to the sum of the squared coefficients (except for the term *piston*). Thus, the normalized Zernike polynomial makes it is easy to calculate total wavefront variance and the relative contribution of each term.

CORNEAL FIRST SURFACE ABERRATION STRUCTURE OF THE NORMAL EYE AS A FUNCTION OF AGE

Investigations of how corneal first surface optics change with aging are still in their early stages. A pioneering study by Oshika, et al[14] of 102 Japanese patients found that for large pupils, total wavefront variance gradually increases with age (Figure 20-3). Oshika, et al's study indicated that asymmetric aberrations increase with age, but symmetric aberrations do not. In a study of 59 Caucasian patients, Guirao, et al[17] also found that total wavefront variance increased with age. However, their work indicated that spherical coma and other higher-order aberrations all correlated with age. Together, the findings suggest possible differences due to race. However, the increase in aberrations is relatively small, particularly in comparison to the aberrations induced by refractive surgery to date.

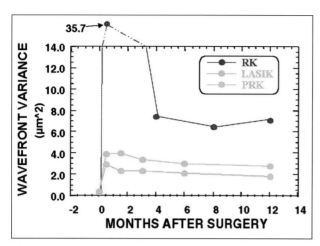

Figure 20-4 Corneal first surface wavefront variance due to the higher-order aberration with respect to a best-fitting sphere to the central cornea as a function of time postsurgery (RK data adapted from Applegate RA, Howland HC, Sharp RP, Cottingham AJ, Yee RW. Corneal aberrations and visual performance after radial keratotomy. *J Refract Surg.* 1998;14:397-407. LASIK and PRK data adapted from Oshika T, Klyce SD, Applegate RA, Howland HC. Comparison of corneal wavefront aberrations after photorefractive keratectomy and laser in situ keratomileusis. *Am J Ophthalmol.* 1999;127:1-7).

Corneal First Surface Aberration Structure Induced by RK, PRK, and LASIK

Refractive surgery is evolving quickly. By the time data have been collected, analyzed, and reported, the surgery being studied has often evolved and in some cases, fallen into disfavor. Nonetheless, the general trends of the 1980s and 1990s are instructive and include:

1. Refractive surgery increases the aberration structure of the corneal first surface.[2,9-11,13,15]

2. The larger the pupil, the larger the surgery-induced corneal first surface aberration.[10,11,13,15]

3. The larger the correction, the larger the surgery-induced corneal first surface aberration.[6,11]

4. Refractive surgery changes the normal distribution of corneal first surface aberration.[10,11,13]

> Refractive surgery is evolving quickly. By the time data have been collected, analyzed, and reported, the surgery being studied has often evolved and in some cases, fallen into disfavor.

In the discussion to follow, we will focus on the corneal first surface aberration over a 7-mm pupil. A 7-mm pupil was chosen because it is a fair representation of the largest pupil diameter (worst case condition) that can be reasonably expected under normal physiologic conditions. The aberration will be less for smaller pupils.

Of the refractive surgeries studied to date, RK induces the largest changes in total corneal first surface aberration.[10,11,13] The aberration is largest immediately after surgery and recovers significantly to stabilize around 23 times presurgical values. LASIK over a 5.5-mm treatment diameter (transition diameter out to 6.5 mm) and PRK over a 5.5-mm treatment diameter (transition diameter out to 7.0 mm) induce less aberration than RK—7.25 times and 5.25 times preoperative values, respectively (Figure 20-4). Newer algorithms for laser ablation treat over a larger area and induce less aberration. In Endl, et al's recent work,[15] PRK with a 5.5-mm surgical zone and transition out to 7.0 mm reported fewer aberrations than a previous study by Martinez, et al of PRK with a 5.0-mm ablation zone with no transition.[11]

In the normal eye, the dominant aberrations are asymmetric (Figure 20-5). Following RK, PRK, and LASIK, the total aberration is increased and dominated by symmetric aberrations.

Corneal First Surface Aberration Structure as a Function of Attempted Correction

The design of refractive surgery changes with the magnitude of the attempted correction. Generally, in RK the larger the attempted correction, the smaller the central surgery-free area. Likewise, in PRK and LASIK, the larger the attempted correction, the smaller the surgical zone designed to fully correct the refractive error. As a consequence, it is reasonable to expect that the corneal first surface aberration structure will vary with the magnitude of the attempted correction. Studies have confirmed this prediction for RK[6] and PRK (Figure 20-6).[11] To our knowledge, similar data have not been reported for LASIK, but we anticipate the results will be similar.

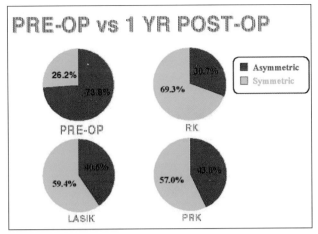

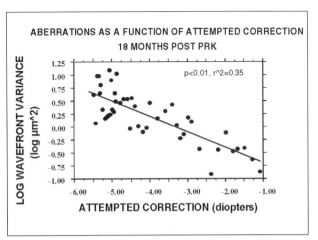

Figure 20-5. The distribution of aberration between asymmetric and symmetric aberrations for eyes before surgery and 1 year after RK, LASIK, and PRK (preoperative and RK figures adapted from Applegate RA, Howland HC, Sharp RP, Cottingham AJ, Yee RW. Corneal aberrations and visual performance after radial keratotomy. *J Refract Surg.* 1998;14:397-407. PRK figure adapted from Martinez CE, Applegate RA, Klyce SD, McDonald MB, Medina JP, Howland HC. Effect of pupil dilation on corneal optical aberrations after photorefractive keratectomy. *Arch Ophthalmol.* 1998;116:1053-1062. LASIK data from Oshika T, Klyce SD, Applegate RA, Howland HC. Comparison of corneal wavefront aberrations after photorefractive keratectomy and laser in situ keratomileusis. *Am J Ophthalmol.* 1999;127:1-7).

Figure 20-6. Total wavefront variance due to the higher-order aberrations (third and fourth order) as a function of attempted correction (for 7-mm pupil) (adapted from Martinez CE, Applegate RA, Klyce SD, McDonald MB, Medina JP, Howland HC. Effect of pupil dilation on corneal optical aberrations after photorefractive keratectomy. *Arch Ophthalmol.* 1998;116:1053-1062).

CORNEAL FIRST SURFACE ABERRATION STRUCTURE AND VISUAL PERFORMANCE

As the aberrations of the eye increase, image contrast decreases (see Chapter Seven). Consequently, visual performance will decrease accordingly. However, since many (but not all) visual tasks in everyday life are well above threshold contrast levels, the cost of having increased ocular aberration is task-dependent. For example, reading high-contrast letters (black letters on glossy white paper, such as *National Geographic* articles) are easier than reading low contrast letters on plain paper (light gray letters on plain paper, such as the back of a credit card statement). Further, as discussed above, corneal topography by itself is not a measure of total ocular aberrations. The problem is further compounded by the fact that aberrations for one optical surface can be compensated by the aberrations of other optical surfaces in a multicomponent system. For example, in the normal eye the aberrations of the cornea are

largely balanced by crystalline lens aberrations. Despite these drawbacks, if the corneal first surface aberrations are large compared to normal ocular aberrations, it is reasonable to assume that they will not be compensated for by the other ocular surfaces and that total ocular aberrations are increased. Consequently, it is not surprising that visual performance decreases as corneal first surface aberrations increase.[18] In Figure 20-7, the area under the contrast sensitivity function decreases as aberrations increase.[18] As can be seen by comparing the functions in Figures 20-8a and 20-8b, high-contrast acuity decreases at a slower rate than low-contrast acuity, as corneal aberrations increase.

CORNEAL TOPOGRAPHY-DRIVEN REFRACTIVE SURGERY

As discussed, corneal topography by itself does not provide adequate information to determine the ideal corneal first surface that would render the eye diffraction limited when combined with the remaining ocular optics. However, if the cornea is severely aberrated (as might occur after penetrating keratoplasty, trauma, high corneal astigmatism, etc), using corneal topography to guide surgery to create a more physiologic surface should improve the optical qual-

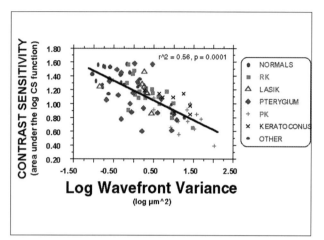

Figure 20-7. Area under the contrast sensitivity function as a function of wavefront variance due to higher-order aberrations (third- through sixth-order aberrations).

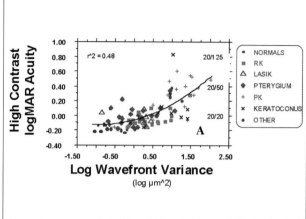

Figure 20-8a. High contrast acuity as a function of wavefront variance due to higher-order aberrations (third- through sixth-order aberrations).

ity of the corneal first surface and improve visual performance in an otherwise normal eye.

The Future

As refractive surgical technique improves to produce smaller and smaller amounts of aberrations or actually reduces inherent aberrations, it will no longer be sufficient to use a spherical fit to the central cornea or the presurgical cornea as a reference surface. Instead, it will be important to use an ideal reference. With the advent of clinically viable wavefront sensing, it is practical to quantify total ocular aberrations over a large aperture and design the ideal corneal first surface that would minimize these aberrations.[19] Deviations between the ideal and the measured surface define the corneal material to be removed to minimize the monochromatic aberrations of the eye.

Even if it is possible to carve and obtain the exact surface we want, it will be impossible to eliminate all ocular monochromatic aberrations. The reason is ocular aberrations are not constant but instead vary with object distance, accommodation, age, tear film construction, etc. However, they can be minimized for a particular set of conditions. Consequently, the correction should be designed to minimize the eye's aberrations for viewing conditions that best meet the needs of the patient. When and if the eye's aberrations or patient needs significantly change (eg, due to aging) and degrade optical performance, a "tune-

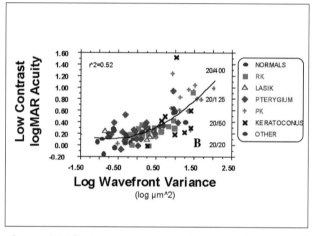

Figure 20-8b. Low contrast acuity as a function of wavefront variance due to higher-order aberrations (third- through sixth-order aberrations).

up" can be performed to re-optimize, assuming adequate corneal tissue remains.

Simply knowing the amount of tissue we wish to remove at each corneal location to achieve the ideal surface shape will not guarantee that the surface shape will in fact be achieved. The cornea is not a piece of plastic.[20] Instead, it is a living biological material under tension. As demonstrated by RK, relieving tension with radial incisions causes the center to flatten and the periphery to steepen.[21] Similarly, in PRK and LASIK the peripheral cornea (outside the ablation area) may steepen as a result of relieving tension centrally (see Chapter Nine).

To the extent that biomechanical responses of the

cornea are predictable across individuals, race, age, etc, refractive surgery can be modified to compensate for the biological response. On the other hand, to the extent that biological response to surgery varies across individuals, so will the surgical outcomes. In either case, the difference between the ideal corneal surface and the surgically obtained surfaces allows us to correctly evaluate how closely we have come to our goal. Further, this difference—if large enough to warrant additional surgery—is the template for the residual correction. To minimize the aberrations, particularly for large corrections, iterative surgery may be required with each successive surgery, removing less material and inducing increasingly predictable corneal response as the ideal is approached. Wavefront sensing will reveal if the aberrations have been minimized but will not reveal if the cornea in fact responded to the surgery as intended. Corneal topography will provide the needed data to determine whether the desired corneal first surface was actually achieved.

> Corneal topography will provide the needed data to determine whether the desired corneal first surface was actually achieved.

ACKNOWLEDGMENTS

Preparation of this chapter was supported by National Institutes of Health (National Eye Institute) grants R01-EY08520 to Dr. Applegate, R01-EY02994 to Dr. Howland, R01-EY03311 to Dr. Klyce, and an unrestricted grant from Research to Prevent Blindness to the Department of Ophthalmology, University of Texas Health Science Center, San Antonio. The authors wish to thank Gene Hilmantel for his assistance in preparation of this chapter and to our collaborators over the past 10 years, especially Jan Buettner, Carlos Martinez, Tetsuro Oshika, and Michael Endl.

REFERENCES

1. Seiler T, Reckmann W, Maloney RK. Effective spherical aberration of the cornea as a quantitative descriptor in corneal topography. *J Cataract Refract Surg.* 1993;19:155-165.

2. Applegate RA, Howland HC, Buettner J, Cottingham Jr AJ, Sharp RP, Yee RW. Corneal aberrations before and after radial keratotomy (RK) calculated from videokeratometric measurements. *Vis Sci Appl Tech Digest (OSA).* 1994;2:58-61.

3. Howland HC, Buettner J, Applegate RA. Computation of the shapes of normal corneas and their monochromatic aberrations from videokeratometric measurements. *Vis Sci Appl Tech Digest (OSA).* 1994;2:54-57.

4. Hemenger RP, Tomlinson A, Oliver K. Corneal optics from videokeratographs. *Ophthalmic Physiol Opt.* 1995;15:63-68.

5. Hemenger RP, Tomlinson A, Oliver KM. Optical consequences of asymmetries in normal corneas. *Ophthalmic Physiol Opt.* 1996;16:124-129.

6. Applegate RA, Hilmantel G, Howland HC. Corneal aberrations increase with the magnitude of radial keratotomy refractive correction. *Optom Vis Sci.* 1996;73:585-589.

7. Schwiegerling J, Greivenkamp JE, Miller JM, Snyder RW, Palmer ML. Optical modeling of radial keratotomy incision patterns. *Am J Ophthalmol.* 1996;122:808-817.

8. Schwiegerling J, Greivenkamp JE. Using corneal height maps and polynomial decomposition to determine corneal aberrations. *Optom Vis Sci.* 1997;74:906-916.

9. Oliver KM, Hemenger RP, Corbett MC, et al. Corneal optical aberrations induced by photorefractive keratectomy. *J Refract Surg.* 1997;13:246-254.

10. Applegate RA, Howland HC, Sharp RP, Cottingham AJ, Yee RW. Corneal aberrations and visual performance after radial keratotomy. *J Refract Surg.* 1998;14:397-407.

11. Martinez CE, Applegate RA, Klyce SD, McDonald MB, Medina JP, Howland HC. Effect of pupil dilation on corneal optical aberrations after photorefractive keratectomy. *Arch Ophthalmol.* 1998;116:1053-1062.

12. Langenbucher A, Seitz B, Kus MM. Interpretation of corneal topography after penetrating keratoplasty with wavefront parameters—comparison between non-mechanical trepanation with excimer laser and motor trepanation (German). *Klin Monatsbl Augenheilkd.* 1998;212:433-43.

13. Oshika T, Klyce SD, Applegate RA, Howland HC. Comparison of corneal wavefront aberrations after photorefractive keratectomy and laser in situ keratomileusis. *Am J Ophthalmol.* 1999;127:1-7.

14. Oshika T, Klyce SD, Applegate RA, Howland HC. Changes in corneal wavefront aberrations with aging. *Invest Ophthalmol Vis Sci.* 1999;40:1351-1355.

15. Endl MJ, Martinez CE, Klyce SD, et al. Irregular astigmatism after photorefractive keratectomy. *J Refract Surg.* 1999;S249-S251.

16. Guirao A, Artal P. Corneal wave-aberration from videokeratography: accuracy and limitations of the procedure. *J Opt Soc Am A.* 2000;17:955-965.

17. Guirao A, Redondo M, Artal P. Optical aberrations of the human cornea as a function of age. *J Opt Soc Am A*. In press.

18. Applegate RA, Hilmantel G, Howland HC, Tu EY, Starck T, Zayac EJ. Corneal first surface optical aberrations and visual performance. *J Refract Surg.* 2000;16:507-514.

19. Klein SA. Optimal corneal ablation for eyes with arbitrary Hartmann-Shack aberrations. *J Opt Soc Am A.* 1998;15:2580-2588.

20. Roberts C. The cornea is not a piece of plastic. *J Refract Surg.* 2000;16:407-413.

21. Howland HC, Rand RH, Lubkin SR. Thin-shell model of the cornea and its application to corneal surgery. *Refract Corneal Surg.* 1992;8:183-186.

Corneal Topography-Guided Ablations

CLINICAL SCIENCE SECTION

Chapter Twenty-One

Customized Ablation Using the Bausch & Lomb Technolas Laser

Michael Knorz, MD

Isn't it nice to wear a suit that was custom tailored? One off-the-rack will also fit most of us but not everybody, and not as well. This comparison may not fit perfectly well, but it certainly describes what customized ablations are all about. There are many ways to "customize" one's treatment. Some of them may be called "art," as they use partial coverage of the ablated area and therefore strongly depend on the surgeon performing them. Others can be called "science," as they use more reproducible ways to achieve the desired result.

I had the opportunity to become involved with customized ablations quite early. When we started, we felt that corneal topography was the ideal source to obtain data on which to base a customized ablation. Corneal topography is readily available and provides a vast amount of data on the most important part of the eye's optical system—the cornea. Our initial study therefore used corneal topography data to calculate a customized ablation. We used several systems, including the C-Scan (Technomed Co, Baesweiler, Germany) and the Orbscan II corneal tomography system (Bausch & Lomb Surgical, Claremont, Calif). We initially treated eyes that had previously undergone refractive surgery ("repair procedures"), then also included so-called normal eyes that underwent a routine laser-assisted in situ keratomileusis (LASIK) procedure. During the last year, we expanded our repertoire by adding an aberrometer that is used to measure the wavefront devi-

ation of the whole eye. The measured wavefront deviation reflects both the refractive error of the eye and higher-order optical aberrations such as coma. Any treatment based on wavefront deviation will theoretically not only treat the refractive error but also optimize the optics of the eye by removing the higher-order optical aberrations.

In this chapter, I will describe the technique using corneal topography and present some examples as well as the results of repair procedures and normal eyes. I will also address the first results obtained with wavefront deviation-guided ablations.

TopoLink Techniques

Spot scanning or flying spot excimer lasers provide the technological platform to perform ablations of any shape.[1] Corneal topography enables us to measure the shape of the individual cornea with great precision, and elevation-based systems like the Orbscan II provide an even better basis for the calculation of the required ablation. Could we combine corneal topography and scanning lasers to create customized ablations? This question posed quite a challenge when we started to treat our first patients with so-called TopoLink LASIK a few years ago.[2] Surgical technique involves the use of the Hansatome microkeratome (Bausch & Lomb Surgical, St. Louis, Mo) and the Keracor 217 (Bausch & Lomb Technolas, Munich, Germany) excimer laser with an active eye tracker. The laser ablation was based on the preoperative corneal topographic map obtained with the Orbscan II corneal analysis system. Three different maps were taken, and the one featuring the least eye movements was used. The maximum movements considered acceptable were 200 μm. Patients who did not comply with this requirement due to poor cooperation were excluded. Once the topography was taken, data were copied and a technician from Bausch & Lomb calculated the ablation profile on site using special software called TopoLink (Version 2.9992TL; Bausch & Lomb Surgical Technolas, Munich, Germany). Input values were manifest refraction in minus cylinder format and corneal thickness as measured by the Orbscan II. The target K-value was determined by the software by subtracting the manifest sphere from the K-value in the steep corneal meridian. The target K-value and a preset shape factor of –0.25 defined the target asphere that we planned to achieve after LASIK.

The TopoLink software basically compares the shape of the target asphere to the corneal shape actually measured. Simplified, the target shape is fitted from beneath to the actual cornea for a given planned optical zone size. The difference between the two shapes is then ablated. Any "overlap"

> Simplified, the target shape is fitted from beneath to the actual cornea for a given planned optical zone size. The difference between the two shapes is then ablated.

between target and actual shape must be outside the planned optical zone, as tissue cannot be "added" — only ablated. The TopoLink software therefore represents a new and different approach that is not based on Munnerlyn's formula. It rather calculates a certain "lenticle" of corneal tissue to be removed, and the scanning laser provides the means to remove this tissue even if its shape is asymmetrical or even irregular. The diameter of the planned optical zone was 6 to 7 mm. Only cases in which the ablation required to achieve these optical zones would have left a residual corneal stromal bed of < 250 μm, the diameter of the planned optical zone was decreased to maintain a residual stromal bed of at least 250 μm. Based on these data, TopoLink calculated a session file that contained information for the scanning laser about which ablation pattern to perform. The session file was transferred via computer disk and loaded into a Keracor 217 excimer laser just prior to treatment. We

used the Keracor 217 excimer laser. This laser uses a 2-mm beam that is scanned across the cornea at a shot frequency of 50 Hz. It was modified by including an aperture that allows the use of both a 1-mm beam and a 2-mm beam.

EXAMPLES OF TOPOLINK

Patient 1. Irregular Astigmatism After Penetrating Injury

This 6-year-old patient had suffered a penetrating injury in her left eye. A light bulb exploded, and glass fragments penetrated her eye, causing corneal lacerations extending from 10 to 12 o'clock peripherally. One year after the initial repair, scar formation caused significant irregular astigmatism. Uncorrected visual acuity was 20/200. With a correction of +0.5 sphere –5.0 cyl axis 170 degrees, an acuity of 20/100 was achieved. Contact lenses were tried but not tolerated by the patient. Corneal topography showed marked irregular astigmatism. We then discussed treatment options with the child's parents. As contact lenses were not tolerated, surgery seemed to be the only option to prevent amblyopia. We considered t-cuts, corneal grafts, and TopoLink LASIK. LASIK was selected as the least invasive and most predictable option. Surgery was performed under general anesthesia. Figure 21-1 shows the topographic workplace on which the ablation is planned. The preoperative topographic map (scale in diopters [D]) is on the upper left, and the ablation profile suggested by the TopoLink LASIK software (scale in microns) is on the upper right. On the lower left, the surgeon can add individual fudge factors, and the expected result is displayed on the lower right side. Comparing maps, we can see that the flat area at the lower right (blue colors) of the preoperative topography map is steepened by the ablation (red color at the lower right of the ablation map). By superimposing the two maps in the upper row, the resulting map, which is displayed at the lower right, should be a perfect sphere (at least theoretically).

The preoperative topographic map and the topographic map 1 day after surgery are shown in Figure 21-2. The color scale is the same in both maps, which can therefore be directly compared. As is clearly visible, the steep area on the upper left is considerably flatter, and visual acuity without correction improved to 20/60 on day 1. Figure 21-2 also shows the differential map. The change map, which visual-

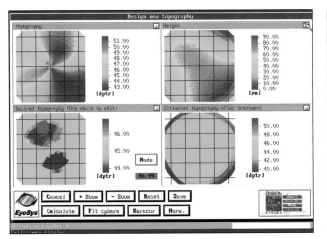

Figure 21-1. Topographic workplace used to design the ablation of patient 1. The preoperative topographic map (scale in diopters) is on the upper left, and the ablation profile suggested by the TopoLink LASIK software (scale in microns) is on the upper right. On the lower left, the surgeon can add individual fudge factors, and the expected result is displayed on the lower righthand side.

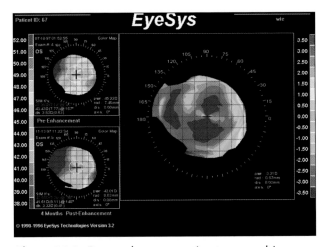

Figure 21-3. Pre- and postoperative topographic maps and differential map of patient 2 (irregular astigmatism after PKP and RK).

izes the ablation that was performed, closely resembles the planned ablation (see Figure 21-1, upper right, for comparison). One year after surgery, visual acuity without correction was 20/80, and with correction of –2 cyl axis 140 degrees, acuity was 20/60. To prevent amblyopia, the right eye was occluded 4 hours a day. Corneal topography at 1 year shows considerable regression of effect. The cornea was still more regular than preoperatively, but most of the effect had regressed. We considered a retreatment

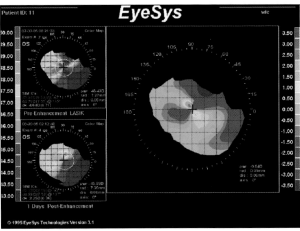

Figure 21-2. Pre- and postoperative topographic maps and differential map of patient 1 (penetrating injury with irregular astigmatism).

and calculated an ablation of 50 µm. Preoperatively, corneal thickness was 587 µm. Flap thickness was 160 µm, and ablation depth during the first TA-LASIK procedure was 86 µm. Central corneal thickness after the first procedure was 430 µm. We therefore decided against a retreatment to avoid possible late keratectasia due to corneal thinning.

Patient 2. Irregular Astigmatism After PKP and RK

This patient had a penetrating corneal graft because of recurrent stromal herpetic keratitis in 1992. He was first referred in 1993. Manifest refraction was +0.25 sphere –6 cyl axis 135 degrees. Corneal astigmatism was –8 D axis 135 degrees and slightly asymmetric. Initially, astigmatic keratotomy (AK) was performed in 1994. After AK, manifest refraction was –2.5 sphere –4 cyl axis 165 degrees. Uncorrected visual acuity (UCVA) was 20/400 and best-corrected visual acuity (BCVA) was 20/60. Corneal topography showed marked irregularity and axis shift (Figure 21-3, upper left). We therefore decided to perform TopoLink LASIK. Average refractive power of the cornea overlaying the entrance pupil was estimated to be 45 D. Spherical equivalent of manifest refraction was –4.5 D. We selected a target K-value of 40.5 D. A 5.4-mm optical zone was used, and ablation depth was 150 µm. Corneal thickness was 610 µm centrally, and both the internal and external margins of the graft were well aligned with the host cornea. It is very important to check alignment prior to the lamellar cut. In poor alignment or localized ectasia at the edge, corneal thickness might

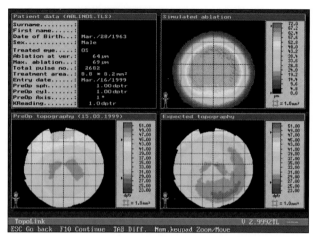

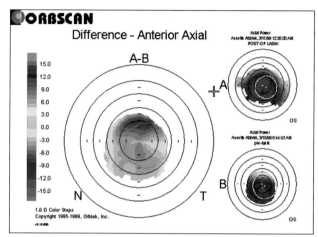

Figure 21-4. Treatment plan for TopoLink LASIK. This plan is shown on the screen of the Keracor 217 excimer laser when the treatment is loaded. It features patient data (upper left), preoperative topography (lower left), simulated ablation pattern (upper right), and the expected postoperative topography (lower right).

Figure 21-5. Orbscan II differential map after treatment. The preoperative map (lower right) shows a decentered ablation. The postoperative map (upper right) shows improved centration. The differential map is shown on the left.

be reduced, and the keratome cut may cause further weakening of the cornea, inducing more ectasia or even a penetration of the anterior chamber. In this patient, alignment was perfect, and the LASIK procedure performed in July 1997 was uneventful. A 160-μm flap was used. One day after TopoLink LASIK, UCVA had improved to 20/30, and BCVA was 20/25 (correction: +0.75 sphere). After 4 months, UCVA was 20/30 and BCVA 20/25, but manifest refraction had changed slightly to +1 sphere −2.0 cyl axis 10 degrees. Corneal topography 4 months after TopoLink LASIK showed marked improvement of the irregularity (see Figure 21-3). Some residual with-the-rule astigmatism was still present, but the irregular astigmatism that was present preoperatively had virtually disappeared, as shown by the differential map (see Figure 21-3).

Patient 3. Decentered Ablation

A 36-year-old woman had LASIK in both eyes in 1998 and was referred to me because of a decentered ablation. The right eye was perfect, but she bitterly complained about permanent monocular diplopia and distorted halos in her left eye. TopoLink LASIK was planned. The corneal topography taken prior to the TopoLink LASIK is shown in Figure 21-4, lower left, and Figure 21-5, lower right. A decentered myopic ablation is visible. The ablation is decentered about 1.5 mm downward and 1 mm temporally. We calculated a customized ablation based on the

Orbscan II topographic map just described. The planned ablation pattern is shown in Figure 21-4, upper right. The scale is in microns. The predicted outcome of corneal topography is shown in Figure 21-4, lower right. The scale is in diopters. I used the Hansatome to create a new flap with a thickness of 160 μm and a diameter of 8.5 mm (8.5-mm suction ring). The surgery was uneventful. The ablation was centered on the center of the entrance pupil, and an eye tracker was used. Figure 21-5 shows the pre- and postoperative maps, as well as the differential map, taken 1 day after surgery. The postoperative map, upper right, shows significantly improved centration and no residual astigmatism. The differential map, left, shows the asymmetric ablation pattern, customized to this individual eye. Visual acuity improved to 20/25 uncorrected, and even more important, monocular double vision and halos were no longer visible. This case indicates that TopoLink LASIK is a valuable tool in the treatment of decentered ablations.

RESULTS OF TOPOLINK IN REPAIR PROCEDURES

In our initial prospective study, we evaluated 29 eyes of 27 patients treated between July 1996 and July 1997. Inclusion criteria were irregular corneal astigmatism due to trauma or previous corneal sur-

Table 21-1

Refraction, Visual Acuity, and Corneal Topography 12 Months After TopoLink LASIK

	GROUP 1 POST-KERATOPLASTY	GROUP 2 POST-TRAUMA	GROUP 3 DECENTERED/SMALL	GROUP 4 CENTRAL ISLANDS
# eyes	n = 6	n = 6	n = 11	n = 6
Cylinder	5.83 ± 1.25 D	2.21 ± 1.35 D	0.73 ± 0.71 D	1.42 ± 1.13 D
Preoperative	(4.00 to 8.00 D)	(1.00 to 5.00 D)	(0 to 2.00 D)	(0 to 3.50 D)
Cylinder at	2.96 ± 1.23 D*	0.50 ± 0.84 D**	0.36 ± 1.05 D	0.50 ± 0.84 D*
12 months	(1.50 to 4.50 D)	(0 to 2.5 D)	(0 to 3.5 D)	(0 to 2.00 D)
Success rate (topo as planned or improved)	66% (n = 4)	83% (n = 5)	91% (n = 10)	50% (n = 3)
Reoperation rate	50% (n = 3)	50% (n = 3)	36% (n = 4)	50% (n = 3)

(UCVA: uncorrected visual acuity; SCVA: spectacle-corrected visual acuity)
*p = 0.01
**p = 0.001

gery. We considered TopoLink LASIK as the last option prior to performing a corneal graft. Eyes were divided into four groups:

- Group 1 (post-keratoplasty) consisted of six eyes (five patients) with irregular corneal astigmatism after penetrating keratoplasty. All grafts were performed more than 2 years ago.
- Group 2 (post-trauma) consisted of six eyes (six patients) with irregular corneal astigmatism after corneal trauma. The trauma dated back more than 2 years in all eyes.
- Group 3 (decentered/small optical zones) consisted of 11 eyes (10 patients) with irregular corneal astigmatism after PRK (one eye) or LASIK (10 eyes) due to decentered or small optical zones. All patients complained about halos and image distortion even during the day.
- Group 4 (central islands) consisted of six eyes (six patients) with irregular astigmatism after PRK (two eyes) or LASIK (four eyes) due to central islands or keyhole patterns. All patients complained of blurred vision or image distortion even during the day.

The results of our initial study using the Corneal Analysis System were presented at the American Academy of Ophthalmology Annual Meeting in New Orleans in 1998 and accepted for publication in *Ophthalmology*. They are shown in part in Table 21-1. In the post-keratoplasty and post-trauma groups, corrective cylinder was significantly reduced, as compared to the preoperative value. The topographic success rate was defined as either the planned correction fully achieved or the attempted correction partially achieved (decrease of irregularity of more than 1 D on the differential map and/or increase of optical zone size of at least 1 mm). The success rate was highest in the decentered/small optical zones group (91%), followed by the post-trauma group (83%). The lowest success rate was observed in the central island group—only 50%. Overall, 14 of the 29 eyes were reoperated (48%) due to regression of effect or undercorrection. The rate of reoperation was lowest in the decentered/small optical zones group at 36% as compared to 50% in all other groups (see Table 21-1).

These results demonstrate that TopoLink LASIK definitely works. We were able to significantly

We were able to significantly reduce irregularities in these extremely irregular corneas. On the other hand, our results demonstrated that most eyes were undercorrected, and we had to adjust the algorithm to take care of the undercorrection.

reduce irregularities in these extremely irregular corneas. On the other hand, our results demonstrated that most eyes were undercorrected, and we had to adjust the algorithm to take care of the undercorrection. Finally, the problem of targeting the right spot on the cornea must be addressed. The results of group 4 (central islands) were poor, which suggests that we may not have hit the right target in these eyes, which featured small and circumscribed irregularities. Ideally, the laser should be locked on a topographic map of the cornea prior to treatment, and that is what we are currently working on to improve the results in the rare cases.

RESULTS OF TOPOLINK IN NORMAL EYES

In a prospective, noncomparative case series, we operated on 203 eyes of 203 patients between January 1999 and July 1999. Results were presented at the American Academy of Ophthalmology Annual Meeting in Orlando in 1999 and accepted for publication in *Ophthalmology*. Inclusion criteria was myopia of -1.00 to –12.00 D with or without astigmatism of up to –4.00 D. The patients were divided into two groups:

- Group 1 (low myopia) consisted of 114 patients with myopia of –1.00 to –6.00 D (mean, -3.83 ± 1.67 D) and astigmatism of 0 to –4.00 D (mean, -1.32 ± 1.06 D).
- Group 2 (high myopia) consisted of 89 patients with myopia of –6.10 to –12.00 D (mean, -7.83 ± 1.38 D) and astigmatism of 0 to –3.50 D (mean, -1.06 ± 0.92 D).

No reoperations were performed in these series and no complications occurred. Three months after surgery, 51 patients of the low myopia group and 40 patients of the high myopia group were available for follow-up. In the low myopia group, 96.1%, and in the high myopia group, 75% were within ± 0.50 D of emmetropia. Uncorrected visual acuity (UCVA) was 20/20 or better in 82.4% of the low myopia group and in 62.5% of the high myopia group; 20/25 or better in 98% of the low myopia group and in 70% of the high myopia group; and 20/40 or better in 100% of the low myopia group and 95% of the high myopia group. In low myopia, spectacle-corrected acuity at the higher levels improved as compared to preoperative values, and 13.7% (n = 7) had a spectacle-corrected visual acuity of 20/12.5 or better; 47.1% (n = 24) saw 20/15 or better after TopoLink LASIK as compared to the preoperative values of 5.9% (n = 3)

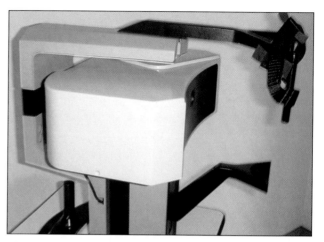

Figure 21-6. Beta version of the Bausch & Lomb Zywave aberrometer. The chin and headrests are visible on the right.

and 37.3% (n = 19), respectively. Differences were statistically significant (p < 0.01). However, comparing mean values (log scale) of spectacle-corrected visual acuity, differences were not significant (p = 0.2). The larger percentage of patients seeing 20/12.5 or 20/15 3 months postoperatively than preoperatively in the low myopia group may indicate an improvement of spectacle-corrected visual acuity due to the customized LASIK. In the high myopia group, no improvement was observed, whereas a one-line improvement should be expected due to higher magnification.[3] The lack of improvement in the high myopia group is most likely due to the fact that corneal refractive surgery in high myopia causes a significant decrease in optical quality of the eye and, consecutively, in quality of vision because of the relationship of optical zone size, reversed asphericity, and pupil size.[4,5]

We were able to demonstrate that the new approach to customize ablation based on corneal topography works clinically at least as well as a standard ablation in normal eyes. This is a significant finding, as our approach is based on a totally different calculation of the ablation: instead of ablations based on Munnerlyn's formula, we defined a target asphere and ablated the differences between it and the actual cornea.

THE BAUSCH & LOMB ZYWAVE ABERROMETER

The Bausch & Lomb Zywave aberrometer (Figure

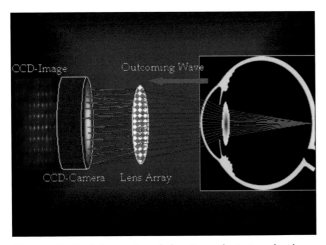

Figure 21-7. Schematic of the Bausch & Lomb aberrometer. A low-intensity laser light is shone into the eye; the reflected light is focused by a number of small lenses (lenslet array) and pictured by a CCD camera. The captured image is shown on the left.

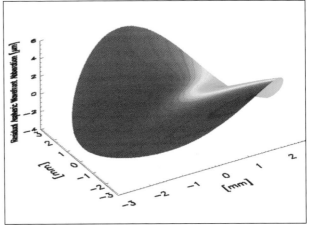

Figure 21-8. Calculated wavefront deformation of an eye with astigmatism (Bausch & Lomb aberrometer). The x and y axes are in millimeters and represent the diameter of the optical zone measured. The z axis is in microns and shows the deviation of the wavefront from plano (residual aspheric wavefront aberration). The "potato chip" pattern is typical in astigmatism.

21-6) uses a low-intensity HeNe laser that is shone into the eye. The pupil is dilated prior to examination to allow for a measured optical zone of at least 6 mm and to prevent accommodation. The reflected light from the fundus is focused by a number of small lenses, a so-called lenslet array, and the resulting picture is captured by a CCD camera (Figure 21-7). Ideally, each of the bright white spots focused by each of the small lenses should have the same intensity and pattern. This would equal a plane wavefront, which means a perfect optical system. As most eyes are not perfect optical systems, the white spots will have different intensities and/or patterns, indicating deviations of the wavefront from plano. The deviations from plano are calculated based on the image captured by the CCD camera, and the actual wavefront deviation is depicted graphically in color-coded maps. Figure 21-8 shows an example of astigmatism. The spherical error was not included. The three-dimensional graph shows the typical "potato chip" pattern of astigmatism. The wavefront deviation is expressed in microns above or below the ideal plane wavefront. The measured deviation, simply multiplied by a constant, can be used to perform the laser ablation. As such, wavefront deviation-guided ablations seem to be a very logical choice. As always, things are not as easy as they look, and my description of the aberrometer technology is certainly considerably simplified.

WAVEFRONT DEVIATION-GUIDED LASIK

The first clinical work using wavefront-guided ablations was done by Dr. McDonald in New Orleans and Dr. Seiler in Dresden, Germany. Some patients showed improvement BCVA, others did not. We started our first treatments using the Bausch & Lomb aberrometer in January 2000 in Mannheim, Germany. Patients were enrolled as part of a prospective study comparing eyes intraindividually. One eye of each patient received standard LASIK, the fellow eye received LASIK using wavefront deviation-guided ablations. Of our first 10 patients treated, three improved by two lines as compared to preoperative spectacle-corrected visual acuity, and seven reached the same visual acuity as preoperatively. Thus, the number of patients treated is still far too small for any conclusions.

SUMMARY

The data presented in this chapter certainly demonstrate that customized ablations have matured and are already being introduced in our daily routine. In their early days, customized procedures were an art dependent largely on the surgeon's skill or luck. The introduction of ablation profiles calculated based on corneal topography was the first step toward a more standardized approach.

TopoLink LASIK, as it was called, was initially used as a repair procedure and showed some promise. Comparative studies also indicated that TopoLink LASIK improved best-corrected visual acuity (BCVA) in a certain number of normal eyes. The final step toward the ultimate goal of perfect customization seems to be the introduction of wavefront deviation-guided ablations. This technology objectively measures the refractive error of the whole eye, plus all the higher-order optical aberrations such as coma. Eliminating the optical aberrations of the eye could mean an improvement on its performance (ie, an increase of visual acuity well above the preoperative level). Statistically, it will also mean a much higher percentage of patients seeing 20/20 or better without correction after LASIK and a much smaller percentage complaining about problems of vision quality in dim light or at night. Customized ablations have finally arrived and are here to stay as an integral part of refractive surgery.

ACKNOWLEDGMENTS

The work presented here is not based on one individual but on the support of many of my colleagues and friends all over the world. Those who contributed significantly include Dr. Maria Clara Arbelaez, Dr. Jorge Alio, Dr. Stephen G. Slade, Dr. Michiel Kritzinger, and Dr. Thomas Neuhann. All were supported by a dedicated team from Bausch & Lomb Technolas in Munich, which included Dr. Kristian Hohla, Dr. Gerhard Yousseffi, Martina Sohr, and many, many others not mentioned by name. I am pleased at the opportunity to thank all of them for their dedication and support.

REFERENCES

1. Knorz MC. Broadbeam versus scanning-beam lasers for refractive surgery. *Ophthalmic Practice.* 1997;15:142-145.
2. Wiesinger-Jendritza B, Knorz MC, Hugger P, et al. Laser in situ keratomileusis assisted by corneal topography. *J Cataract Refract Surg.* 1998;24:166-174.
3. Applegate RA, Howland HC. Magnification and visual acuity in refractive surgery. *Arch Ophthalmol.* 1993;111:1335-1342.
4. Holladay JT, Dudeja DR, Chang J. Functional vision and corneal changes after laser in situ keratomileusis determined by contrast sensitivity, glare testing, and corneal topography. *J Cataract Refract Surg.* 1999;25:663-669.
5. Pallikaris IG. Quality of vision in refractive surgery. *J Refract Surg.* 1998;14:551-558.

Chapter Twenty-Two

Corneal Interactive Programmed Topographic Ablation Using the Lasersight Laser

Giovanni Alessio, MD
M. Gabriella La Tegola, MD
Carlo Sborgia, MD

INTRODUCTION

The rationale for photorefractive surgery is that there is a close correlation between the optical properties of the cornea and its shape. Hence, surgical manipulation to correct the shape can alter the refractive status of the eye. However, although this premise is undoubtedly true, the relationship between the shape of the cornea and its performance status is much more complex than is generally believed. In reality, each cornea has unique characteristics in regard to diameter, dioptric power, width, curve, aspheric index, meridian profile, and shape.

One of the limits of refractive surgery is the fact that it is difficult to correct irregular forms of astigmatism, either idiopathic or postsurgical, and there is even a risk of worsening irregular astigmatism.[1,2] This is because the most common software used to manage photoablation takes into account only the refractive correction desired, and very few programs consider the mean keratometric power calculated on an ideal corneal model. In this way, a standard ablative pattern is extended to different corneas. This may result in variable outcomes.

Although in most cases corneal surgery leads to an excellent outcome in terms of visual acuity (corrected or uncorrected) and refraction, some patients complain of poor visual quality. The cause of onset of this poor quality vision is not easily identifiable. We have found it helpful to use corneal topography in such cases, as this will often reveal alterations of the corneal surface (central islands, irregular astigmatism) that might offer a plausible explanation of the patient's problems. Irregular astigmatism causes distorted vision that can only be partially corrected by the use of spectacles. While this is a cause of complaint in patients with native irregular astigmatism, it is more pronounced in postrefractive surgical patients who had not suffered from this problem prior to refractive surgery.

These circumstances have led to recognition of the need to study new surgical regimens aimed at smoothing the corneal surface and correcting both ametropia and irregularity of the anterior surface of the eye. The best chance of achieving this aim seemed to be by exploiting the diagnostic and imaging possibilities offered by altimetric (height mapping) topography and the treatment potential of flying spot excimer lasers.

METHODS

On this basis, in January 1996 in collaboration with Ing. D'Ippolito at the LIGI Company in Taranto, Italy, we developed a software program called Corneal Interactive Programmed Topographic Ablation (CIPTA), which couples a corneal elevation topograph (Orbscan) with a flying spot laser (Laserscan 2000, Lasersight, Orlando, Fla), by means of an interface to support topography-assisted photoablative treatments.[3]

The Orbscan is an optical topograph featuring special characteristics that set it apart from the other topographs available on the market; the system uses a placido and slit projection system. The topographic systems based on a placido disc enable maps to be drawn that provide information on the corneal curve (axial and tangential) derived from mathematical calculations. Programs have recently been added that make it possible to represent the altimetric (height) differences of the anterior corneal surface as compared with a reference sphere. The latter sphere is calculated by integral calculations on the measurements of the corneal curve (ie, from axial topography).[4,5]

The slit projection system offers a number of advantages for the purposes of topographic ablation as compared with the placido disc system.[6-9] The main one is the possibility of acquiring extremely precise altimetric topographic data and reconstructing the actual shape of the corneal surface, thus identifying even minimally irregular areas. Moreover, Orbscan can supply this precise information on the shape of the cornea regardless of its orientation with respect to the instrument.

Laser Delivery

To perform customized photoablative treatment, we used a flying spot laser—the Laserscan 2000 up to 1998—and the LSX (Lasersight, Orlando, Fla) thereafter. The latter is a software-driven ablation system regulated by internal scanning that does not require additional devices (masks, rotating discs, etc). It employs a small diameter spot (800 to 1000 μm) with a gaussian energy distribution guided by the software over the surface to be treated with a frequency of 100 to 200 Hz (ie, it emits 100 to 200 spots per second). The energy used by the laser is 3 to 5 mJ at the source and only 0.7 to 1.2 mJ at the cornea.[10] An infrared active/passive eye tracker was used; we put it in active form with movement up to 1.2 mm and passive over this diameter. Thanks to these properties, the laser can perform treatments on any shape and achieve ablations of variable depth during the same treatment. It can also reach all points of the cornea—even the most peripheral—until 10 mm.[2]

Corneal Shape Design

The normal cornea has an *aspheric surface* with a more pronounced curve in the central portion and gradually flattening out toward the periphery. The most faithful reproduction of all the corneal asym-

> The normal cornea has an aspheric surface with a more pronounced curve in the central portion and gradually flattening out toward the periphery.

metries and anomalies is achieved by altimetric height maps that use a sphere as the reference system. The Orbscan expresses the difference in height between the reference sphere and the eye surface being examined as the radial distance from the center of the sphere. It is displayed as a color scale to enable immediate reading.

CIPTA software is based on the same principle as altimetric topography, but instead of comparing the cornea being examined with a reference sphere it compares it with an aconic ellipsoid with an adjustable coefficient of asphericity to preserve the patient's physiological astigmatism and prolate shape. Descartes' work taught us that the surface that produces the best image is the so-called "Cartesian ellipsoid."[11] The aconic ellipsoid is the ideal shape the cornea should have in order to provide the patient with optimal qualitative and quantitative vision. The two shapes are compared and a map is built which, starting from the difference in height of the two profiles, provides precise data (in microns) on the shape and depth of the ablation to be performed at each point.

This ideal corneal model is "built" with the aid of the CIPTA software by the surgeon, who can study the various possible types of ablations and choose the one best suited. The software was deliberately planned to be interactive to enable the surgeon to take an active part in the decision-making process and select the best solution at each step. The altimetric topography of the cornea is first acquired by the Orbscan. The software then asks whether the current visual axis should be preserved or another one chosen. If we choose to preserve the actual visual axis, the theoretical shape of the "new" cornea will be forced to move up or down on the visual axis; if we change this axis, the new corneal shape will be forced to move on the normal at the point chosen as center of the treatment. At this stage, the center of the hypothetical ablation should be identified. There are many different possibilities:

- The pupil (ie, the pupil centroid), which is most commonly chosen as the center of ablation because this is the laser eye tracker's automatic default setting.
- The fixation point (ie, the corneal reflex of the fixation target of the Orbscan [or patient's topo-

graphic visual axis—the ideal line between the topography telecamera lens and the patient's macula]). This is the point chosen in hypermetropic treatments in which the patient has a high kappa angle. Postoperatively, the corneal apex will coincide with the topographic visual axis.

- The apex, which is the most protruding point of the cornea (ie, the nearest to the topography lens). This is generally close to the previous two points, but in cases of irregular corneas with asymmetrical astigmatism, the treatment can be centered on this point.
- The pachymetric point. The software allows a point of given thickness to be chosen as the ablation center. The topograph can indicate the thinnest corneal point to guide such a choice.
- The cursor, which enables selection of any point on the cornea, judged by the surgeon to be best suited as the center point by moving the cursor over the topographic image.
- The input, which is a function that enables location of a given point on the cornea selected on the basis of its mathematical coordinates.

Once the ablation center has been chosen, the ablation diameters are decided. The first diameter the computer asks for is the minimal optical refractive zone. This is the minimal optical zone that includes all the desired refractive corrections (it is not equal, therefore, to the effective treatment diameter). This should always be the diameter of the patient's pupil in scotopic conditions to ensure good visual quality even in low light conditions. The maximum diameter will, instead, be chosen to delimit the extent of the treatment. For example, in treatments for myopic astigmatism the ablation shape provided by the computer is a cylinder that covers the whole cornea, whereas by inserting the maximum diameter it is possible to limit the extension of the cylinder. Then, after having chosen the width of the cylinder (the ablation optical zone) on the basis of the pupil diameter, we can limit its length to the zone of interest (this diameter will also be less than the real diameter of the treatment, which includes a transition zone).

The next step, in cases where the surgeon decided in the previous step to choose the option of changing the visual axis, is to define the ablation axis. As mentioned above, ablation is calculated on the basis of the micrometric difference between the "ideal shape" and the actual shape of the cornea.

Choice of Ablation Axis (Axial or Floating)

There are two possible alternatives for the choice of ablation axis: axial or floating. The former axis will necessarily coincide with that of the true shape of the cornea as well as the resultant postoperative axis. The floating axis, on the other hand, approximates the best match between the axis of the ideal shape and that of the true shape of the cornea, maintaining the same center and external diameters. The latter choice is particularly useful in cases of corneas with a highly irregular profile to enable maximal tissue sparing by limiting the quantity of energy applied.

> The floating axis, on the other hand, approximates the best match between the axis of the ideal shape and that of the true shape of the cornea, maintaining the same center and external diameters.

Refractive Data Display

The program displays the refractive data. Three columns of data will appear, showing (from left to right) the preoperative data, the treatment parameters, and the postoperative data. The first column includes:
- Preoperative keratometric data.
- Astigmatism value and its axis.
- Aspheric coefficient.

The data inserted in the central column will express:
- The spherical defect (myopia or hyperopia) expressed in diopters.
- The cylindrical defect expressed in negative diopters and its respective axis. The software always suggests total correction of the cylindrical corneal error. It is then up to the operator to choose how much cylinder to correct.

The third column will show:
- The estimated postoperative keratometric values.
- The estimated postoperative astigmatism value and its axis.
- The postoperative aspheric coefficient.

Apart from the postoperative data, all other values can be set as required although they are interdependent and a change in one value will automatically alter the others. Cylindrical correction is always evaluated according to a vectorial calculation.

Insertion of the refractive data is a particularly important step because at this stage the results of the previous clinical examination can be imported into the program to enable the best correction. In other words, the topographic assessments can be combined with the patient's cycloplegic and/or subjective refractive values.

Ablation design can then be chosen, which can be calculated as superficial (PRK) or intrastromal (LASIK) according to the surgical technique to be adopted.

Blend Transition Zones and Laser Epithelial Debridement

Next, the diameter and depth of the blend zone is defined. A transition zone is needed to blend the ablated corneal surface with the nontreated surface. Its extent will be directly proportional to the amount of alteration made in the corneal profile. The software advises a certain ablation diameter and depth, but these can be modified as the surgeon sees fit. Unlike traditional corneal surgery, with this technique the blend zone has a constant slope and will therefore be wider in deeper treatment areas and narrower in more superficial treatment areas. A constant slope in the blend zone reduces the risk of regression.

In the case of superficial ablation, the software proposes epithelial laser debridement to a depth of 50 μm and a diameter of 0.5 mm greater than the diameter of the blend zone. These parameters can be modified by the operator; other forms of debridement can also be chosen.

Final Treatment Variables

A window will then appear on the monitor displaying the ablation scheme in the form of three rings, the inner and outermost corresponding to the minimal and maximal ablation optical zones and the middle ring to the blend zone. The statistical data for the ablation are then displayed, including:

- The ablation volume (expressed in millimeters^3): this provides the information on the quantity of energy required and the time needed.
- Ablation surface (expressed in millimeters^2): this indicates the surface extension to be prepared for treatment.
- The maximal ablation depth and its Cartesian coordinates.
- The residual corneal thickness after photoablative treatment in the thinnest part and its coordinates.
- The diameter of the optical zone (minimum).
- The distance between the center of ablation and

the pupil centroid, expressed in Cartesian coordinates; these coordinates are entered into the laser eye tracker.

Finally, the ablation topographic map is displayed. The warm colors show the treatment areas: the ablation depth will range from yellowish-green for more superficial points to deeper and deeper red for greater-depth treatment areas. By moving the cursor over the screen, the depth of ablation of each single point can be checked; its values are displayed on the right of the screen.

The treatment data are transferred to a diskette, then directly to the software of the flying spot excimer laser, which will perform the predefined treatment.

> The warm colors show the treatment areas: the ablation depth will range from yellowish-green for more superficial points to deeper and deeper red for greater-depth treatment areas.

RESULTS

We started to perform topographic ablation using CIPTA at our institute in 1997. The first cases we treated had irregular astigmatism following refractive surgical treatment (PRK) or trauma (perforating corneal wounds). All were difficult cases to manage and could not have resulted in satisfactory visual acuity even with the aid of contact lenses. After our first encouraging results, further indications were added.

We treated 206 eyes with topographic ablation up to December 1999. Of these, 90 eyes were affected by myopia or regular myopic astigmatism, 64 by irregular myopic astigmatism (idiopathic, post-ECCE, post-traumatic; post-PRK retreatments, post-LASIK, post-RK), 22 by regular hypermetropic astigmatism, and 30 by irregular hypermetropic astigmatism (idiopathic or post-PRK) (Table 22-1). Patients' mean age was 35.5 ± 8.2 years and mean follow-up at the time of this study was 13.2 months (range: 3 to 29 months).

Myopia and Myopic Astigmatism

The 90 eyes with regular myopia or myopic astigmatism all underwent their first refractive surgery. The preoperative spheric equivalent was -7.23 ± 3.96 D (range: -1 to -14.50), whereas at the last postoperative control the mean spheric equivalent was -0.10 ± 0.8 D (range: -2.50 to +2). The percentage of spheric

Table 22-1								
Uncorrected Visual Acuity Before and After Treatment								
	REG HYPEROPIC N=22		IRREG HYPEROPIC N=30		IRREG MYOPIC N=64		REG MYOPIC N=90	
Visual Acuity	Preop	Postop	Preop	Postop	Preop	Postop	Preop	Postop
> 20/40	6 (27.7)	16 (72.7)	3 (10)	22 (73.3)	4 (6.3)	56 (87.5)	8 (8.9)	80 (88.9)
= 20/20	0 (0)	7 (22)	0 (0)	15(30)	0 (0)	33 (51.6)	0 (0)	52 (57.8)

correction was 99.6% (range: 97% to 126%). The preoperative astigmatism value ranged from -0.75 to -6 D. To correct this, we performed vectorial analysis according to Alpins' method.[12] Mean target induced astigmatism (TIA) was 3.29 ± 1.32, and surgical induced astigmatism (SIA) was 3.14 ± 1.29, with an index of success (directly proportional to the difference vector and inverse to the TIA vector; ideal result = 0, showing achievement of the targeted astigmatism correction) of 0.05.

Irregular Myopic Astigmatism

The group of 64 eyes with irregular myopic astigmatism included eyes previously subjected to refractive surgery (PRK 50 eyes, LASIK 10 eyes, RK two eyes that presented with decentering associated with undercorrection, and two eyes with corneal scarring). The mean preoperative spheric equivalent was -3.24 ± 2.4 D (range: -0.373 to -6.87), whereas postoperatively it was 0.127 ± 0.85 D (range: -2.50 to +1.50). The percentage of spheric correction was 94.7% (range: 57.14% to -156.6%). The range of preoperative astigmatism was between -0.75 and -6.75 D. Mean TIA was 2.058 ± -1.57 and SIA 1.92 ± 1.47, with an index of success of 0.14.

Hyperopic (Hypermetropic) Astigmatism

The group of eyes with regular hyperopic astigmatism (22 eyes) consisted of patients being treated for the first time. The mean preoperative spherical equivalent was 3.57 ± 1.30 D (range: -0 to 5.75) versus 0.66 ± 0.78 D (range: -0.25 to +2.25) postoperatively. The percentage of spherical correction was 81.94% (range: 33% to 114%). Preoperative astigmatism ranged from +1.75 to +5 D. Mean TIA was 3.03 ± 1.22 and SIA 2.6 ± 1.22, with an index of success of 0.22.

Irregular Hyperopic Astigmatism

Finally, the 30 eyes with irregular hyperopic astig-

matism (idiopathic in six, post-phaco in two, post-hypermetropic PRK in 16, post-myopic PRK in 6) presented a preoperative spheric equivalent of 2.58 ± 1.19 D (range: 0 to +4.50) and a postoperative equivalent of 0.68 ± 1.08 D (range: -0.50 to +3). The percentage of spheric correction was 85.9% (range: 42.8% to 114.2%). Postoperative astigmatism ranged from +0.75 to +4 D. Mean TIA was 2.35 ± 1.32 and SIA 1.62 ± 0.95, with an index of success of 0.33.

The good refractive results led to an improvement in natural and corrected visual acuity. The results for natural acuity are shown in Table 22-1. We noted that only one patient in the group with irregular hyperopic astigmatism lost one Snellen line of best-corrected visual acuity (BCVA). In all the other cases, an improvement by one, two, or even three Snellen lines BCVA or no change was noted compared to preoperative BCVA.

Retreatments

Retreatment had to be performed in a total of eight patients: haze appeared in one eye in the group with irregular myopic astigmatism. Four eyes subjected to myopic LASIK (regular myopic astigmatism group) were found to be undercorrected and three eyes regressed after hypermetropic treatment.

Clinical Examples

Case 1. One month after myopic PRK of sph –8.25, a patient presented with a plano refraction and UCVA of 20/20 but with glare and halos due to a small optical zone (Figure 22-1). A CIPTA, centered on pupil centroid (center), was carried out to enlarge the optical zone (Figure 22-2). Two months after treatment, UCVA was 20/20 with no subjective symptoms (Figure 22-3).

Case 2. A 43-year-old woman had a hyperopic astigmatism of sph +2.25 cyl +2 x 65 degrees (Figure 22-4) and BCVA of 18/20. A CIPTA treatment, cen-

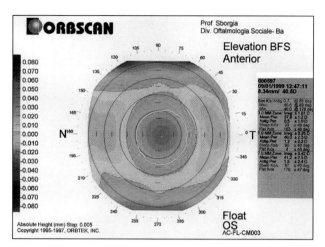

Figure 22-1. Case 1: Orbscan elevation corneal topography of -8.25 post-myopic PRK patient with a plano refractive error who complained of glare and halos. Note the small effective optical zone.

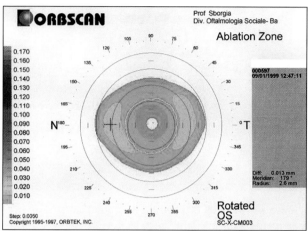

Figure 22-2. Ablation plan of Case 1 using CIPTA treatment centered on the pupil centroid (center) to enlarge the effective optical zone.

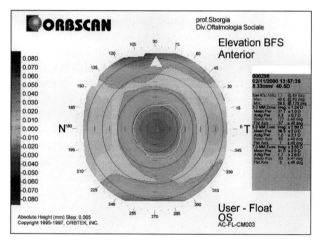

Figure 22-3. Case 1: Orbscan elevation corneal topography demonstrating enlarged optical zone 2 months after retreatment to enlarge the optical zone. The patient's symptoms resolved and he retained 20/20 vision.

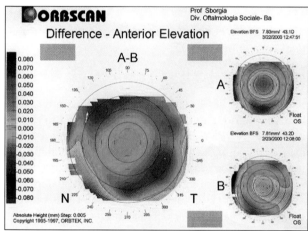

Figure 22-4. Case 2: Orbscan corneal topography demonstrating post- and preoperative maps (A and B), as well as a subtraction map (A-B).

tered on the line of sight, was performed (Figure 22-5). One month after CIPTA, UCVA improved to 20/20 with plano refraction (see Figure 22-4A).

Case 3. One patient had BCVA of 20/20 with sph –5.00 cyl –1.00 x 160 degrees (Figure 22-6). A CIPTA treatment was performed on the pupil centroid (Figure 22-7). Postoperatively, UCVA was 20/20 and plano refraction (see Figure 22-6A) with no halos/glare.

Case 4. A CIPTA treatment was performed for a myopic astigmatism of sph –6.50 cyl –0.80 x 15 degrees (Figure 22-8). Preoperatively, BCVA was

20/20 (Figure 22-9), but the patient had irregular astigmatism. One month after treatment, UCVA was 20/20 with plano refraction (see Figure 22-9A) and without subjective symptoms.

Case 5. Two years after myopic PRK of sph –9, a 43-year-old male patient presented with an decentered treatment (Figure 22-10). His refraction was plano –1.75 x 95 degrees. A CIPTA (Figure 22-11) centered on the pupil was performed to correct the refractive error and to reposition the new refractive area in the center of the cornea. Postoperatively, UCVA was 20/20 with a plano refraction, with a

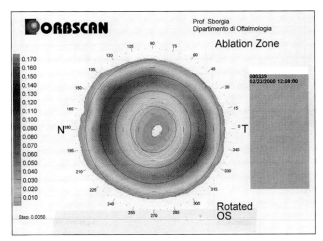

Figure 22-5. Case 2: Orbscan ablation zone map showing height change produced by the CIPTA program.

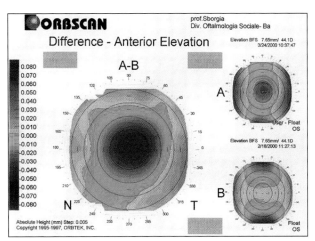

Figure 22-6. Case 3: Orbscan corneal topography demonstrating postoperative (A) compared to preoperative (B) maps for a patient with a refraction of -5.00 - 1.00 x 160. Postoperatively, the patient was 20/20 without correction.

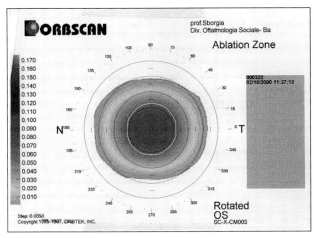

Figure 22-7. Case 3: Orbscan CIPTA treatment showing change in height for a patient treated for -5.00 - 1.00 x 160.

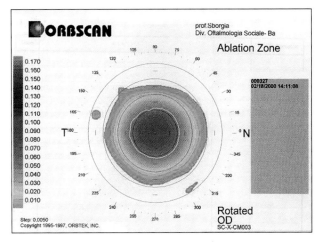

Figure 22-8. Case 4: Height map of post-CIPTA treated eye for myopic astigmatism for a refractive error of –6.50 -0.80 x 15 degrees.

recentered treatment (Figure 22-12). This result is stable after 1 year (Figure 22-13), as evident on the differential elevation map between 1-month (see Figure 22-13A) and 1-year postoperatively (see Figure 22-13B).

DISCUSSION

The results of our study suggest that coupling topographic altimetric data with a computer that can process and control laser ablation is a valid solution for correcting ametropia and irregular forms of astigmatism.

Before this work, some authors had already performed topography-assisted ablation. Seitz, et al[13] corrected irregular astigmatism using Zernike's method of decomposition of topographic height data. Wiesinger-Jendritza, et al[14] recently published a work about the results of LASIK performed with the aid of topographic imaging for irregular astigmatism. However, no other study used height maps using the Orbscan[6-9] prior to our introduction of this technique. The reasons for patient satisfaction and the absence of complications and regression observed in our experience can be attributed to the principles underlying the design of the CIPTA software. In other words:

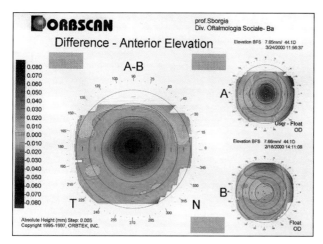

Figure 22-9. Case 4: Height difference map demonstrating 1-month postoperative (A) and preoperative (B) maps on the right side as well as the difference map on the left (A-B).

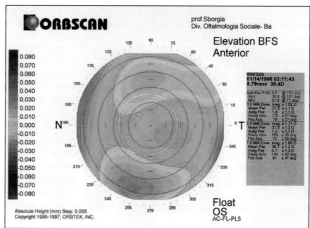

Figure 22-10. Case 5: A decentration pattern on postoperative elevation corneal topography of an eye that was treated 2 years previously for –9.00 D of refractive error. His postoperative refractive error was plano –1.75 x 95 degrees. Note the decentration.

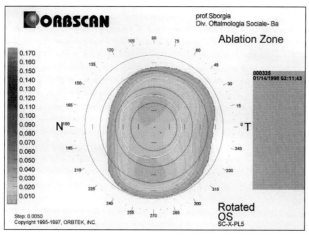

Figure 22-11. Case 5: Height Orbscan topography centered on the pupil to correct the decentration noted in Figure 22-10.

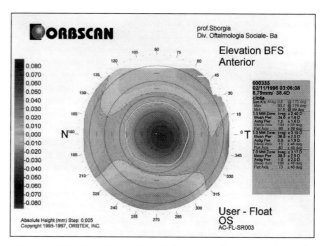

Figure 22-12. Case 5: Orbscan elevation best-fit sphere elevation map showing good centration. The patient's UCVA was 20/20 with plano refraction.

1. The ablation takes into account the true shape of the cornea using height mapping rather than a mathematical model.
2. The ablation software minimizes the ablation volume and, at the same time, creates an adequate ablation optical zone defined on the basis of pupil diameter.
3. The blend (transition) zone has a constant slope in all directions, making the ablation profile very gradual and thus reducing the risk of regression.

Moreover, this software aims to solve the divergence between treatments performed only on the basis of topographic data and those based only on refractive data by combining the two. In fact, the interactive process makes it possible, while inserting the ablation data, to place a greater emphasis on one or the other, as judged best in each single case. This is more important in cases of irregular astigmatism in which topographic and refractive data are unlikely to coincide.

Longer follow-up may confirm the value of this new technique, but we feel this is a step forward in refractive surgery because it enables "customized" treatment of each cornea and each type of ametropia.

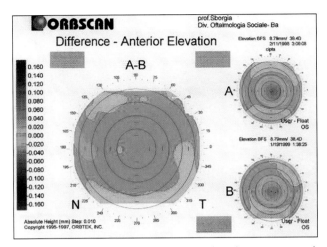

Figure 22-13. Case 5: Stability of Orbscan corneal topography comparing 1-month (A) and 1-year (B) anterior elevation topography. The subtraction map (A-B) reveals no change over this period.

REFERENCES

1. Buzard KA, Fundingsland BR. Treatment of irregular astigmatism with a broadbeam excimer laser. *J Refract Surg*. 1998;13:624-636.

2. Buzard KA. Optical aspects of refractive surgery. In: R Elander, L Rich, J Robin, eds. *Principles and Practice of Refractive Surgery*. Philadelphia, Pa: WB Saunders Co; 1997.

3. Sborgia C. Topographic-assisted PRK: a working hypothesis. Symposium on Cataract, IOL and Refractive Surgery Congress on Ophthalmic Practice Management. Boston, Mass; April 26-30, 1997.

4. Roberts C. Characterization of the inherent error in a spherically-biased corneal topography system in mapping a radially aspheric surface. *J Refract Corneal Surg*. 1994;10:103-111.

5. Roberts C. The accuracy of power maps to display curvature data in corneal topography system. *Invest Ophthalmol Vis Sci*. 1994;35:3525-3532.

6. Friedlander MH, Granet NS. Non-placido disk corneal topography. In: R Elander, L Rich, J Robin, eds. *Principles and Practice of Refractive Surgery*. Philadelphia, Pa: WB Saunders Co; 1997.

7. Schultze RL. Accuracy of corneal elevation with four corneal topography systems. *J Refract Surg*. 1998;14:100-104.

8. Snook R. Pachymetry and true topography using the Orbscan system. In: J Gills, D Sanders, S Thornton, eds. *Corneal Topography: The State of the Art*. Thorofare, NJ: SLACK Incorporated; 1995:89-103.

9. Sborgia C. Usefulness of the Orbscan machine in the management of photorefractive keratectomy. IRSS/AAO Orbscan Clinical Topography Symposium. Chicago, Ill; October 24-26, 1996.

10. Vetrugno M, Alessio G, Sborgia C. Scanning excimer laser: caratteristiche tecniche e prime esperienze cliniche. *Estratto da: Annali di Oftalmologia e Clinica Oculistica*. 1996;CXXII(1).

11. Weingeist T, Lieregang TJ, Slamovits TL. Optics, refraction, and contact lenses, 1997-1998; Chapter II: 47, American Academy of Ophthalmology.

12. Alpins NA. New method of targeting vectors to treat astigmatism. *J Cataract Refract Surg*. 1997;23:65-67.

13. Seitz B, Langenbucher A, Kus MM, Naumann GOH. Topography-based flying-spot mode correction of irregular corneal astigmatism using the 193 nm excimer laser. *Invest Ophthalmol Vis Sci*. 1997;4(Suppl):S537-544.

14. Wiesinger-Jendritza B, Knorz MC, Hugger P, Liermann A. Laser in situ keratomileusis assisted by topography. *J Cataract Refract Surg*. 1998;24:166-174.

Chapter Twenty-Three

Computerized Topography-Controlled Ablation Using the Meditec Laser

Klaus Ditzen, MD
Stefan Pieger, Dipl Ing

INTRODUCTION

For the computerized topographic ablation, it is necessary to combine the advantages of a special topographic device showing the irregularities and decentrations after myopic and hyperopic refractive ablation in an elevation map with the advantages of a flying spot excimer laser system such as the MEL 70 (Aesculap Meditec, Jena, Germany) with gaussian profile and 35 Hz repetition rate. The target will be a smooth stromal and corneal surface with a spherical shape in order to improve visual acuity and reduce glare and halo caused by the asymmetric corneal surface. Possible indications are the correction of decentrations seen after primary myopic, astigmatic, or hyperopic ablations, or as a procedure for a primary aspherical ablation.

PROCEDURE

The ablation has to be done with an active eye tracking system. In the case of the MEL 70, the active eye tracker uses the limbus or a limbus-fixed tracking ring as a target. Therefore, it is not necessary to widen the pupil, but it will be necessary to center the Purkinje reflex in the pupillary area with a needle. The red tracking centration point has to be adjusted before the flap is lifted. For the topography-guided ablation, we used the elevation maps of the Technomed C-Scan (Technomed GmbH, Baseweiler,

Germany) and the Tomey TMS II or III (Tomey and Erlanger, Tennenloke, Germany).

In order to minimize the risk of incorrect topography data, the results of three measurements were compared. The keratometric and elevation map data are used to calculate the best-fit sphere (Figure 23-1). If necessary, the target sphere can be modified in order to achieve a certain change in refraction by shifting the z axis of the ablation. The data of the highest points referring to the refraction (~13 μm per diopter [D]) is checked. After shifting the z axis, it is absolutely necessary to simulate the different ablations. The special data will be checked again on the ablation. At this point, the calculation can be adjusted. After this procedure, the keratometric map will show the simulated outcome, and the data will be automatically transferred into a laser shot file. This file will be loaded via computer zip disk into the MEL 70. After centration of the active eye tracker to the Purkinje reflex, the flap can be reopened and the active eye tracker can be locked in on the limbus ring target. The TOSCA (topographic simulated customized ablation) ablation can be started by pressing the foot switch, similar to a normal ablation.

METHODS

From January 1999 to July 1999, 21 eyes of 21 patients were treated (11 females, 10 males). The mean age was 39 ± 8.6 years (range: 30 to 48 years).

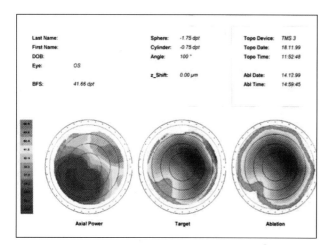

Figure 23-1. Preoperative axial power, target and ablation map display of the Meditec TOSCA software.

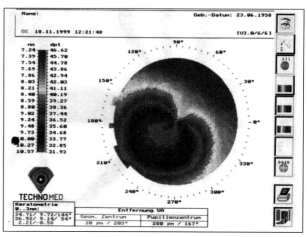

Figure 23-2. Example 1: preoperative topography of patient LM, OS. Note the decentered ablation inferior-nasally.

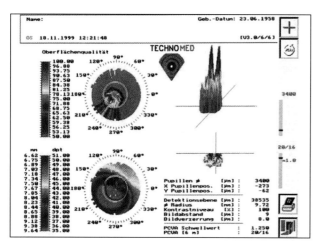

Figure 23-3. Example 1: preoperative ray tracing of patient LM. The ablation is decentered inferior-nasally.

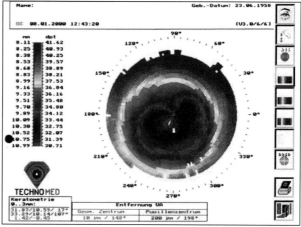

Figure 23-4. Example 1: postoperative topography of patient LM demonstrating improvement in corneal topography.

All eyes suffered from glare and reduced contrast sensitivity caused by decentered ablation after myopic or hyperopic laser-assisted in situ keratomileusis (LASIK). Fifty percent of the eyes had monocular diplopia.

The target of the study was to improve best spectacle-corrected visual acuity (BSCVA) with hard contact lenses as opposed to glasses, and to treat residual refractive errors.

All patients had to sign a release about the experimental nature of this new enhancement procedure.

After reopening the flap, a stromal ablation was done with the MEL 70 gaussian-profile flying spot system (1.8-mm spot size and 35 Hz repetition rate). The excimer laser ablation was planned based on videokeratography images taken with the TMS II/2, TMS III, or Technomed C-Scan.

Every eye was examined for subjective refraction, objective refraction, slit lamp biomicroscopy, funduscopy, central keratometry with the pre- and postoperative intraocular pressure.

Results

Follow-up data were taken after 1 week, 1 month, 3 months, and 5 months after surgery. The ray trace module of the Technomed C-Scan was used to simulate blurring and contrast sensitivity for different pupil sizes pre- and postoperatively. Figures 23-2 through 23-19 show pre- and postoperative data for four selected cases. Tables 23-1 through 23-4 contain the corresponding refractive data.

In these eyes we showed the keratometric maps

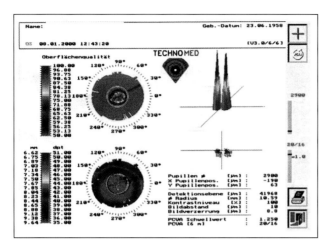

Figure 23-5. Example 1: postoperative ray tracing of patient LM noting improvement in ray tracing.

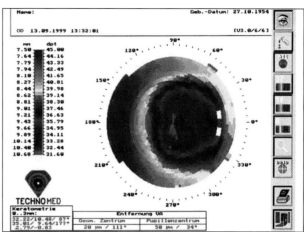

Figure 23-6. Example 2: preoperative topography OD of patient GM demonstrating temporal decentration.

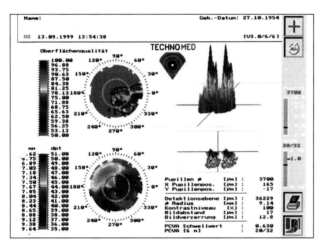

Figure 23-7. Example 2: preoperative ray tracing OD of patient GM.

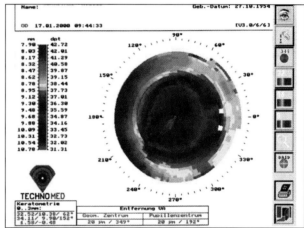

Figure 23-8. Example 2: postoperative topography OD of patient GM. The corneal topography is now more symmetric.

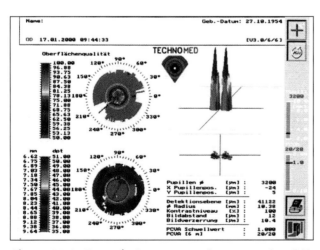

Figure 23-9. Example 2: postoperative ray tracing OD of patient GM with improved ray tracing.

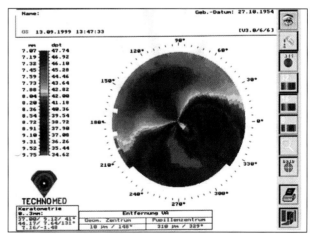

Figure 23-10. Example 3: preoperative topography OS of patient GM showing inferotemporal decentration.

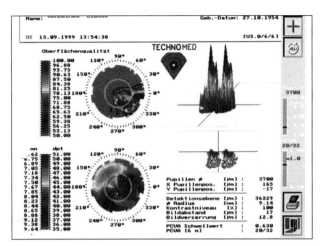

Figure 23-11. Example 3: preoperative ray tracing OS of patient GM.

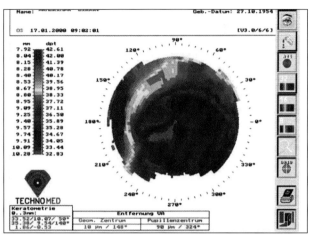

Figure 23-12. Example 3: postoperative topography OS of patient GM showing improved centration.

taken with the Technomed C-Scan. For the last case, we showed the elevation map of the Tomey TMS III as well. This elevation map is the key for the planned calculation of how much tissue at which location must be ablated. The color in the elevation map in the last case shows the deviation from a perfect spherical surface (yellowish-brown = hill, blue = valley, green = nominal surface). The perfect sphere (reference surface—best-fit sphere) is an automatic selection of the best K-value. This K-value is optimal for the patient's corneal shape but not necessarily for the subjective refraction. The correct definition of the target K-value is very important for the surgeon.

Follow-up data were analyzed with the Datagraph Med outcomes analysis software version 1.12. Graphs for stability, predictability, safety, and efficacy where produced from the postoperative data (Figures 23-16 through 23-19).

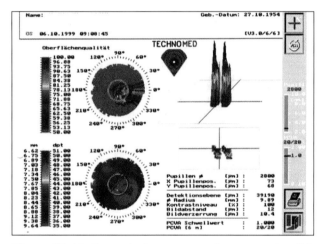

Figure 23-13. Example 3: postoperative ray tracing OS of patient GM. The ray tracing shows definite improvement from the pre-retreatment status.

DISCUSSION

Irregularities with small, steep valley and hill structures should be treated with foreign filling materials.[1,2] Irregularities with steep hill and valley profiles are mostly flattened through the leveling effect of the epithelium. Therefore, the topography image seems to be smoother on the corneal surface

> Irregularities with steep hill and valley profiles are mostly flattened through the leveling effect of the epithelium. Therefore, the topography image seems to be smoother on the corneal surface than in reality on the cut and reopened stromal surface.

than in reality on the cut and reopened stromal surface. Residual irregularity will remain over larger areas. The true flap thickness is also uncertain.

It is difficult for elevation maps to show the real central irregularities if they are working based on a placido disc system. Incorrect fixation of the patient's eye can especially produce wrong data. Little differences in fixation change the position of the pupillary center, and it is possible to get different topography images of the same eye (Figures 23-20 and 23-21). Additionally, there may be unknown differences between the measured corneal surface and the treated stromal surface, because in the LASIK technique there is an intrastromal ablation and not a superficial corneal ablation, as in PRK.[3] Currently there is no

Table 23-1
Example 1: Results of Patient LM*

	REFRACTION	UCVA	BSCVA
Preoperative	-1.75 sph -1.75 cyl x 150°	20/50	20/50
1 day postoperative	-0.75 sph -0.75 cyl x 40°	20/50	20/40
1 month postoperative	-0.50 sph -0.75 cyl x 40°	20/50	20/40

Improved ray-tracing (contrast sensitivity) after 1 month. Loss of monocular diplopia.
*41 years old LA.

Table 23-2
Example 2: Results of Patient GM,* OD

	REFRACTION	UCVA	BSCVA
Preoperative	+ 5.0 sph -3.0 cyl x 90°	20/50	20/40
1 day postoperative	+ 0.5 sph -1.0 cyl x100°	20/50	20/40
3 month postoperative	+2.75 sph -1.0 cyl x 60°	20/40	20/30

Improved ray tracing (contrast sensitivity) after 3 months. Loss of monocular diplopia.
*46 years old, RA

Table 23-3
Example 3: Results of Patient GM,* OS

	REFRACTION	UCVA	BSCVA
Preoperative	-6.5 sph -6.0 cyl x 50°	<20/50	20/50
1 day postoperative	+1.0 sph -2.0 cyl x 45°	20/40	20/50
3 months postoperative	+0.5 sph -0.5 cyl x 0°	20/30	20/40

Improved ray tracing (contrast sensitivity). Loss of monocular diplopia.
*46 years old, OS.

intraoperative topography-guided ablation possible because of the rough stromal surface.

The 21 ablated eyes in the cases of decentration after myopic and hyperopic LASIK procedures are probably too small a group to make a final statement about efficacy of topography-guided LASIK. In all these cases, this method was able to reduce the side effects of decentrations, as shown in the Datagraph Med analysis of efficacy, safety, stability, and predictability. In this study, we could see postoperative improvements of such cases for the first time. As opposed to older studies for myopic PRK and myopic and hyperopic LASIK,[4-7] there is now a possibility of correcting decentrations and irregularities with the new gaussian-profile 1.8-mm spot size MEL 70 excimer laser.[8]

This technique is very promising, as topography-guided corneal ablations could also be done in primary aspheric corneas that we treat only with a spherical ablation. Finally, aberration-guided abla-

Table 23-4
Example 4: Results of Patient VJ, OD

	REFRACTION	*UCVA*	*BSCVA*
Preoperative	+3.0 sph -1.25 cyl x 50°	20/40	20/30
1 day postoperative	-4.0 sph -1.0 cyl x 30°	20/50	20/40
1 month postoperative	+0.75 sph -0.75 cyl x 0°	20/40	20/25
5 months postoperative	+1.0 sph -1.0 cyl x 20°	20/40	20/25

Nearly no improvement in ray tracing (contrast sensitivity), continued blurring, loss of monocular diplopia.

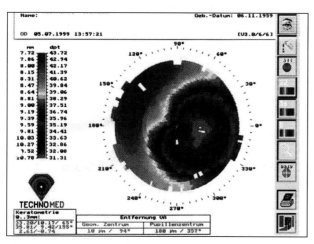

Figure 23-14. Example 4: preoperative topography of patient VJ.

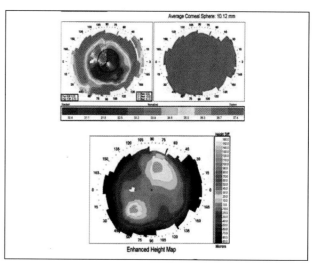

Figure 23-15. Example 4: preoperative Tomey target and height map of the desired ablation for patient VJ.

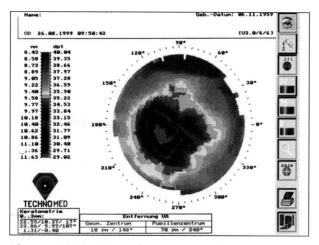

Figure 23-16. Example 4: 1-month postoperative topography of patient VJ.

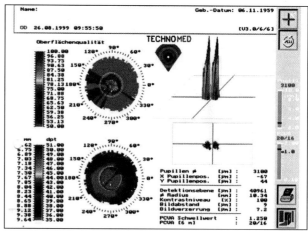

Figure 23-17. Example 4: 1-month postoperative ray tracing of patient VJ.

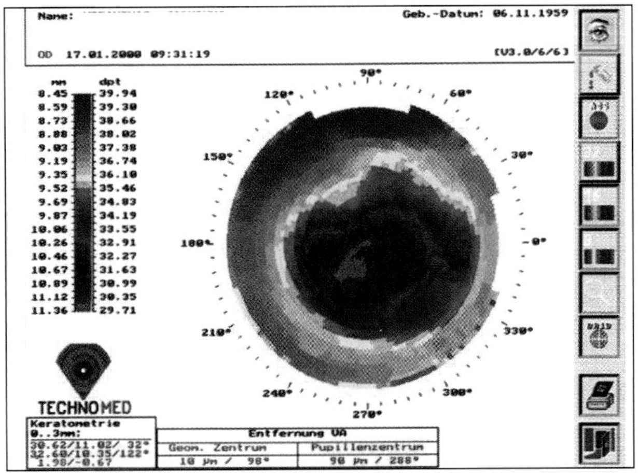

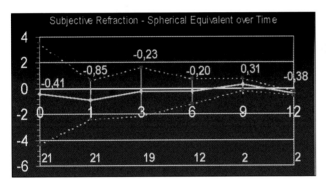

Figure 23-18. Example 4: 5-month postoperative topography of patient VJ.

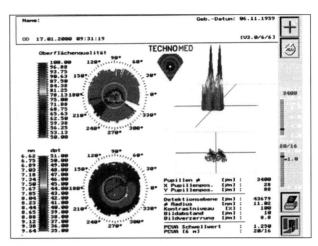

Figure 23-19. Example 4: 5-month postoperative ray tracing of patient VJ. Note improvement from the preoperative ray tracing.

Figure 23-20. Preoperative topography of patient HM.

tions will be able to improve BSCVA and increase the quality of the vision, reduce glare, and improve contrast sensitivity.[9-11]

CONCLUSION

This technique is still at an early stage of development. One has to consider that the surgeon is absolutely depending on the topography system's images, precision, and reproducibility. There will be a wider acceptance of this method when different techniques are standardized, either in PRK or LASIK. It will then be possible to see real improvements. The biggest discrepancy is the current measurement of corneal topography (corneal surface) and the different situations for ablation after reopening of the flap.

Still, there were satisfying results independent from the corneal topography system in BSCVA, UCVA, stability, and predictability. In all eyes we

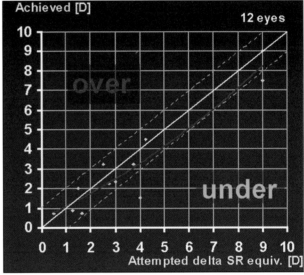

Figure 23-21. Different preoperative topography of the patient in Figure 23-20.

reached an enlargement of the optical zone and a reduction of monocular diplopia. Further studies have to be done.

REFERENCES

1. Dausch D, Schroeder E. Die Behandlung von Hornhaut-und Skleraerkrankungen mit dem Excimer laser. *Fortschr Ophthalmol.* 1990;87:115-120.

2. Sher N, Bowers RA, Zabel RW, et al. Clinical use of 193 nm excimer laser in the treatment of corneal scars. *Arch Ophthalmol.* 1991;109:491-498.

3. Wiesinger-Jendritza B, Knorz M, Hugger P, Liermann A. Laser in situ keratomileusis assisted by corneal topography. *J Cataract Refract Surg.* 1998;24:168-174.

4. Dausch D, Smecka Z, Klein R, Schroeder E, Kirchner S. Excimer laser photorefractive keratektomy for hyperopia. *J Cataract Refract Surg.* 1997;23:169-176.

5. Ditzen K, Anschuetz T, Schroeder E. Photorefractive keratectomy to treat low, medium and high myopia: a multicenter study. *J Cataract Refract Surg.* 1994;20(Suppl):234-238.

6. Ditzen K, Huschka H. Laser in situ keratomileusis (LASIK) for myopia. In: T Tokoro, ed. *Myopia Updates.* Tokyo, Japan: Springer Verlag; 1998:169-180.

7. Ditzen K, Huschka H, Pieger S. Laser in situ keratomileusis for hyperopia. *J Cataract Refract Surg.* 1998;24:42-47.

8. Dausch D, Schroeder E, Dausch S. Topography-controlled excimer laser photorefractive keratectomy. *Arch Ophthalmol.* 2000;118(1):17-21.

9. Seiler T, Kaemmerer M, Mierdel P, Krinke HE. Ocular optical aberrations after photorefractive keratectomy for myopia and myopic astigmatism. *Graefes Arch Clin Exp Ophthalmol.* 1999;237(9):725-729.

10. Mierdel P, Kaemmerer M, Krinke HE, Seiler T. Effects of photorefractive keratectomy and cataract surgery on ocular optical errors of higher order. *Am J Ophthalmol.* 1999;127(1):1-7.

11. Oshika T, Klyce SD, Applegate RA, Howland HC, El Danasoury MA. Comparison of corneal wavefront aberrations after photorefractive keratectomy and laser in situ keratomileusis. *Am J Ophthalmol.* 1999;127:1-7.

Chapter Twenty-Four

Computerized Topographic Ablation Using the VisX CAP Method

Gustavo E. Tamayo, MD

Mario G. Serrano, MD

INTRODUCTION

The Contoured Ablation Patterns (CAP) method (VisX, Inc, Santa Clara, Calif) was officially launched in April 1999 at the American Society of Cataract and Refractive Surgery (ASCRS) meeting in Seattle, Wash. This method was a step forward in the treatment of irregular astigmatism, as it created a "link" between a topographical corneal map and the excimer laser. However, it is the surgeon who controls the ablation and sets the treatment parameters, such as shape, depth, location, and size, as well as the number based on the topographical map and his or her own clinical judgment.

Background

The milestone of the VisX approach to the treatment of irregular astigmatism was a paper published in *Ophthalmology* in May 1994 by Gibralter and Trokel.[1] This paper suggested that decentration of the excimer beam to ablate the "steepest" areas of the irregular corneas as shown by conventional, axial, or tangential topographical maps may improve decentration. The experiment used off-axis treatments by manually moving the laser to the approximate location of the irregularity, rather than treating only the center. This global approach was the first step in the search for a formula to treat this extremely disabling problem.

Following these guidelines, we treated several patients, resulting in some improvement but less than we expected, which we attributed to the inaccurate location of the steepest area on the corneal surface and, therefore, misplacement of the excimer beam. In 1996, we produced the prototype of a "grid corneal marker," patented the following year—an instrument designed to translate the steepest area of the topography map onto the corneal surface. Once properly marked and aligned with the visual axis, the grid pattern enabled us to more precisely localize the steepest area derived from the preoperative topography map. This point became the center of the ablation zone, even though it was off-center from the visual axis. Unfortunately, our results did not improve with this method.

Buzard and Fundingsland[2] demonstrated that by treating only the refractive defect in irregular corneas, poor results were obtained in refraction, visual acuity, and quality of vision. In 1997, we came to realize the wide difference between steepness and elevation with the development of the concept of slope of a mountain (steepness) as opposed to the top of the mountain (most elevated area). We found that the steepest area in a curvature map is never located at the highest area in an elevation map (Figure 24-1).

Our treatment was changed to ablate the highest

> Our treatment was changed to ablate the highest or most elevated areas, as determined by elevation topography.

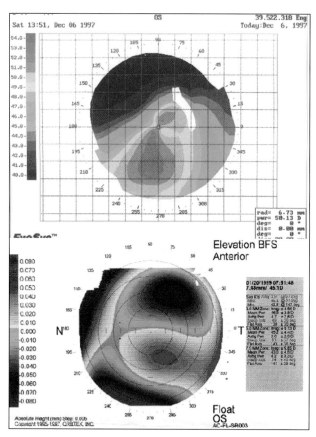

Figure 24-1. In this keratoconus patient, the most elevated area of the cornea (top) is geographically distinct from the steepest area (bottom), depicting the wide difference between the two topography methods.

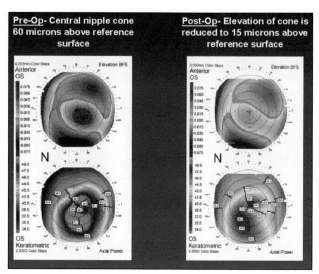

Figure 24-2. Left: preoperative elevation map of keratoconus treated with manual decentration. Right: excellent postoperative result 18 months after surgery.

or most elevated areas, as determined by elevation topography (Figure 24-2). We manually decentered the excimer beam and our results improved dramatically. After gaining extensive experience with this "manual" method, on March 30, 1999, the first three patients in the world were treated by us with the CAP method from the VisX Star S2 system. The CAP method allows beam size, shape, depth, and location to be exactly programmed into the laser to match the corresponding irregularities on the topography map. The beam can vary in size from 1.2 to 6.5 mm in diameter and can be offset in any direction from the visual axis (Figure 24-3). This eliminated the need for manual decentration of the excimer beam and allowed us to input the specific X and Y offsets of the corneal elevation from the topography map into the laser. The laser automatically decentered the beam relative to the visual axis. This was a big step forward toward a "TopoLinked" ablation. Since its launch, hundreds of corneas have been treated successfully with the CAP technique.

CAP METHOD DEFINITION

The CAP method is a software upgrade for the VisX Star S2 system, with wider flexibility when compared to other software platforms. It enables the surgeon to program the excimer beam relative to shape, size, depth, and location. The CAP method allows surgeons to treat any corneal irregularity using seven treatment options that can be centered or decentered. They are: myopia, myopic astigmatism, hyperopia, hyperopic astigmatism, multipass multizone treatments, phototherapeutic keratectomy (PTK), and standard ablations (Table 24-1). It is also possible to program as many as 20 sequential ablations within one treatment sequence.

For the purposes of this book, we will concentrate this chapter on the decentration properties of the excimer beam of the VisX Star S2 with the CAP method (see Figure 24-3). With this capability we are able to produce topography-assisted excimer laser ablations (ie, the use of corneal topography to plan treatments with the intention of regulating the contour of any cornea regardless of shape, asymmetry, or irregularity).

Table 24-1
CAP Method Treatment Options

- Myopia
- Myopic astigmatism
- Hyperopia
- Hyperopic astigmatism
- Multipass multizone treatments
- PTK
- Standard

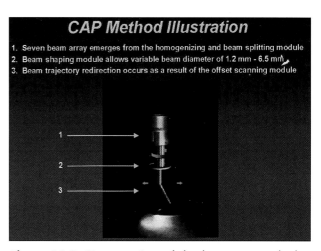

Figure 24-3. Decentration of the beam to reach the most elevated area in an irregular cornea, from the VisX Star S2 system (SmoothScan) CAP method.

CLINICAL APPLICATIONS OF THE CAP METHOD

The CAP method is very flexible software, suited for the treatment of any corneal defect: regular or irregular.

Regular Defects

1. Myopia
2. Myopic astigmatism
3. Hyperopia
4. Hyperopic astigmatism
5. Mixed astigmatism with cross cylinder technique:
   - Hyperopic astigmatism component first
   - Residual myopic astigmatism component
6. PTK

One of the most important features of this method is the treatment of irregular astigmatism, a very disabling refractive problem that can be classified as either nonacquired or acquired.

Irregular Defects

Nonacquired:
1. Keratoconus
2. Pellucid marginal degenerations
3. Congenital asymmetrical astigmatism
4. Corneal dystrophies

Acquired:
1. From previous refractive surgery
   - Decentration in LASIK surgery
   - Decentration in PRK surgery
   - Incisional refractive surgery
2. From other types of corneal surgeries
3. From corneal trauma

CAP ABLATION TECHNIQUE

Topography-Assisted Excimer Laser Ablations

Excimer laser beams can only remove tissue from the cornea. They cannot add tissue to it. Therefore, regularization of a corneal contour with an excimer laser is based on resection of some amount of tissue from the top of the elevated areas and resection peripherally around the depressed areas to produce their desired elevation.

The surgical plan for a custom ablation with CAP is usually subjective and individual. Every cornea with irregular astigmatism has a unique condition, therefore generalization is not possible. These types of treatment cannot be left to a fixed nomogram. Rationale behind every treatment has to be developed. We do not believe an isolated topography map can be treated without analysis by the refractive surgeon. CAP ablation planners, presented in this chapter, are an advancement that gives the refractive surgeon a more systematic approach to analyze and decide the treatment in these difficult, unique cases.

The Technique

A three-step method was developed in order to produce better and more consistent results with the CAP method.

First step: Elevation topography is mandatory

- Any type of elevation topography can be used: Placido disc-based topographers with elevation software such as Humphrey or Dicon, or slit scan elevation topographers like Orbscan.
- Conventional refractive power topography indicates the curvature of the cornea and does not distinguish between power and elevation. If we erroneously remove tissue from the steepest area, we may increase the slope of the elevation and compromise rather than improve the visual quality of that particular cornea.

Second step: Analysis of the elevation topography

We determine the critical ablation parameters from the preoperative elevation topography by:

- Locating the most elevated areas of the cornea, as measured in millimeters in distance between the center of the pupil and the highest point of the area on both the horizontal and vertical meridians. The grid pattern from the preoperative topography map is used for this purpose.
- Defining the shape and size of the most elevated areas. The ablation can be spherical, cylindrical, or elliptical to match the shape of the treatment areas. If ablation is elliptical or cylindrical, the axis has to be determined by finding the major axis of the irregularity and translating it to the center of the pupil.
- Defining very precisely the elevation in microns of the zones to be ablated, as measured from the preoperative topography map. The elevation in the map is always related to an "ideal" or best-fit curvature to the overall corneal surface. An example of this elevation subtraction is demonstrated in Figure 24-2.

Third step: Program the laser

The treatment of irregular astigmatism using the VisX Star S2 system with the CAP method is based on decreasing the height of the "bumps" of the corneal surface. The amount of tissue resected is what is important in this type of treatment. As a result, the preoperative refractive error is measured with the primary intent to smooth the irregularities in the context of the objective refraction. With this analysis, we are able to determine the refractive power of specific areas of the cornea in a similar manner as wavefront technology.

In topography-assisted excimer laser ablation with the CAP method, only the dioptric power of the ablation is changeable, which dictates the depth of the treatment. The other ablation parameters were predetermined and fixed by analysis of the preoperative elevation topography map: diameter, size, shape, and number of microns to resect. Therefore, the final dioptric calculated power of the ablation is irrelevant.

The exact position of the excimer treatment is programmed into the computer using the x and y offsets relative to the visual axis in a Cartesian coordinate format. Finally, as many as 20 different ablations for one corneal surface can be programmed in a sequential mode in any order as decided by the surgeon, with or without a pause in between them.

LASIK versus PRK

Both types of surgery can be done with CAP. The type of surgery to perform on any particular cornea is personally decided by the surgeon after a serious analysis of every case. Some general considerations should be taken into account.

LASIK is always the first option, provided that:

- Stromal residual tissue is at least 250 microns after the ablation.
- A complete flap can be produced by the microkeratome. Beware of too steep corneas or corneas with many incisions or previous surgeries.
- The size of the flap fits the decentered ablation. Be cautious when a hyperopic treatment is going to be undertaken.

In corneal ectasias such as keratoconus we strongly advise PRK.

CLINICAL RESULTS

Results of treatment of irregular astigmatism with the VisX Star S2 system CAP method have been encouraging. Although it is not a refractive procedure, the goal is to do away with glasses or contact lenses, and we have obtained reduction in topographic and keratometric astigmatism, reduction in manifest refractive error, and, of course, marked improvement in visual acuity. Visual symptoms such as glare, halos, burst, monocular diplopia, ghost images, etc, decreased in the subjective evaluation in the majority of our patients. It is important to men-

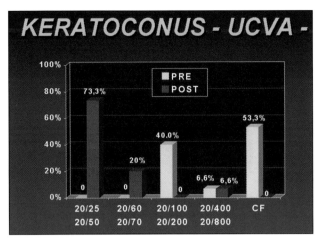

Figure 24-4a. Preoperative elevation map of keratoconus treated with "manual " decentration.

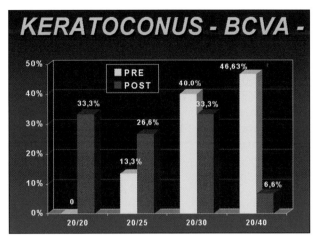

Figure 24-4b. Postoperative elevation map of keratoconus shows the excellent result 18 months after the surgery.

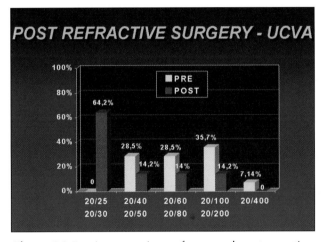

Figure 24-5a. A comparison of pre- and postoperative UCVA in the post-refractive group.

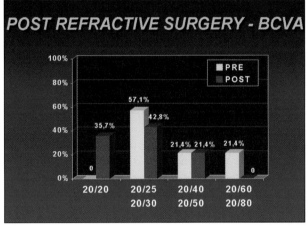

Figure 24-5b. A comparison of pre- and postoperative BCVA in the keratoconic group.

tion that these symptoms are the key factor in the process of deciding to have another surgery for most of the patients with irregular astigmatism after other refractive procedures. However, evaluation of the improvement in quality of life is difficult and subjective. Therefore, we measure the success of the treatment with conventional analysis. A complete ophthalmological evaluation pre- and postoperatively was undertaken. The following criteria were recorded for statistical purposes: uncorrected visual acuity (UCVA), best-corrected visual acuity (BCVA), keratometry readings, manifest refraction, and elevation topography maps.

For analysis, because of the large differences in etiology and symptomology, we have divided the results into two main groups: one group of keratoconus patients and another group of postrefractive surgery patients. The latter group includes incisional refractive surgery and excimer laser surgery. The results of UCVA and BCVA are presented in Figures 24-4a and b (keratoconus) and Figures 24-5a and b (postrefractive surgery).

Keratoconus Group

Marked improvement in all the parameters were obtained in this group, with a mean follow-up of 9 months and stability after the third month (Figure 24-6). All cases were treated with the PRK CAP method. Although longer follow-up is needed, surgery was decided after the development of contact es. The only other option was a corneal transplant, with all the risks involved in this type of surgery.

Before treatment, 67% of the eyes were 20/400 or worse uncorrected. Postoperatively, 75% of the eyes have 20/60 or better UCVA and 58.3% are 20/40 or better (see Figure 24-4a). Fifty-six percent of the eyes gained lines of vision, with 18% of the eyes gaining two or more lines of BCVA. This is noted in Figure 24-3b, which shows that 50% of the eyes were 20/30 or better BCVA preoperatively; this number improves to 75% after treatment. A temporary loss of one line of vision was reported in one patient due to the development of a bacterial corneal ulcer. After several months, this patient's vision returned to his original BCVA.

We noted in our refractive results that astigmatism was reduced from 4.93 D preoperatively (range: 1.0 to 8.0) to 3.25 D (range: 0 to 6.0). Keratometry mean power was also reduced from 48.12 D (range: 41.70 to 55.00) to 45.46 D (range: 38.75 to 50.75).

Postrefractive Surgery Group

The presence of bothersome symptoms derived from the irregularity, as well as the overall poor quality of vision, was the key factor motivating this group to decide on surgery. Figures 24-7a and b show a patient with irregular astigmatism treated with the CAP method. Mean follow-up was again 9 months, and stability was achieved earlier than in the keratoconus group (1.2 months) due to the fact that 85% of the cases were treated with the LASIK CAP method.

All patients reported subjective improvement in visual symptoms (in different degrees according to their own judgment). Satisfaction was generally rated high, although 25% of the patients reported "less improvement than expected." None of the patients complained of worsened symptoms, and all stated they would repeat the surgery if needed.

UCVA improved from 80% of the cases preoperatively in the 20/200 or worse group to 82% in the 20/60 group postoperatively, and 72% in the 20/40 group (see Figure 24-4a). When BCVA was recorded, 27% of the patients were 20/25 preoperatively. This number increases to 55% in the postoperative eyes (see Figure 24-4b). Fifty-four percent of the eyes gained one line of BCVA. No loss of lines were reported.

Although mean keratometry readings did not change significantly (36.7 preoperatively to 37.9 postoperatively), the manifest refraction markedly changed. Mean preoperative astigmatism was 5.27 D (range: 3.5 to 10.0) to 2.20 D postoperatively (range:

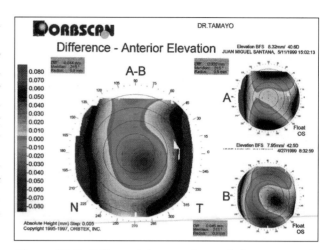

Figure 24-6. Differential map of case 1 (keratoconus). Note the nice regularization of the corneal contour postoperatively and the location of the ablation at the top of the cone. A: postoperative map; B: preoperative map; A-B: subtraction map.

0.25 to 3.0).

CLINICAL EXAMPLES

Case 1

Male, 22 years of age, with bilateral keratoconus. Intolerant to contact lenses, very unhappy with glasses correction. Desired some type of surgery in his left eye.

- Dx: Keratoconus left eye

Preoperative evaluation: UCVA left eye 20/100 (ghost image)

- BCVA left eye 20/40 (ghost image)
- Keratometry: 43.00/51.00/150
- Manifest refraction: -1.00 -5.00 x 155°

Surgical procedure: CAP ablation with PRK in the left eye

- Myopic ellipse 5.0 x 3.0 mm 40 microns, x:-0.7; y:-1.0
- (-4.49 -7.86 DC x 36°)

Postoperative evaluation: 11 months follow-up

- UCVA left eye 20/40 (no ghost image)
- BCVA left eye. 20/20^{-1}
- Keratometry: 43.00/45.00/160
- Manifest refraction: +1.25 -1.75 x 140°

Topography evaluation: see Figure 24-6.

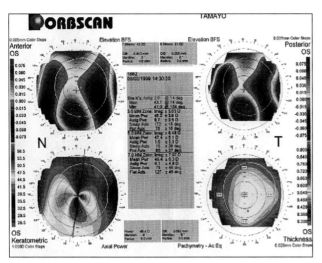

Figure 24-7a. Case 2: preoperative elevation topography map, who had previous incisional surgery. Note the marked steepening inferiorly.

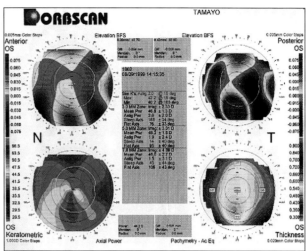

Figure 24-7b. Case 2: postoperative elevation topography map after CAP method treatment. The visual axis is now relatively free of irregularities, which correlated with significant improvement in acuity and quality of vision.

Case 2

Female, 34 years of age, underwent astigmatic radial keratotomy with trapezoidal incisions plus radial incisions 10 years earlier. Wanted surgical correction of the left eye because of monocular diplopia, glare, and halos.

- Dx: Irregular astigmatism postincisional surgery

Preoperative evaluation: UCVA left eye counting fingers 3 meters

- BCVA left eye 20/30 (symptoms)
- Keratometry: 44.75/38.75 x 60°
- Manifest refraction: +5.00 -3.00 x 55°

Surgical procedure: CAP method correction in left eye with LASIK

- Hyperopic cyl 5.0 x 6.5 mm 28 microns (pl +3.0 x 10°)
- Myopic ellipse 4.0 x 3.2 mm 41 microns, x:-0.5; y:-3.0
- (-7.30 -3.95 x 80°)
- Myopic cyl 6.0 x 4.5 mm 14 microns, x:-0.5; y: 0.0
- (Pl –1.95 DC x 80°)

Postoperative evaluation: 7 months after surgery

- UCVA left eye 20/30 (no diplopia, continued glare)
- BCVA left eye 20/25
- Keratometry: 40.00/42.00 x 2°
- Manifest refraction: +1.50 -1.75 x 20°

Topography evaluation: see Figures 24-7a and b.

Case 3

Female, 25 years old, in the third postoperative month after bilateral LASIK surgery. Complained of blurred vision, halos, and ghost images.

- Dx: Irregular astigmatism post decentered LASIK treatment.

Preoperative evaluation: UCVA right eye 20/60

- BCVA right eye 20/30
- Keratometry: 47.25/45.50/45″
- Manifest refraction: +3.75 -0.75 x 45°

Surgical procedure: Relifting the flap to correct with CAP method

- Myopic ellipse 5.0 x 2.7 mm 45 microns, x:-2.0; y: -2.0
- (-5.00 -12.00 x 35°)
- Myopic sphere 3.0 mm 15 microns, x: -2.0; y: +1.0
- (-5.00)
- Hyperopia +1.5 D 14 microns centrated 8.0 to 5.0 mm

Topography evaluation: see Figures 24-8a and b.

CAP Planners

Improvement in the treatment of irregular astigmatism will come from the improvement in the way we look at the corneal surface using corneal topography systems. The majority of excimer lasers are capable of regularizing the corneal contour. The VisX Star

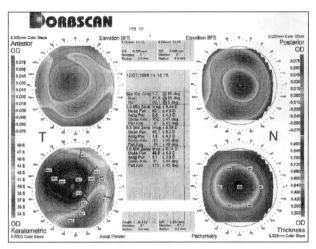

Figure 24-8a. Case 3: decentered LASIK treatment noted. Above left: preoperative elevation topography map. Lower left: axial topography demonstrates the asymmetric astigmatism.

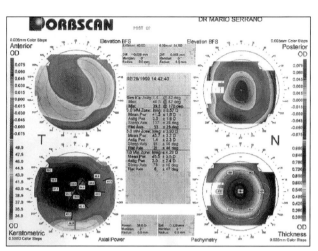

Figure 24-8b. Case 3: post CAP treatment. Elevation topography noted. There is regularization of the corneal surface, explaining the improved vision in this eye postoperatively.

S2 system with the CAP method is capable of improving corneal contour. This excimer laser system has a scanning beam that can go anywhere in the cornea with any shape and any size. However, to program the laser, information coming from the preoperative corneal map is needed. Therefore, more accurate maps are necessary to improve planning the ablation in irregular corneas.

Since 1847, when Henry Goode[3] invented a disc of concentric circles, later modified by Antonio Placido,[4,5] ophthalmologists have used them to evaluate the corneal curvature, taking advantage of the reflecting properties of the cornea. The first videokeratography systems were based on the computerized analysis of a placido disc image. In 1987, Maguire, et al[6] introduced a color-coded topographical map based on placido disc images. Since then, manufacturers have used various proprietary algorithms to produce graphic representations of corneal topography. Those companies developed specific programs for the adaptation of contact lenses that were in fact elevation topography maps inferred from the reflection on the cornea of those concentric rings. Those maps used the concept of best contact lens fit, which is the way to produce an "ideal" corneal curvature and find elevated and depressed zones related to this "ideal" contour.

Because of the high refractive power of the cornea, little changes in shape can produce large changes in refraction and reflection. Therefore, an excellent way to detect small changes in the corneal curvature utilizes its reflective properties. As a result, placido disc-based topography units are well-suited for the production of more precise and accurate elevation topography maps. They will need further refinement with more exact mathematical algorithms.

Topography ablation planning software allows surgeons to preoperatively visualize the effect of the planned ablation on the topography map and make the necessary adjustments prior to surgery until the postoperative map shows regularization of the corneal contour and fulfills the goal of the surgery. Today, two companies are working independently of VisX in the production of a very precise CAP planner: Humphrey and Dicon Paradigm. These companies produce an elevation map derived from the reflection on the corneal surface of placido discs. They enable the surgeon to judge the effect and make the necessary changes to a planned ablation, predicting a postoperative topography map (Figures 24-9a and b). This simulation can be used as a guide in performing the actual topography-assisted excimer laser ablation.

> Topography ablation planning software allows surgeons to preoperatively visualize the effect of the planned ablation on the topography map and make the necessary adjustments prior to surgery.

CONCLUSION

The CAP method from VisX Star S2 is a powerful, surgeon-controlled tool with the capability of treating localized irregular areas on the cornea. The suc-

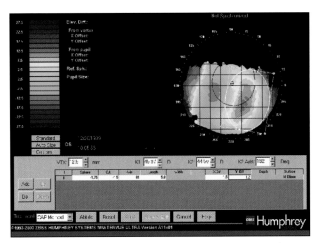

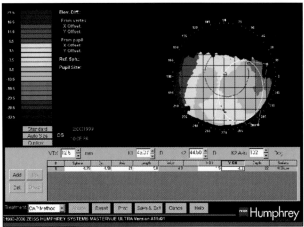

Figure 24-9a. An elliptical ablation using the new CAP ablation planner from Humphrey. The shape can be drawn onto the map and position, size, and shape will be automatically calculated. The surgeon enters the depth.

Figure 24-9b. A cylindrical ablation using the new CAP ablation planner from Humphrey.

cess of this technique is dependent upon determining an exact calculation of the shape, location, size, and depth of the ablation as extracted from elevation topography maps. The reported results show an accurate technique with improvement of visual symptoms, as well as uncorrected and corrected visual acuity. The technique has also proved to be safe, as no permanent lost lines of BCVA have been measured. On the contrary, more than 50% of the eyes treated with this technique gained one or more lines of vision.

In the near future, CAP ablation planners from Humphrey and Dicon will allow the surgeon to see the predicted postoperative topography map before surgery and, therefore, make the necessary changes to the ablation parameters until the goal of the surgery is achieved.

REFERENCES

1. Gibralter R, Trokel SL. Correction of irregular astigmatism with the excimer laser. *Ophthalmology.* 1994;101:1310-1315.

2. Buzard KA, Fundingsland BR. Treatment of irregular astigmatism with a broadbeam excimer laser. *J Refract Surg.* 1997;13:624-636.

3. Goode H. *Trans Cambridge Phil Soc.* 1847;8:495.

4. Placido A. Novo instrumento de esploracao da cornea. *Periodico Oftalmol Practice.* 1880;5:27-30.

5. Placido A. Novo instrumento para analyse immediate des irregularidades de curvatura da cornea. *Periodico Oftalmol Practice.* 1880;6:44-49.

6. Maguire LJ, Singer DE, Klyce SD. Graphic presentation of computer-analyzed keratoscope photographs. *Arch Ophthalmol.* 1987;105:223-230.

7. Wilson SE, Wang JY, Klyce SD. Quantification and mathematical analysis of photokeratoscope images. In: DJ Schanzlin, JB Robin, eds. *Corneal Topography: Measuring and Modifying the Cornea.* New York, NY: Springer-Verlag; 1992.

8. Tamayo G, Serrano M. Grid corneal marker. New surgical approach for the treatment of irregular astigmatism. Poster presented at the Panamerican Congress, Cancun; May 1997.

Surgeon-Guided Customized Ablation

Chapter Twenty-Five

Management of Decentered Ablations

Ioannis G. Pallikaris, MD
Vikentia J. Katsanevaki, MD

INTRODUCTION

Corneal ablation with the 193-nm excimer laser for the correction of refractive errors has excellent precision with insignificant thermal side effects. In general, the tissue beneath the ablation site remains transparent and smooth. Decentration, a photoablation-related complication of refractive surgery, can produce many detrimental visual effects. What is most important is the range of decentration. Gross decentration, with the transition zone surrounding the flat ablated zone over the entrance pupil, may be associated with troublesome nighttime symptoms of halos and glare, especially in younger individuals with large pupils.

A decentered ablation < 0.5 mm from the pupil center is graded as mild, from 0.5 to 1.0 mm moderate, and more than 1.0 mm severe.[1]

DECENTERED ABLATIONS

Risk Factors for Decentered Ablations

Factors that may contribute to decentration include poor patient fixation, improper alignment of the ablation zone by the surgeon, and optics misalignment of the laser delivering systems. Laser beam inhomogeneity as well as nonuniform corneal hydration may also play a role.

Clinical Implications of Decentered Ablations

Although rare, eccentric ablation after photorefractive procedures is a vision-threatening complication. In more severe cases, decentered ablations can induce line loss, irregular astigmatism, and monocular diplopia. Even without affecting high-contrast visual acuity (Figure 25-1) in moderate and mild cases, eccentric ablations can decrease contrast sensitivity, causing subjective symptoms such as glare and halos.[2-4]

> Even without affecting high-contrast visual acuity in moderate and mild cases, eccentric ablations can decrease contrast sensitivity, causing subjective symptoms such as glare and halos.[2-4]

Incidences of Decentrations After Photorefractive Procedures

Ablation zone decentration was reported as < 0.7 mm after photorefractive keratectomy (PRK) in the majority of reports.[5-9] In an initial study, Sher, et al reported up to 32% of 48 eyes treated for moderate and high myopia exhibited decentration > 1.0 mm.[7] The percentage of eyes reporting decentered ablation of 0.5 mm or more after laser-assisted in situ keratomileusis (LASIK) was up to 16%.[10-14]

Pallikaris and Siganos (Meditec) reported comparable centration in the PRK and LASIK groups.[10]

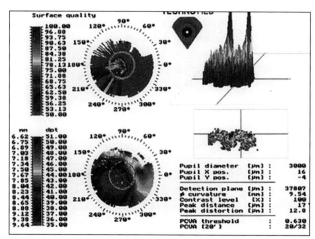

Figure 25-1. Ray tracing analysis maps representing a visual effect of –15 D eccentric ablation after LASIK simulating photopic (up, 3-mm pupil aperture) and scotopic (down, 6-mm pupil aperture). Patient's refraction after the operation is plano with no line loss. He complained of ghost images and difficulty in driving at night.

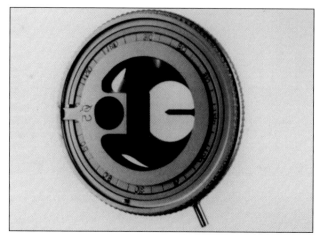

Figure 25-2. Arcutome: an instrument specially designed for the performance of arcuate cuts in several optical zones as well as customized length and depth of the corneal incision.

Condon, et al (Summit) found worse centration in the LASIK group.[14] The authors attributed this to three factors:

1. Fixation differences between lasers (patient fixation versus suction mask).

2. Longer duration of LASIK treatments for high refractive errors as well as poorer fixation of higher ametropic LASIK patients.

3. More difficult marking at the stromal bed of the interface.

Using the latest generation laser systems with active tracking during photoablation reduced decentrations of > 1 mm from 0%[1] to 6%[15] of treated eyes reported. Some authors suggest that ablation zone decentrations of 1.0 mm or slightly more may be tolerated with minimal or no subjective visual disturbance.[2,10] Doane, et al comparing two subgroups—one with decentration < 0.5 mm and the other with > 0.5 mm—that failed to show any statistical significance between groups in terms of halo, glare, and night driving problems. The authors concluded that decentrations of < 0.89 mm from the pupillary center are unlikely to produce significant visual symptoms.[9]

MANAGEMENT OF DECENTERED ABLATIONS

To date, few reports deal with the management of

eccentric ablations.[16-23] Proposed techniques include incisional and photorefractive procedures.

Incisional Techniques

Arcuate Cuts

Performing arcuate cuts is the technique of choice for the management of mild symptoms due to eccentric ablations before more invasive procedures implicating the optical zone. Arcuate cuts using customized diamond knives (Figure 25-2) can be performed according to special nomograms across the axis of decentration 180 degrees from the center of the prior ablation.

In a series of 10 patients (with eccentric ablations of 1.9 to 2.4 mm and ablation zone sizes of < 4 mm), the performance of a single arcuate cut (see Figure 25-2) has resulted in a topographic shift of a small central part of the ablation zone by 0.2 to 0.8 mm toward the side of the cut. This topographic "nipple shift" resulted in moderate to marked improvement of patients' asthenopic and subjective symptoms (Figure 25-3).[16,17]

Photorefractive Techniques

Masking Techniques

Photoablation of an irregular corneal surface will simply reproduce the irregularity in deeper stroma. Masking agents can protect deeper areas during pho-

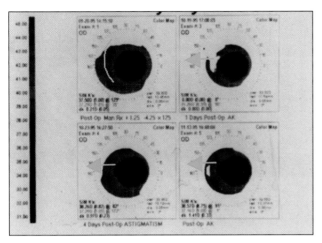

Figure 25-3. Serial profile maps of an eye treated with a temporal arcuate cut for optical zone enhancement. Induced "nipple shift" reduced the patient's asthenopic symptoms.

toablation, allowing more elevated focal areas to be excised and thus smoothing the corneal surface.

Masking techniques refer to photorefractive procedures utilizing various masking means to protect flatter corneal areas while steeper areas are excised with the excimer laser.

Masking Fluids

Masking fluids of varying viscosities have been investigated. Kornmehl, et al[24] investigated the ability of several fluids of different viscosities to mask deeper tissues while exposing protruding irregularities during phototherapeutic keratectomy (PTK) procedures. They reported that a fluid of moderate viscosity (between that of saline and 1% carboxymethylcellulose) is most desirable for this procedure. Very viscous fluids do not cover irregular surfaces uniformly, whereas laser viscosity fluids tend to run off quickly, exposing both peaks and valleys, thus resulting in irregular surfaces after ablation.

To further define optimal parameters for surface smoothing with the excimer laser, Fassano and colleagues[25] reported smoother corneal surfaces using low repetition rates. They assumed that relatively lower repetition rates (2 Hz compared to 10 Hz) allow time for the applied fluid to flow over the corneal surface, filling deeper depressions in the cornea as necessary (hertz rate refers to ablation cycles per second).

Epithelial Masking

In primary photorefractive procedures, the epithe-

> The technique of corneal smoothing utilizes the epithelium to act as a natural masking agent for the underlying stroma.

lium is usually mechanically removed assuming that the uneven thickness, as well as the differential ablation rates of the nucleus and the cytoplasm, may lead to irregular surfaces. The technique of corneal smoothing utilizes the epithelium to act as a natural masking agent for the underlying stroma. The epithelium has also been successfully used as a masking agent for the treatment of eccentric ablations.

Talamo and colleagues described a combined technique of transepithelial photoablation along with masking using 0.3% methylcellulose in flatter areas[21] to restrict the stromal ablation to the steeper areas evident on the topographic map.

Transepithelial ablation for the correction of corneal irregularity after LASIK was also reported in two LASIK cases with complicated flaps resulting in irregular corneas and associated scarring.[26] These authors stress the need for sufficiently high residual myopia to allow complete ablation of the flap. Total corneal thickness should also be taken into account in eyes that have inadequate thickness.

The PALM Technique Using Collagen Gel

Ideally the masking should[1] have the same ablation rate as that of the cornea,[2] be biocompatible,[3] and adhere well to the cornea.[25] Applicability of collagen solutions as masking agents for corneal photoablation was examined in experimental models of animal and cadaver eyes.[27-30]

The photoablatable lenticular modulator (PALM) technique refers to the use of a modified collagen gel for the photorefractive correction of corneal surface irregularities. The PALM gel has all the physical properties mentioned above. The ablation rate of the PALM gel was equivalent to that of the cornea using irregular porcine corneas in a model described by Englanoff, et al.[27] Examining the biocompatibility of the gel, light and transmission electron microscopy did not reveal differences of corneal ultrastructure between experimental and control specimens of rabbit corneas.

PALM gel is fully thermoreversible. When heated to 49°C it is in liquid form, solidifying to gel within minutes after being applied to the corneal de-epithelialized surface.

When still in liquid form, a customized rigid contact lens is used as a mold for the lenticle's upper sur-

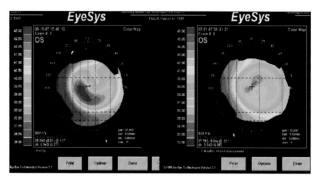

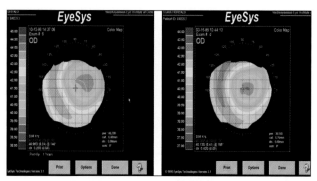

Figure 25-4. Preoperative (left) and postoperative (right) videokeratography maps of a patient treated with the PALM technique for the management of eccentric ablation. Treatment improved visual acuity and resolved the patient's reported monocular diplopia.

Figure 25-5. Corneal topographies of a patient treated for myopia (-6 D) complicated with eccentric ablation (videokeratography on the left). Two years after treatment, the patient's UCVA was 20/32 and BCVA 20/20 (-1.0 x 60 degrees) with no line loss but severe monocular diplopia and glare. The patient was treated with diagonal ablation (-2 D at 6-mm optical zone, centered 1.5 mm temporally on the 60-degree meridian). Two months after treatment (videokeratography on the right) the patient retains her BCVA and reports elimination of her subjective symptoms.

face. Removal of the lens after 4 minutes results in a stable lenticle that is well adhered onto the cornea. Full removal of the gel lenticle with photoablation reproduces the lenticle's upper surface to the cornea. The PALM technique can be applied to a de-epithelialized cornea or onto bare stroma under a flap for the treatment of eccentric ablations after both procedures.

As currently used at the University of Crete for the treatment of eccentric ablations, the PALM technique has produced very encouraging results (Figure 25-4).

Diametral (Eccentric) Ablation

Diametral ablation[18-20] is one of the few photorefractive techniques proposed to treat prior decentered ablations. This technique utilizes a combination of transepithelial PTK, followed by a second decentered photorefractive procedure based on preoperative corneal topography and marks on the cornea. The second photorefractive ablation is topographically centered, eccentric by the identical distance to the center of the pupil but opposite to the initial procedure. During this spherical photorefractive procedure, the residual epithelium over the previously treated zone acts as a shield for further ablation. The alteration of this technique as opposed to Talamo's report[21] is that the second PRK is not centered over the pupil and uses only the epithelium as a natural masking agent.

Diametral (eccentric) ablation is also reported with good results after LASIK.[20] We performed diametral ablation in seven eyes of seven patients for the management of prior eccentric ablations. Maximum decentration was 2 mm, 1.44 ± 0.5 (mean

± standard deviation) as estimated by corneal topography subtraction maps.[10] All patients suffered severe subjective symptoms such as ghost images and monocular diplopia. Attempted correction ranged from –7.5 to -2 D (-4.44 ± 1.74 D, mean ± standard deviation). Uncorrected visual acuity was improved in all but one eye after treatment, with the spherical equivalent ranging from –0.5 to +3.25 D (1.09 ± 1.28 D, mean ± standard deviation). Subjective symptoms were improved in all eyes and were completely alleviated in two patients. Results are summarized in Table 25-1 (our own previously unpublished data). Although good results were achieved in terms of high-contrast Snellen visual acuity, this method, which is highly dependent on the videokeratography subtraction maps, is unlikely to produce a regular spherocylindrical refracting corneal surface affecting the optical zone's homogeneity. An example of this technique is shown in Figure 25-5.

Nizzola-Vinciguerra Technique

The Nizzola-Vinciguerra technique[23] achieves an asymmetric ablation complementary to the prior decentered treatment utilizing PTK through a series of metallic diaphragms of varying apertures. The metallic diaphragms is used instead of a masking fluid to protect flatter areas from further photoablation. The series of these metallic diaphragms are suc-

Table 25-1

Change in BSCVA and Reported Subjective Symptoms after Diametral Ablation

BSCVA*				*SUBJECTIVE SYMPTOMS*	
	Preop	Pre Diagonal	Post Diagonal	Pre Diagonal	Post Diagonal
1	20/20	20/20	20/25	Severe	mild
2	20/25	20/32	20/25	Severe	moderate
3	20/25	20/32	20/25	Severe	mild
4	20/20	20/20	20/20	Severe	mild
5	20/20	20/25	20/25	Severe	mild
6	20/40	20/40	20/40	Severe	Relieved
7	20/32	20/32	20/32	Severe	relieved

cessively used during treatment, starting with the larger and ending with the smallest one. The diaphragms are put in a specially designed suction mask that must be centered on the axis of decentration at the beginning of the procedure.[3]

TopLinked Ablation

Topography-assisted software programs have been recently incorporated in the latest generation of laser delivery systems. Based on elevation maps, they selectively guide the ablation of irregular corneas. TopoLinked ablation, currently under clinical evaluation apart from its other applications, holds a promise for the future treatment of decentered ablation. Clinical results of the various systems being developed are described in detail in Section III.

SUMMARY

We have seen the development of a number of techniques including incisional, photorefractive, masking, and more recently corneal TopoLink techniques to alleviate decentered ablations. These techniques have improved many patients' vision, but refinements with preventing and treating this problem are rapidly evolving. Future developments such as corneal TopoLink and wavefront sensing hold great promise in the management of decentration.

REFERENCES

1. Tsai Y, Lin JM. Ablation centration after active eye-tracker-assisted photorefractive keratectomy and laser in situ keratomileusis. *J Cataract Refract Surg.* 2000;26:28-34.

2. Mulhern MG, Foley-Nolan A, O' Keefe M, Condon PI. Topographical analysis of ablation centration after excimer laser photorefractive keratectomy and laser in situ keratomileusis for high myopia. *J Cataract Refract Surg.* 1997;23:488-494.

3. Terrel J, Bechara SJ, Nesburn A, et al. The effect of globe fixation on ablation zone centration in photorefractive keratectomy. *Am J Ophthalmol.* 1995;119:612-619.

4. Pande M, Hillman JS. Optical zone centration in keratorefractive surgery; entrance pupil center, visual axis, coaxially sighted corneal reflex, or geometric corneal center? *Ophthalmology.* 1993;100:1230-1237.

5. Talley AR, Hardten DR, Sher NA, et al. Results one year after using the 193 nm excimer laser for photorefractive keratectomy in mild to moderate myopia. *Am J Ophthalmol.* 1994;118:304-11.

6. Maguen E, Salz JJ, Nesburn AB, et al. Results of excimer laser photorefractive keratectomy for the correction of myopia. *Ophthalmology.* 1994;101:1548-57.

7. Sher NA, Hardten DR, Fundingsland B, et al. 193 nm excimer photorefractive keratectomy in high myopia. *Ophthalmology.* 1994;101:1575-82.

8. Schwartz-Goldstein BH, Hersh PS. Corneal topography of phase III excimer laser photorefractive keratectomy: optical zone centration analysis. *Ophthalmology.* 1995;102:951-62.

9. Doane JB, Cavanaugh TB, Durrie DS, Hassanein KH. Relation of visual symptoms to topographic ablation zone decentration after excimer laser photorefractive keratectomy. *Ophthalmology.* 1995;102:42-7.

10. Pallikaris IG, Siganos DS. Excimer laser in situ keratomileusis and photorefractive keratectomy for correction of high myopia. *J Cataract Refract Surg.* 1994;10:498-510.

11. Bas AM, Omnis R. Excimer laser in situ keratomileusis for myopia. *J Refract Surg.* 1995;11:S229-233.

12. Pallikaris IG, Siganos DS. Laser in situ keratomileusis to treat myopia: early experience. *J Cataract Refract Surg.* 1997;23:39-49.

13. Fiander DC, Tayfour F. Excimer laser in situ keratomileusis in 124 myopic eyes. *J Refract Surg.* 1995;11:S234-238.

14. Condon PI, Mulhern M, Fulcher T, et al. Laser intrastromal keratomileusis for high myopia and myopic astigmatism. *Br J Ophthalmol.* 1997;81:199-206.

15. Coorpender SJ, Klyce SD, Mc Donald MB, et al. Corneal topography of small beam tracking excimer laser photorefractive keratectomy. *J Cataract Refract Surg.* 1999;25:675-684.

16. Pallikaris IG, Siganos DS. LASIK complications and their management. In: J Talamo, RR Krueger, eds. *The Excimer Manual.* Boston, Mass: Little Brown and Co; 1997:227-244.

17. Pallikaris IG, Siganos DS. A new optical effect of arcuate keratectomy. In: IG Pallikaris, DS Siganos, eds. *LASIK.* Thorofare, NJ: SLACK Incorporated; 1998:297-302.

18. Seiler T, Schmidt-Petersen H, Wollensak J. Complications after myopic PRK primarily with the Summit laser. In: JJ Salz, PJ McDonnel, MB McDonald, eds. *Corneal Laser Surgery.* St Louis, Mo: CV Mosby; 1995:131-142.

19. Alkara N, Genth U, Seiler T. Diametral ablation—a technique to manage decentered photorefractive keratectomy for myopia. *J Refract Surg.* 1999;15:436-40.

20. Seiler T, McDonnell P. Excimer laser photorefractive keratectomy. *Surv Ophthalmol.* 1995;40:89-118.

21. Talamo JH, Wagoner MD, Lee SY. Management of ablation decentration following excimer photorefractive keratectomy. *Arch Ophthalmol.* 1995;113:706-707.

22. Pallikaris I, Panagopoulou S, Katsanevaki V. The PALM technique: photoablated lenticular modulator. In: IG Pallikaris, DS Siganos, eds. *LASIK.* Thorofare, NJ: SLACK Incorporated; 1998:277-278.

23. Vinciguerra P, Nizzola GD, Airaghi P, Ascari A, Nizzola F, Azzolini M. A new technique for the excimer laser correction of decentration after PRK and LASIK. In: IG Pallikaris, DS Siganos, eds. *LASIK.* Thorofare, NJ: SLACK Incorporated; 1998:281.

24. Kornmehl EW, Steinert RF, Puliafito CA. A comparative study of masking fluids for excimer laser phototherapeutic keratectomy. *Arch Ophthalmol.* 1991;109:860-863.

25. Fassano PA, Moreira H, McDonnel PJ, Sinbawy A. Excimer laser smoothing with model of anterior corneal surface irregularity. *Ophthalmology.* 1991;98:1782-1785.

26. Kapadia MS, Wilson SE. Transepithelial photorefractive keratectomy for treatment of thin flaps or caps after complicated laser in situ keratomileusis. *Am J Ophthalmol.* 1998;126(6):827-829.

27. Englanoff JS, Kolandouz-Isfahani AH, Moreira H, Cheung DT, Trokel SL, McDonnel PJ. In situ collagen mold as an aid in excimer laser superficial keratectomy. *Ophthalmology.* 1992;99:1201-1208.

28. Margaritis AG, Pallikaris IG, Siganos DS. Properties of a new two component gel material as an aid in PRK corneal remodeling. *Invest Ophthalmol Vis Sci.* 1994;35(4):3553.

29. De Vore DP, Scott JB, Nordquist RE, Hoffman RS, Nguyen H, Eifferman RA. Rapidly polymerized collagen gel as a smoothing agent in excimer laser photoablation. *J Refract Surg.* 1995;11(1):50-55.

30. Stevens SX, Bowyer BL, Sanchez-Thorin JC, Rocha G, Young DA, Rowsy JJ. The BioMask for treatment of corneal surface irregularities with excimer laser phototherapeutic keratectomy. *Cornea.* 1999;18(2):155-63.

Chapter Twenty-Six

Topographic Steep Central Islands

Weldon W. Haw, MD
Edward E. Manche, MD

INTRODUCTION

Topographic steep central islands have been reported following photorefractive keratectomy (PRK), laser-assisted in situ keratomileusis (LASIK), and automated lamellar keratoplasty (ALK).[1-13] These islands may result from spatial variance of tissue removal with relative central undercorrection.[14] Islands may result in visual symptoms, undercorrections, loss of best spectacle-corrected visual acuity (BSCVA), poor contrast sensitivity, and poor visual performance.

PREVALENCE OF CENTRAL ISLANDS

The prevalence of topographic steep central islands in the current literature is dependent on the definition of "island," the postoperative duration, amount of preoperative correction, and the type of topography system used to identify islands. Topographic steep central islands are commonly diagnosed in symptomatic patients with an island ≥ 1.0 to 3.0 mm diameter and ≥ 1.0 to 3.0 diopters (D) in height. Krueger characterized a steep central island as a topographic area of steepening at least 3.0 D in height and at least 1.5 mm in diameter.[5] The central zone had to be 3.0 D steeper than the midperiphery in all four quadrants and at least 1.5 mm in diameter when scaling the videokeratograph with the eye. In this retrospective study of 39 eyes treated with a broadbeam excimer laser, 20% at 3 months and 11% at 6 months had topographic islands when using this criteria.

The prevalence of steep central islands is also dependent upon the type of topography system used to identify the island. In one study, steep central islands were identified 1 month following PRK in 50 eyes (81%) that were treated with the Technomed C-Scan (Technomed, Baesweller, Germany) as compared to 22 eyes (35%) with the EyeSys CAS (EyeSys, Houston, Tex).[15]

Most of the published studies on central islands have evaluated islands following PRK. The incidence of steep central islands has varied from 0% to 4.7% of eyes up to 12 months following LASIK.[11-13] In higher level corrections, central islands may be observed in up to 17% of eyes for spherical and 16% of eyes for toric corrections despite pretreatment using the broadbeam Keracor 116 excimer laser following LASIK.[16]

THE ETIOLOGY OF CENTRAL ISLANDS

Multiple theories have been proposed to explain the origin of topographic steep central islands. Fundamentally, steep central islands develop from less central photoablation relative to the immediate surrounding area (or peripheral overablation).[14] Although the development of steep central islands is likely to be multifactorial, the most prevalent theo-

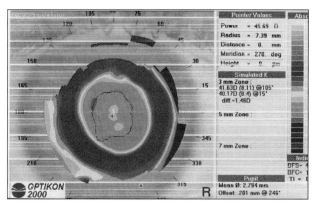

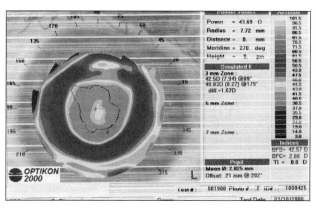

Figure 26-1a. This figure demonstrates an example of a steep central island following LASIK with a broadbeam excimer laser system. The axial curvature map is shown. Note the central steepening characteristic of a topographic central island. Elevation data can be obtained by taking the height difference between the cursor reading at the steepest point at the apex of the island and the flatter area at the edge of the island. This elevation difference should be used to plan the treatment of steep central islands.

Figure 26-1b. This figure demonstrates an example of a steep central island following LASIK with a broadbeam excimer laser system. The meridional (also called "true" or tangential) curvature map is shown.

ries include the differential hydration/acoustic shockwave theory and the vortex plume theory.[5] The differential hydration theory proposes that each pulse of energy results in an acoustic shockwave that results in intraoperative central stromal hydration. Since hydrated stroma is more resistant to photoablation, a steep central island results. The vortex plume theory proposes an ejected central cloud of debris from each laser pulse interferes with energy delivery to the underlying stroma. Other mechanisms include laser optics deterioration and postoperative focal central epithelial hyperplasia (following PRK). Notably, steep central islands are a product of flat, broadbeam excimer laser profiles. Significant topographic islands have not been reported with smaller beam scanning or spot lasers.

In order to avoid steep central islands, current broadbeam excimer lasers have incorporated anticentral island software that increases the delivery of pulses to the center of the ablation profile. Most pretreatment anticentral island protocols apply 1 to 2 microns per diopter at an optical zone of 3.0 mm or less to avoid postoperative islands with broadbeam

excimer lasers.[17] Blowing nitrogen gas and aerosol over the cornea during the ablation and cleaning fluid from the cornea have been shown to reduce the incidence of steep central islands.[8]

RISK FACTORS FOR CENTRAL ISLANDS

Several risk factors for the development of steep central islands have been reported. The use of a broadbeam excimer laser delivery system has already been described. Commercially available broadbeam excimer lasers include VisX, Summit, Schwind, and Technolas Keracor 116. Additional risk factors include a larger ablation zone and higher attempted level of correction.[14]

CLINICAL OBSERVATIONS ON CENTRAL ISLANDS

The typical presentation of a steep central island occurs in a patient with myopia who underwent excimer laser photoablation with a broadbeam laser and who complained of poor quality of vision, monocular diplopia, or "ghosting" in the early postoperative period. Slit lamp examination is unremarkable. Uncorrected visual acuity may be poor. Manifest refraction may demonstrate significant undercorrection with loss of BSCVA. Computerized corneal videokeratography is used to confirm the clinical diagnosis. The topography reveals a central elevated area shown as a red, yellow, or green island (warmer colors) surrounded by a peripheral flat-

> In order to avoid steep central islands, current broadbeam excimer lasers have incorporated anticentral island software that increases the delivery of pulses to the center of the ablation profile.

tened area shown as a sea of blue (cooler colors) on computerized corneal topography color maps (Figures 26-1a and 26-1b).

Following LASIK for high myopia, keratectasia may be misdiagnosed as a topographic "steep central island." Both conditions may present with symptoms of monocular diplopia, poor uncorrected visual acuity, loss of BSCVA, and a localized steepening on videokeratography. However, it is important to correctly distinguish between iatrogenic keratectasia and a steep central island since treatment of keratectasia with further ablation may exacerbate the ectatic process. In addition, photoablation of a thin cornea during LASIK retreatment may result in corneal perforation.[18] The progressive nature of serial topography may help establish the correct diagnosis of keratectasia.[19] This further supports the treatment strate-

> We suggest observing the eyes 3 to 6 months prior to retreatment, particularly in thin corneas.

gy of observing eyes with central islands for at least 3 to 6 months prior to retreatment, particularly in thin corneas. A 250-micron minimal posterior stromal bed should be preserved to maintain long-term corneal integrity and avoid postoperative iatrogenic ectasia.[17] Classic corneal topography systems only provided information from the anterior corneal surface. The Orbscan topography system uses a scanning slit measurement system (Orbtek, Inc, Bausch & Lomb, Salt Lake City, Utah), which is able to measure the posterior corneal curvature, and thus can directly identify posterior corneal ectasia.

MANAGEMENT OF CENTRAL ISLANDS

Some patients with symptomatic steep central topographic islands may not desire further refractive surgical interventions. These patients may be managed conservatively with observation and reassurance. The topographic elevation of the steep central island may decrease rapidly over time. Following PRK with a broadbeam excimer laser, steep central islands >3.0 D and >1.5 mm were found to occur in 71% of eyes at 1 week, 51% of eyes at 1 month, 20% at 3 months, and 1% at 6 months.[5] In a prospective study by McGhee, 90% of topographic islands following PRK resolved by 6 months and 100% resolved by 1 year without surgical intervention.[7] A rigid gas permeable contact lens is a reasonable

option to maximize the immediate visual rehabilitation.

The natural history of central islands following LASIK has not been well documented. In our experience, islands following LASIK appear to resolve more slowly and incompletely as compared to islands following PRK.

Treatment of Central Islands Following PRK

Since many islands will spontaneously resolve over time, a symptomatic topographic island should be observed a minimum of 3 to 6 months prior to consideration for surgical intervention. Persistent steep central islands can be considered for treatment with multiple laser alternatives. The diameter of the ablation zone can be calculated from the diameter of the island on computerized videokeratography. The amount of correction can also be calculated from the height of the island on the elevation or "true" topographic map. Using Munnerlyn's formula (see case 1), the ablation depth can be directly calculated.[20] The ablation depth and ablation zone is programmed into the excimer laser. Both PRK and PTK modes have been described to successfully treat topographic islands.[6,9]

PRK mode offers the advantage of an adjustable iris diaphragm that delivers more pulses centrally over the apex of the topographic island. Theoretically, this should provide a smoother ablation of the island when compared to the ablation through a fixed iris diaphragm, as in the PTK mode (equal ablation to the center and periphery of the island). However, the PTK mode has the advantage of allowing the surgeon to specify the number of pulses and size of the ablation zone. Unfortunately, at the time of printing of this text, all current US Food and Drug Administration (FDA)-approved broadbeam excimer lasers in the United States have nonadjustable ablation zones in PRK mode. Thus, the surgeon must request the laser manufacturer to specifically program the laser to allow for central island treatments using the PRK mode.

In order to avoid excessive hyperopic shift, it is advisable to adjust the depth of the ablation. We typically program 60% to 70% of the full correction into the laser. As epithelial hyperplasia and remodeling occur, the topography may continue to regularize.

Treatment of Central Islands Following LASIK

For steep islands following LASIK, the flap is lifted (as in a retreatment procedure), and the photoab-

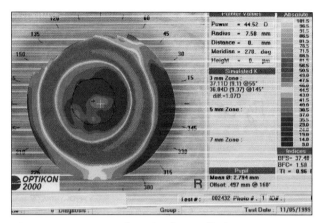

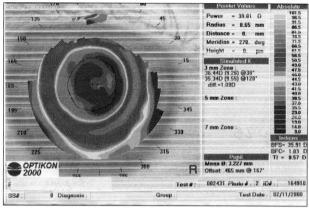

Figure 26-2a. Meridional (also called "true" or tangential) computerized corneal topography map 3 months following LASIK for myopia. Note the 6.0-D steep central island.

Figure 26-2b. Elevation map 3 months following treatment of the steep central island with PTK mode under the primary keratectomy flap. Note the improvement in the central island.

lation is centered over the island. For islands following PRK, the epithelium is removed and the ablation is centered over the island. In a case series by Manche, eight eyes underwent reablation with either PTK or PRK for a symptomatic topographic island following PRK, LASIK, or myopic keratomileusis in situ using the methods described above.[6] All eight eyes experienced a reduction of topographic central islands, 75% an improvement in uncorrected visual acuity, and 100% of eyes returned to within one line of their preoperative level of BSCVA. Similar improvements in BSCVA have been reported by Castillo in three patients with steep central islands managed with PRK reablation.[9] Although we have had success in treating significant topographic steep central islands using the method described by Manche,[6] we recommend that clinicians uncomfortable with this method wait for improvements in excimer laser technology.

Further improvements in excimer laser technology are expected to result in alternative treatment options for eyes with steep central islands. Promising technology includes the use of customized or corneal topography-guided ablations. Currently, these options have not been approved by the FDA. However, VisX is currently investigating the use of contoured ablation pattern (CAP) technology for the treatment of irregular corneas.

CAP technology is a software upgrade to the VisX Star S2 excimer laser system that uses a beam-shaping module that narrows and redirects a seven-beam scanning array to customize an ablation. This technology allows the refractive surgeon to specify the size, depth, and location of the ablation based on computerized corneal topography.[21] Other companies such as Bausch & Lomb, Nidek, Meditec, and Lasersight are also developing corneal topography-based customized ablations that may be helpful in the treatment of steep central islands. This is further detailed in the corneal topography-guided ablation section of this book.

Preoperative corneal topography is important in planning the ablation pattern. The corneal elevation map is the most useful in defining the characteristics of corneal irregularities since conventional curvature maps do not distinguish between elevation and curvature. In addition, topography ablation planning software (TAPS) is also being developed to enhance postsurgical outcomes. This software will allow the surgeon to design and simulate the effects of different ablation patterns *before* treating the eye.

Cases Examples

Case 1

A 54-year-old male underwent uncomplicated LASIK OD for high compound myopic astigmatism with the VisX S2 SmoothScan using a 6.0-mm zone. Preoperative cycloplegic refraction was -11.50 +0.75 x 050, which yielded a visual acuity of 20/40 (amblyopia). At the 3-month postoperative visit, the patient was complaining of poor vision OD. UCVA was 20/100. BSCVA was 20/30 with -2.50 +0.75 x 020. Videokeratography revealed a 6.0 keratometric diopter topographic island that was 2 mm in diameter (Figure 26-2a).

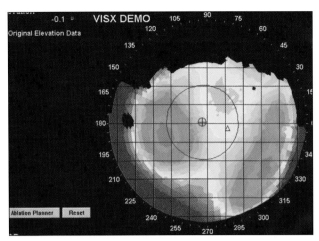

Figure 26-3a. Computerized corneal topography elevation map following a decentered myopic ablation. Note the paracentral steep central island (courtesy of VisX, Inc).

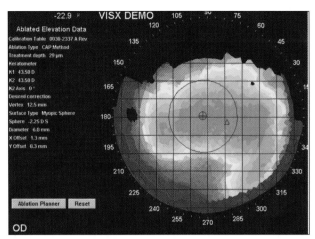

Figure 26-3b. Computerized corneal topography elevation map following treatment of the paracentral central island and decentered ablation with VisX CAP technology. Note the improvement in the island (courtesy of VisX, Inc).

The Munnerlyn equation can be used to determine the required tissue ablation to achieve a refractive correction.[20] The depth (height) of tissue ablation (microns) is given by:

$$\frac{\text{diopter power of the island} \times (\text{diameter of island})^2}{3}$$

Applying the Munnerlyn formula to the above example yeilds:

$$\frac{6.0 \text{ D} \times (2 \text{ mm})^2}{3} = 8 \text{ microns}$$

By the Munnerlyn equation, 8 microns of tissue were required to completely correct the steep central island.[20] In order to avoid overcorrection, 5 microns of PTK x 2.0 mm was programmed into the VisX S2 SmoothScan excimer laser. The flap was lifted, the ablation was centered over the island, and the treatment was performed without complications. The patient's UCVA was 20/30 3 months following the central island retreatment. Symptoms of distortion and blurring had resolved. BSCVA was 20/30 (amblyopia persisted but improved) with -0.25 + 0.75 x 40. Videokeratography revealed marked improvement in the steep central island (Figure 26-2b).

Case 2

The elevation topography map of a decentered myopic ablation with a paracentral steep central island is shown in Figure 26-3a. The topography is regularized following customized ablation using the VisX CAP technology (Figure 26-3b). Further details on this technique are provided in Chapter Twenty-Four.

SUMMARY

In summary, steep central topographic islands may result in a suboptimal visual outcome following broadbeam excimer laser ablation. Current treatment options include the use of PRK or PTK mode with the depth and size of the treatment parameters adjusted by the topographic characterization of the island. Reasonable outcomes have been demonstrated using these methods. However, future technology using customized ablation software and topography ablation planning software is expected to improve these results and offer new treatment alternatives to patients with this problematic condition.

REFERENCES

1. Price F. Central islands of corneal steepening after automated lamellar keratoplasty for myopia. *J Refract Surg.* 1996;12:36-41.

2. Colin J, Cochener B, Gallinaro C. Central steep islands immediately following excimer photorefractive keratectomy for myopia (letter). *J Refract Corneal Surg.* 1993;9:395-6.

3. Lin DTC. Corneal topographic analysis after excimer

photorefractive keratectomy. *Ophthalmology.* 1994;101:1432-9.

4. Levin S, Carson CA, Garrett SK, Taylor HR. Prevalence of central islands after excimer laser refractive surgery. *J Cataract Refract Surg.* 1995;21:21-6.

5. Krueger R, Saedy NF, McDonnell PJ. Clinical analysis of steep central islands after excimer laser photorefractive keratectomy. *Arch Ophthalmol.* 1996;114:377-81.

6. Manche EE, Maloney RK, Smith RJ. Treatment of topographic central islands following refractive surgery. *J Cataract Refract Surg.* 1998;24:464-70.

7. McGhee CN, Bryce IG. Natural history of central topographic islands following excimer laser photorefractive keratectomy. *J Cataract Refract Surg.* 1996;22:1151-8.

8. Forster W, Clemens S, Bruning, et al. Steep central islands after myopic photorefractive keratectomy. *J Cataract Refract Surg.* 1998;24:899-904.

9. Castillo A, Romero F, Martin-Valverde JA, et al. Management and treatment of steep islands after excimer laser photorefractive keratectomy. *J Refract Surg.* 1996;12:715-20.

10. Abbas UL, Hersh PS. Early corneal topography patterns after excimer laser photorefractive keratectomy for myopia. *J Refract Surg.* 1999;15:124-31.

11. Salchow DJ, Zirm ME, Stieldorf C, Parisi A. Laser in situ keratomileusis for myopia and myopic astigmatism. *J Cataract Refract Surg.* 1998;24:175-82.

12. Salchow DJ, Zirm ME, Stieldorf C, Parisi A. Laser in situ keratomileusis (LASIK) for correction of myopia and astigmatism. *Ophthalmologe.* 1998;95:142-7.

13. Knorz MC, Liermann A, Wiesinger B, Seiberth V, Liesenhoff H. Laser in situ keratomileusis (LASIK) for correction of myopia. *Ophthalmologe.* 1997;94:775-9.

14. Shimmick JK, Telfair WB, Munnerlyn CR, Bartlett JD, Trokel SL. Corneal ablation profilometry and steep central islands. *J Refract Surg.* 1997;13:235-45.

15. Krueger R, Seiler T. PRK postoperative and complication management. In: JH Talamo, RR Krueger, eds. *The Excimer Manual: A Clinician's Guide to Excimer Laser Surgery.* Boston, Mass: Little Brown and Co; 1997:249-63.

16. Knorz MC, Wiesinger B, Liermann A, Seiberth V, Liesenhoff H. Laser in situ keratomileusis for moderate and high myopia and myopic astigmatism. *Ophthalmology.* 1998;105:932-40.

17. Probst LE, Machat JJ. Mathematics of laser in situ keratomileusis for high myopia. *J Cataract Refract Surg.* 1998;24:190-5.

18. Joo CK, Kim TG. Corneal perforation during laser in situ keratomileusis. *J Cataract Refract Surg.* 1999;25:1165-7.

19. Seiler T, Koufala K, Richter G. Iatrogenic keratectasia after laser in situ keratomileusis. *J Refract Surg.* 1998;14:312-7.

20. Munnerlyn CR, Koons SJ, Marshall J. Photorefractive keratectomy: a technique for laser refractive surgery. *J Cataract Refract Surg.* 1988;14:46-52.

21. VisX. *Quick Guide to Performing Variable Ablations Using the VISX CAP Method.* VisX CAP Training Manual; 2000.

Chapter Twenty-Seven

Customization of Ablation Optical Zone Sizes in LASIK

Barrie D. Soloway, MD, FACS
Ronald R. Krueger, MD, MSE

INTRODUCTION

Predictability, stability, and safety have been listed as factors that are required for refractive surgical procedure success. Unlike any refractive surgical procedure in the past, excimer laser reshaping of the cornea (either with photorefractive keratectomy [PRK] or laser-assisted in situ keratomileusis [LASIK]) satisfies these requirements. It is being accepted by ophthalmologists and patients as a method to reduce people's dependence on optical aids such as glasses or contact lenses. The market for these procedures in the United States has doubled every year since US Food and Drug Administration (FDA) approval of excimer lasers for PRK in 1995. Despite the overwhelming success of LASIK in the majority of patients, reports are beginning to appear in the medical literature, on the Internet, and in the news media that even with a result of 20/20 uncorrected distance visual acuity, issues such as the quality of vision in low light settings can cause patient dissatisfaction with their results. Nonacuity-related symptoms such as decreased contrast sensitivity, glare, starburst, and halo may interfere with the quality of vision that patients experience after surgery. There are numerous reasons implicated as causes of these problems, such as decentration of the ablation optical zone, irregular topography or refraction in the ablation optical zone, areas of treatment and nontreatment in the ablation optical zone, and

haze or scarring in the optical zone. Another cause of poor acceptance of the outcome from excimer refractive surgery occurs when the patient's scotopic (dark light) pupil size is greater than the ablation optical zone treated by the laser. It has been suggested that the use of larger ablation optical zones in patients who have larger scotopic pupil sizes might diminish the amount of nonacuity-related symptoms these patients might experience. Evidence based on postoperative wavefront analysis of the increase in optical aberrations within the pupil with undersized ablation optical zones, as well as ray tracing algorithms used in topography over the entire surface of the cornea for different pupil sizes, tend to confirm this. Until recently, however, excimer laser technology was unable to treat a larger ablation optical zone (> 6 mm), and this remained an issue to be determined.

The wavefront map created with the Alcon Summit Autonomous CustomCornea wavefront measurement device (Figure 27-1) shows only the higher-order aberrations created in the peripheral portion of the red reflex pupillary zone of a postoperative LASIK patient (lower right side of figure). This patient had a "standard" ablation optical zone (6.0 mm) treatment for a prescription of –3.25 –1.75 x 170 degrees. Due to the small ablation optical zone treatment along the 80-degree meridian and the typical smaller size of the effective optical zone obtained with LASIK, spherical aberration of 0.32 root mean

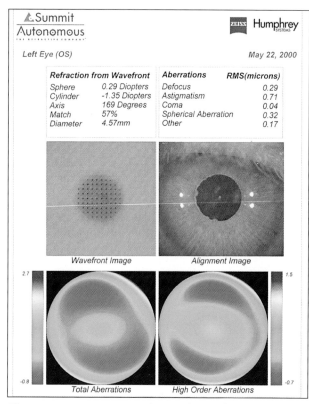

Figure 27-1. Post-LASIK photo of wavefront aberration map demonstrating induced higher-order aberrations.

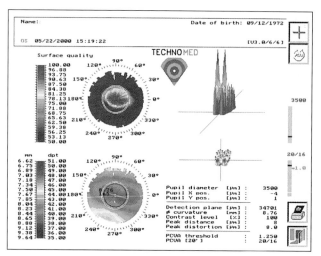

Figure 27-2. Photo of Technomed ray tracing topography at 3.5-mm pupil size in a postoperative LASIK patient.

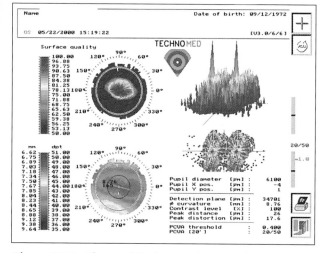

Figure 27-3. Photo of Technomed ray tracing topography at 6.1-mm pupil size in a postoperative LASIK patient.

square (RMS) microns is present in this patient even with a mesopic pupil size of 4.57 mm at the time of measurement.

Figure 27-2 shows the Technomed C-Scan ray tracing resolution in the same patient when pupil size is 3.5 mm. Here, good resolution is evident in the patient's ability to resolve two image points with a close peak difference of 8.0, a peak distortion of 8.0, and a potential corrected visual acuity of 20/16. Figure 27-3 shows the same patient's pupil size of 6.1 mm. Once again, the aberrations due to optical zone negative clearance with pupil size, particularly in the 80-degree meridian, show up in the increase in peak distance to 26, peak distortion of 17.6, and potential corneal visual acuity reduction to 20/50.

HISTORY OF ABLATION OPTICAL ZONE SIZES

The keratomileusis procedure originally developed by Dr. José Ignacio Barraquer used a variety of methods to create the required refractive change.[1,2] Originally, the refractive change was affected with hand dissection, later shaped on a cryolathe, and finally treated the cap or bed with a second pass of the microkeratome. With each technique, the effective optical zone diameter depended on the refractive change required. The maximum diameter was limited to the size of the cap produced with early styles of microkeratomes. Patients' nonacuity-related complaints of glare were related to the use of smaller effective optical zones, as well as decentration of the effective optical zone and irregular astigmatism.

Radial Keratotomy

Radial keratotomy (RK) used the incisional optical zone size measurement in a nomogram format based on the amount of correction desired. Incisional optical zone sizes of < 3.00 mm were not recommended due to the high likelihood of nonacuity-related complaints. Even in many patients with larger incisional optical zones, nonacuity-related symptoms limited their satisfaction with the surgery. In these patients, a starburst pattern around light was one of the frequent complaints, apparently resulting from scarring from the incision within the entrance pupils.

Excimer Laser Ablation

In the early 1980s, Trokel learned of the excimer laser and began its development as a tool for reshaping the eye.[3] The original work envisioned the laser as a computerized scalpel that could more accurately perform the RK incisions.[4] By adjusting the number of pulses, the depth of the cut could be controlled; and by adjusting the excursion to the laser treatment, the length of the incision could be controlled. Subsequently, the lamellar approach of tissue removal gained favor. This approach allowed for a larger ablation optical zone, and because it did not require as deep an ablation, it maintained the structural integrity of the cornea. In 1987, McDonald performed the first PRK treatments on sighted eyes. Ablation optical zone diameters were limited in size (4.5 to 5.5 mm) due to the limitations of the lasers available at that time. Through the 1990s, optical zone sizes have increased to the 6 mm standard size originally approved by the FDA.[5] Six millimeters was generally accepted as large enough to avoid nonacuity-related problems and was within the technologic reach of the broadbeam lasers available at that time. As a greater number of people underwent excimer laser treatment for refractive disorders, problems of glare and other nonacuity-related issues began to surface in the medical literature.[6,7] Maintaining or improving the quality of vision can be added to the list of basic requirements of any refractive surgery procedure if we are to continue to successfully treat greater numbers of people.

THE TECHNICAL CHALLENGE OF LARGER ZONES

There are limitations in our ability to appropriately widen the effective optical zone in every patient.

In order to safely and accurately treat patients with larger ablation optical zones, we must fully understand the following three concepts.

As the ablation widens:
1. The depth of the ablation increases according to Munnerlyn's formula.
2. The keratome must expose a corneal bed diameter that is properly sized, as well as properly placed.
3. The treatment time increases, changing the hydration characteristics of the corneal stroma.

In addition, the limited ablation optical zone size of the broadbeam excimer laser limits the surgeon. It is also critical to accurately measure scotopic pupil size in order to treat the patient with an appropriate ablation optical zone size. We will discuss these issues in the next section.

DEPTH OF THE ABLATIONS

Munnerlyn's formula gives us a generalized way of calculating the depth of a single zone myopic ablation.[8] It shows how the depth of the ablation increases linearly as the dioptric strength of the treatment increases. Since we are treating an increased area when we enlarge the diameter of the optical zone, the ablation depth increases in an exponential fashion.

> The depth of ablation increases linearly with dioptric strength and exponentially with the diameter of the optical zone.

$$\frac{(\text{optical zone diameter in mm})^2 \times \text{diopters}}{3}$$

With single zone treatments, the Alcon Summit Autonomous LADARVision laser ablation depths are listed in Table 27-1.

The safety and stability of the refractive result depends on the tectonic integrity of the cornea. Results of keratomileusis for hyperopia showed that corneal ectasia occurs with thinning of the cornea below 200 microns. The comprehensive refractive surgery (CRS) study used 250 microns as a lower limit for the residual corneal bed. During the period of this study of thousands of patients, no occurrences of iatrogenic corneal ectasia occurred. Preoperative pachymetry for surgical planning becomes a requirement in all patients treated with larger optical zones.

Table 27-1

LADARVision Ablation Depths

OPTICAL ZONE SIZE	MICRONS REMOVED PER DIOPTER
6.0 mm	12 microns
6.5 mm	14 microns
7.0 mm	17 microns
7.5 mm	20 microns
8.0 mm	24 microns

Intraoperative pachymetry or microkeratomes producing measured and reproducible flap thickness allow the surgeon to reliably predict residual stromal bed pachymetry and avoid this complication. As no reliable method to increase the thickness of the patient's cornea in myopia treatment currently exists, we are limited in our ability to widen some patients' optical zone due to this lower limit. Two methods that will allow additional residual corneal thickness are to:

1. Cut a thinner flap.
2. Adjust the ablation to use a multizone strategy that blends the periphery of the optical zone.

By cutting a thinner flap, more tissue is available in the corneal bed for ablating. However, there are risks, such as a thinner flap's greater difficulty in replacement and potential to heal without striae. Additionally, more care must be taken to relift it should an enhancement procedure be required. Using a multizone technique to blend the optical zone in the periphery may also result in less tissue removal at the expense of a decrease in the prescription change in that area and potential for an increase in nonacuity-related symptoms.[9] Future treatments such as CustomCornea wavefront measurement-based treatments might help to further reduce tissue removal with improved laser algorithms used for corneal reshaping.

THE MICROKERATOME FLAP DIAMETER AND POSITION LIMITATIONS

With 5- and 6-mm optical zone laser treatments, the size and position of the keratectomy bed were not typically limiting to the treatment. The Chiron Automated Corneal Shaper (Claremont, Calif) was the predominant microkeratome in use in the United States during the first years of the excimer lasers' FDA approval, and flap sizes greater than 7 mm were generally able to be obtained in all but the flattest eyes. As the flap does not have refractive significance, it could be decentered slightly toward the hinge to allow treatment without ablation of the hinge. In the United States, FDA approval of excimer laser PRK treatment for hyperopia occurred in November 1998. Due to the transition zone required in a hyperopic ablation, surgeons were now ablating out to 9.0 mm diameters on the corneal surface. As surgeons used these hyperopic algorithms for hyperopic LASIK treatments, there was a need for new microkeratomes that could reliably produce flaps > 9.0 mm. Microkeratomes such as the Summit-Krumeich-Barraquer microkeratome, the Moria LSK One, and Carriazo Barraquer, and the Bausch & Lomb Hansatome became available with multiple suction rings, allowing the creation of larger flaps.

The relationship of the suction ring to flap size is illustrated in Table 27-2.

In general, each of these three items is related to the fact that when there is more corneal tissue exposed to the cutting plane of the microkeratome, the corneal flap will be larger.

The size of the flap that can be produced is not the only problem the surgeon must contend with when attempting to treat larger optical zones. Another microkeratome-related issue is the surgeon's ability to position the flap in the correct position on the cornea in order to have the greatest amount of stromal bed centered in the treatment area. Here, the use of an adjustable reticule can help the surgeon align the suction ring in the proper position—slightly decentered toward the hinge prior to engaging suction. An example is the Alcon Summit Autonomous LADARVision (yellow cross-hatched area in Figure 27-4), showing the position and size of the area to be treated projected on the cornea.

Table 27-2		
LASIK Flap Diameter		
	LARGER DIAMETER FLAP ASSOCIATED WITH:	*SMALLER DIAMETER FLAP ASSOCIATED WITH:*
Corneal diameter	Smaller corneal diameter	Larger corneal diameter
Corneal curvature	Steeper corneal curvature	Flatter corneal curvature
Suction ring axial height	Thinner or shorter ring height	Thicker or taller ring height

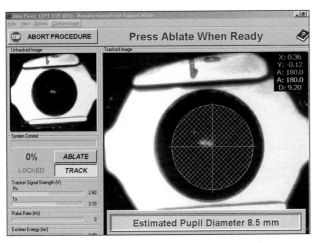

Figure 27-4. The treatment zone image from the LADARVision system.

The fit of the suction ring to the globe, as well as the speed with which it attains suction, are two factors that will help to reduce suction ring drift and subsequent malposition of the suction ring and flap produced. The applanation window of the Summit-Krumeich-Barraquer microkeratome further confirms the proper centration of the expected stromal bed prior to the keratectomy.

The ability to adjust the thickness of the resulting flap, as discussed previously when residual stromal bed pachymetry is an issue, should factor into the surgeon's decision-making process when choosing a microkeratome. The microkeratomes that were used for automated lamellar keratomileusis, such as the Chiron Automated Corneal Shaper, were available with an adjustable plate that determined flap thickness. If a plate was not placed into the microkeratome or was positioned incorrectly, perforation into the anterior chamber of the pressurized eye could occur with severe consequences. Most current microkeratomes have a fixed depth to prevent this compli-

cation. Microkeratome manufacturers have produced new heads that will cut different flap thicknesses, such as the Moria 130 and 150 heads, and the Hansatome 160 and 180 heads. Alcon Summit Autonomous is developing a different microkeratome blade to use in their existing SKBM head to allow the surgeon to produce different thickness flap sizes without the expense of a totally new head.

Strategies to avoid having the hinge limit the ability to ablate a larger optical zone include decentering the flap toward the hinge or changing the orientation of the hinge depending on the ablation desired.

It is also important to remember that the hinge will decrease the diameter of the flap perpendicular to it. The effect is to diminish the size of the ablation zone. Strategies to avoid having the hinge limit the ability to ablate a larger optical zone include decentering the flap toward the hinge or changing the orientation of the hinge depending on the ablation desired. With-the-rule astigmatism typically produces an oval-shaped ablation with the minor axis in the vertical position. Against-the-rule astigmatism will produce an oval with the minor axis in the horizontal position. The use of a superior hinge for with-the-rule astigmatism and a nasal hinge for against-the-rule astigmatism can also limit the possibility that the hinge will be in the ablation area.

As indicated in Figure 27-5, the Alcon Summit Autonomous LADARVision system uses a mask feature for treatment of larger optical zones.

This square or arc-shaped area (red) is able to be positioned over the hinge when it lies within the treatment zone (yellow) by the laser system operator prior to the start of the ablation on the tracked image. It is a software guard that will prevent the laser from firing pulses in that area, thereby preventing ablation

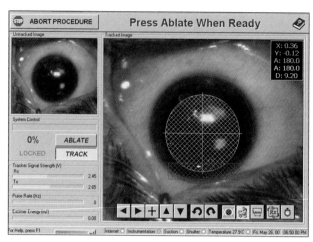

Figure 27-5. The mask feature on the LADARVision system.

Table 27-3
Nomogram Adjustment for Optical Zone Increases*

6 to 6.9 mm	No additional nomogram adjustment
7 to 7.9 mm	Additional 2% nomogram reduction
8 mm or greater	Additional 5% nomogram reduction

*Found to be required by the author. Similar adjustments have been noted by others using other lasers. (MacRae, ARVO, 1999).

of the underside of the flap at the hinge. Other options include mechanically masking the flap with an instrument or cellulose sponge. Ideally, one could prevent inadvertent hinge treatment by a customized ablation design.

ABLATION TREATMENT TIME

With a larger volume of tissue needing to be removed to create the corneal profile change over a larger corneal area, treatment times increase. The state of hydration of the corneal stroma continues to decrease as the time of exposure increases. With this relatively drier cornea, the excimer laser removes more stromal tissue per pulse. Due to this dryness, as we increase the optical zone size, nomogram adjustments are typically required. Table 27-3 demonstrates the nomogram adjustment plan of one of the authors (BDS). The other author uses a greater, more conservative nomogram adjustment of 3% to 5% reduction of the spherical equivalent refraction for each 0.5 mm increase in zone size, up to 15%. An individual surgeon should use this beginning information to develop his or her own nomogram adjustment.

LASER LIMITATIONS

The first excimer lasers used for refractive surgery were broadbeam lasers. The initial beam from all excimer lasers is gaussian in its energy distribution, with a greater amount of energy centrally. In order to allow these broadbeam lasers to be used for precise reshaping of the cornea, the beam must be homogenized, producing a beam profile that distributes the energy evenly.[10] These lasers require a large amount of laser energy and therefore more argon fluoride gas to produce a beam that will cover the full area of the ablation, thus lowering the repetition rate of the laser. This beam is then sent through an aperture to modify its shape or size, which will affect the desired optical result. Current broadbeam lasers available in the United States are only recently capable of increasing the optical zone diameter of up to 6.5 mm for myopic corrections. With astigmatism, this size may be reduced to as low as 5 mm. With the advent of small spot scanning lasers such as Bausch & Lomb, Nidek, Lasersight, and the Alcon Summit Autonomous LADARVision system, optical zones as large as 8 mm with treatment zones up to 10 mm are capable of being produced. Here, the laser produces a small (1.0 to 0.8 mm) diameter spot that does not require optical homogenization. It is then positioned on the surface of the eye by small servomirrors that can direct the beam further into the periphery of the cornea than had previously been possible.

THE MEASUREMENT OF PUPIL SIZE

The measurement of the patient's scotopic pupil size is the starting point for determining if the patient is at risk for nonacuity-based complaints from standard optical zone excimer laser surgery. Customization of the optical zone size to that of the scotopic pupil size or 1 mm larger can reduce these

> The measurement of the patient's scotopic pupil size is the starting point for determining if the patient is at risk for nonacuity-based complaints from standard optical zone excimer laser surgery.

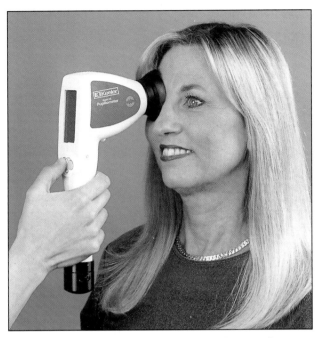

Figure 27-6a. Clinical use of the Keeler Pupilscan II pupillometer.

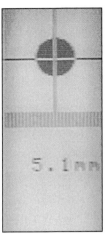

Figure 27-6b. Automatic measurement reading to the nearest tenth of a millimeter with the Keeler Pupilscan II.

risks. Customization of the ablation optical zone size based on scotopic pupil size can also minimize unnecessary tissue removal and increase the treatment range. Conservation of tissue by reducing the ablation optical zone size in older individuals may increase the range of treatment available without exceeding ablation depth limitations (personal communication, Scott M. MacRae, 1999). This is discussed further in Chapter Eight. Accuracy in these measurements is dependent on the ability to adequately visualize the pupil in order to measure it, but at the same time not cause the pupil to constrict by reaction to visible light or accommodation. Methods available for pupil size determination range are numerous, as noted below. Originally, many patients were measured with standard pupil size measurement cards in mesopic conditions. This method was limited to 1- mm steps and adequate lighting for the observer to see the pupil card was necessary. Measurement using the reticule from the slit lamp with a thin cobalt blue light in a dark room is one method of scotopic pupil measurement. This method, however, is dependent on the observer's skill in thinning the light down and observing for maximum physiologic pupillary dilation. The Oasis Colvard pupillometer uses night vision technology to visualize the pupil in darkness. With this instrument, the observer must line up the measuring reti-

cule to determine the pupil's size. Reticule marks in millimeter increments limit this instrument's ability to accurately measure the pupil to tenths of a millimeter.

Keeler's Pupilscan II model 12A (Figures 27-6a and b) uses multiple infrared diodes to measure the pupil under scotopic conditions and automatically provides the measurement reading to the nearest tenth of a millimeter without the need for subjective interpretation.

ENLARGED ABLATION OPTICAL ZONE STUDY

Do larger ablation optical zone treatments customized for scotopic pupil size really result in better patient satisfaction and less glare? This was the simple question we asked when the larger treatment zones became available in October 1999. Prior to that time, only wavefront data and ray tracing with different treatment zone sizes seemed to confirm this as true. Since previously we were unable to treat these larger optical zones, no valid answer was known. During the next 3 months at the New York Eye and Ear Infirmary's Vision Correction Center, patients with large scotopic pupil sizes were recruited for LASIK treatment with large optical zones. The purpose of this study was to answer that question.

Methods

Entry Criteria

Four major criteria were used for patients to be enrolled in this study. First, the scotopic entrance pupil had to be ≥ 6.0 mm. The patient's pachymetry needed to be sufficient to allow for the larger zone's ablation depth and allow for at least 280 microns of residual stromal thickness should the patient need further laser ablation enhancement. The corneal diameter and curvature needed to be sufficient to predictably allow for an adequate flap size and position. Lastly, the eyes were targeted for distance correction, and monovision near eyes were not included in the data.

Preoperative Testing and Treatment

Preoperative measurements were manifest and cycloplegic refraction, scotopic pupil size, ultrasonic pachymetry, topography, keratometry, and corneal diameter. The patient's informed consent was obtained. Minor axis optical zone diameter treatments were chosen according to the predicted flap diameter and residual pachymetry, and ranged from equal to the scotopic pupil size to 1 mm larger. The Moria LSK One or Bausch & Lomb Hansatome microkeratome was used, depending on the desired corneal flap diameter and thickness required.

A total of 274 eyes of 163 patients underwent correction with the LADARVision excimer laser using the available Geneva version software to allow for optical zone treatment sizes up to 8.0 mm and transition zone sizes up to 10.0 mm in diameter. The mean spherical correction of the patients treated was –2.59 diopters (D) (range: 0.00 to –5.00 D). The mean cylindrical correction of the patients treated was –1.10 D (range: 0.00 to –4.00 D). The minimum postoperative follow-up was 3 months.

Results

Postoperative topographic analysis of these patients typically showed large diameter central corneal flattening (Figure 27-7).

Patients who achieved 20/15 or better uncorrected visual acuity without enhancement totaled 11.3%. Patients who achieved 20/20 or better uncorrected visual acuity without enhancement totaled 86.1%. The percentage of patients' eyes that had uncorrected visual acuity of 20/40 or better was 98.5%. No patients lost two or more lines of visual acuity. Patients were questioned about their night vision at the 1-week and 3-month postoperative visits. The percentage of patients who reported an improvement in night vision as compared to preoperatively with glasses or contact lenses was 23.3%. Although no patients reported debilitating nonacuity-related night vision symptoms and patient satisfaction levels

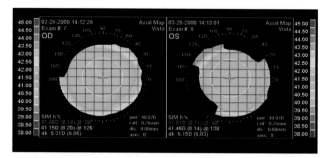

Figure 27-7. Topography of large zone treatment.

> The percentage of patients who reported an improvement in night vision as compared to preoperatively with glasses or contact lenses was 23.3%.

were high, 3.7% of patients enrolled reported an increase in night vision nonacuity-related symptoms.

CONCLUSION

Customizing the laser treatment to the scotopic pupil size or larger with the LADARVision system excimer laser in patients with pupil sizes ≥ 6.0 mm resulted in minimal subjective glare. The need to measure patients' scotopic pupil size and customize the ablation optical zone treatment size are important factors in reducing subjective reports of nonacuity-related night vision problems.

REFERENCES

1. Barraquer JI. Queratoplastia refractiva. *Estudios Inform.* 1949;10:2-21.

2. Barraquer JI. Keratomileusis for the correction of myopia. *Arch Soc Am Oftal Optom.* 1964;5:27-48.

3. Trokel SL. Srinivasan R, Braren B. Excimer laser surgery of the cornea. *Am J Ophthalmol.* 1983;96:710-715.

4. Cotliar AM, Schubert HD, Mandel ER, Trokel SL. Excimer laser radial keratotomy. *Ophthalmology.* 1985;92:206-208.

5. O'Brart DPS, et al. The effects of ablation diameter on the outcome of excimer laser photorefractive keratectomy: a prospective, randomized double-blind study. *Arch Ophthalmol.* 1995;113:438-443.

6. O'Brart DPS, Lohmann CP, Fitzke FW, et al. Disturbances in night vision after excimer laser photorefractive keratectomy. *Eye.* 1994;8:46-51.

7. Della Russo J. Night glare and excimer laser ablation diameter. *J Cataract Refract Surg.* 1993;19:565.

8. Munnerlyn CR, Koons SJ, Marshall J. Photorefractive keratectomy: a technique for laser refractive surgery. *J Cataract Refract Surg.* 1988;14:46-52.

9. Krueger RR, et al. Clinical analysis of excimer laser photorefractive keratectomy using a multiple zone technique for severe myopia. *Am J Ophthalmol.* 1995;119:263-274.

10. Mandel E, Krueger R, Puliafito C, Steinert R. Excimer laser large area ablation of the cornea. *Invest Ophthalmol Vis Sci.* 1987;28(Suppl):275.

Chapter Twenty-Eight

Cross Cylinder Ablation

Paolo Vinciguerra, MD
Fabrizio I. Camesasca, MD

Regression, corneal haze, and functional symptoms secondary to optical aberrations are possible complications of astigmatism correction with the excimer laser, either using photorefractive keratectomy (PRK) or laser-assisted in situ keratomileusis (LASIK). The main cause of these complications lies in the great dioptric gradient induced by the commonly used ablation strategies in the transition area along the steepest topographical meridian (Figure 28-1).[1,2]

Such a relevant dioptric gradient located in a small topographic area appears to cause midperipheral corneal multifocality inducing glare, night halos, and reduced contrast sensitivity. A sharp change in curvature of the corneal surface may stimulate cell-mediated regression and haze after PRK, as well as regression, visual acuity loss, and striae after LASIK.

TREATMENT FOR ASTIGMATISM AND POSTOPERATIVE CORNEAL SHAPE

It is well known that regular astigmatism is characterized by the presence of two "main" orthogonal meridians, the steepest and the flattest meridians. We are less prone to remember that countless meridians with decreasing curvatures from the steepest to the flattest are interposed between these two main meridians (Figure 28-2).

The presently available techniques for the correction of myopic astigmatism are adequate on the

> A standard ablation appears to be adequate on the steepest meridian but actually overcorrects the oblique ones, leading to a hyperopic shift.

steepest meridian but create overcorrection on the oblique meridians, which have a lower dioptric power. For example, if we treat for 5 diopters (D) of cylindrical ablation with an ablation optical zone (OZ) of 5 mm, we plan 30 microns ablation on 126-degree axis. The real ablation is instead 40 microns, with an overcorrection of 10 microns. A standard ablation appears to be adequate on the steepest meridian but actually overcorrects the oblique ones, leading to a hyperopic shift. A spherical overcorrection of $\geq$ 20% with an irregular "four-leaf" astigmatism on the oblique meridian occurs (Table 28-1 and Figures 28-3 and 28-4).

Perfect ablation for myopic astigmatism should completely correct the steepest meridian as well as the oblique ones in proportion to their curvatures. The flattest meridian should remain unchanged. In order to avoid regression, a dioptrically progressive corneal shape is determined.

Epithelial layering follows a superficial tension law.[3] When it meets irregular surfaces, corneal epithelium becomes thicker in order to fill gaps. A thicker epithelium induces scar tissue formation underneath. Therefore, corneal irregularities are partially compensated by deposition of scar tissue. This mechanism, unfortunately, leads to regression of an

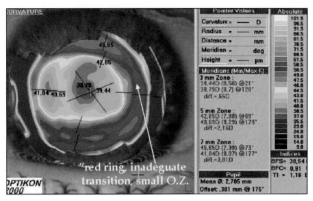

Figure 28-1. Inadequate transition on the steep meridian postoperatively.

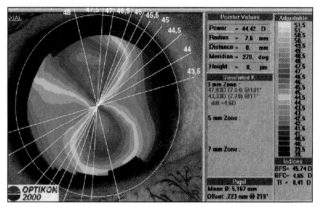

Figure 28-2. Progressive change in dioptric power of the astigmatism from one axis to the other.

Table 28-1

Myopic Cylindrical Ablation

Axis	Theoretic Ablation (Microns)	Real Ablation (Microns)	Resulting Overcorrection (D)
90	50	50	0
108	40	47.5	+0.75
126	30	40	+1
144	20	29	+0.9
162	10	15.5	+0.55
180	0	0	0

imparted correction.[4] Corneal scarring and epithelial thickening can also lead to midperipheral flattening. In order to avoid regression and visual acuity decrease, a regular and progressive change of corneal curvature is mandatory.

It is commonly thought that a large ablation diameter (ie, 6.5 mm) is not associated with regression, while a small ablation diameter (ie, 4 mm) is. This is not completely true: by studying topographical maps, we notice that with large ablations we have changes of the ablation edge due to scar tissue formation and/or epithelial hyperplasia. Changes take place at the edge of the ablation and far from the pupillary area, thus the OZ remains homogeneous and patients are asymptomatic. In small ablations, on the contrary, OZ edge modifications are within the pupillary area, thus the OZ becomes nonhomogenous with multifocality and optical aberration. Patients note night halos, visual loss, and glare. Regression leads to a new myopic astigmatism on

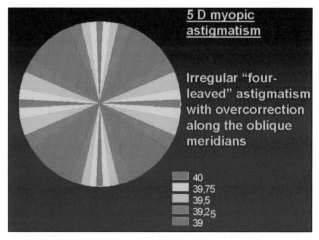

Figure 28-3. Outcome of 5 D myopic astigmatism correction causing overcorrection along the oblique meridians.

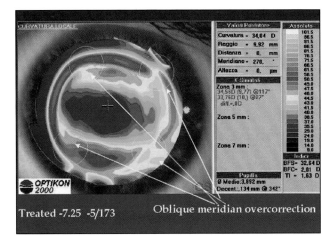

Figure 28-4. A practical example of the theoretical pattern presented in Figure 28-3. Note the oblique meridian overcorrection.

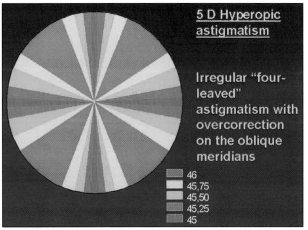

Figure 28-5. Outcome of 5 D hyperopic astigmatism correction causing overcorrection along the oblique meridians.

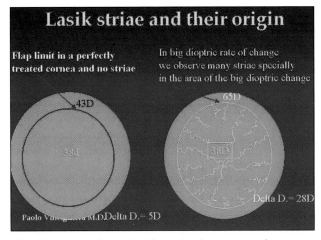

Figure 28-6. When the dioptric change rate between the corneal center and periphery is relevant and the curvature is not progressively changing, the flap cannot adequately follow the changes in curvature, thus striae may occur.

the steepest meridian and a positive spherical equivalent because of hypercorrection on the oblique meridian. Eventually, we will have a mixed astigmatism, which is more difficult to retreat.

Exactly the opposite situation can be observed in the correction of hypermetropic astigmatism. There is an overcorrection on the oblique meridians: when regression takes place we will have a mixed astigmatism (Figure 28-5).

Epithelium hyperplasia covering corneal irregularities may lead to regression after LASIK.[5] The surgeon can eliminate regression by scraping hyperplastic epithelium, but as weeks go by the epithelium grows again, following the superficial tension law.

Regression leads to a new myopic astigmatism on the steepest meridian and a positive spherical equivalent because of hypercorrection on the oblique meridian.

Striae formation after LASIK represents another example of the importance of a regular corneal surface. After excimer ablation, striae occur when there is a great dioptric gradient between the OZ and the peripheral "red ring" (see Figure 28-1), evidenced by topography.[6,7] Curvature variation from a flat to steep cornea is remarkable and reversed with respect to the physiological corneal curvature. The flap cannot lie evenly on this irregular stromal surface (Figure 28-6), and striae will occur.

Maintaining a physiologically prolate cornea after excimer ablation (avoiding creation of an oblate cornea) is the goal of the refractive surgeon. The excimer laser performs a toric ablation by the movement of two parallel blades progressively away one from the other.

The flattest meridian, parallel to the blades, does not change its curvature because it is homogeneously ablated. The steepest meridian—orthogonal to the blades—is flattened, receiving an ablation maximal at the corneal center and decreasing in the periphery.

Similar to myopic astigmatism, hyperopic astigmatism is corrected with the ablation of two adjacent concave cylinders. In this way, within the pupillary area, a "positive" cylinder is created. Hyperopic astigmatism ablation aims to increase steepness on the flatter meridian while minimizing treatment of the steepest one. Following the same reasons discussed for myopic astigmatism, in this case the end

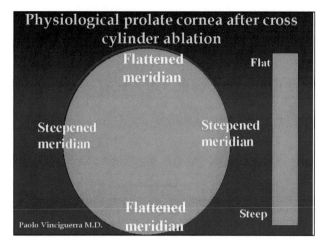

Figure 28-7. Overlap of cross cylinders leads to a prolate, physiologically aspherical cornea in myopic, hyperopic, or mixed astigmatism.

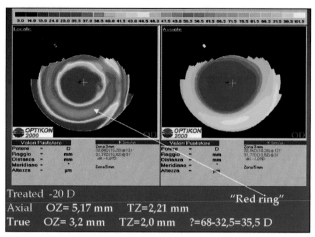

Figure 28-8. The "red ring" is the expression of a non-constant change in midperipheral curvature.

> Hyperopic astigmatism ablation aims to increase steepness on the flatter meridian while minimizing treatment of the steepest one.

result is also an irregular "four-leaf" astigmatism with overcorrection along the oblique meridians and a myopic shift (see Figure 28-5). The aberration induced by the myopic and the hyperopic astigmatism ablation are diametrically opposed and almost perfectly symmetric. It is important to remark how overlap of cross-cylinders leads to a prolate, physiologically aspherical cornea either in myopic, hyperopic, or mixed astigmatism (Figure 28-7).

OPTICAL ZONE SHAPE—SPLITTING TECHNIQUE

Commonly, topographic maps after excimer ablation show in local scale, a blue area in the center of the effective optical zone and a red ring in midperiphery, representing a hypercurvature on the ablation edge. A normal myopic excimer ablation with a single ablation optical zone and a small transition area increases the midperipheral curvature, creating the typical topographic "red ring." This is an oblate cornea (Figure 28-8).

It is important to notice how a 5-mm ablation optical zone treatment does not correspond to a real 5-mm effective optical zone on the topographic map because the OZ edge is included in red ring. We usually obtain a different effective optical zone than the programmed ablation area (see Figure 28-8). High myopia with small programmed ablation areas will have a "red ring" close to the pupillary area, so these patients complain of night halos, loss of vision quality due to multifocality, and optical aberration.

In order to avoid this midperipheral hypercurvature, myopia correction requires the application of several optical zones. This necessity to achieve a more continuous-shaped transition zone (TZ) has led to development of solutions such as the multiple zone technique.[8] This technique implies a constant dioptric gradient for each ablation optical zone, not a constant ablation depth.

The splitting technique consists of dividing the entire spherical and cylindrical myopic ametropia in optical zones that are dioptrically constant (Table 28-2).[9] We program seven or eight ablation optical zones in high myopia. Every ablation optical zone corrects the same amount of spherical diopters, as well as the same amount of cylindrical defect. The first ablation optical zone is the largest one, and the others are progressively smaller. There is a progressive dioptric gradient from the center to the periphery of the ablated area. We recommend remaining within a maximum of 3 D and a minimum of 0.50 D of correction for each ablation optical zone.

The splitting technique avoids creation of a topographical "red ring" in the midperiphery zones and

> The splitting technique avoids creation of a topographical "red ring" in the midperiphery zones and therefore leads to effective optical zones larger than planned ablation areas.

		Table 28-2			
		Ablation Strategy for Case 1*			
ZONE	SPHERE (D)	CYLINDER (D)	AXIS	OPTICAL ZONE DIAMETER (MM)	TRANSITION ZONE DIAMETER (MM)
1	—	+2	70	5.5	9
2	-1.50	-0.50	160	6.5	8.5
3	-1.50	-0.50	160	6	8
4	-1.50	-0.50	160	5.5	7.5
5	-1.50	-0.50	160	5	7
6	-1.50	—	—	4.5	6.5
7	-1.50	—	—	4	6

*Preoperative refraction -7 D sph -4 D cyl (160°)

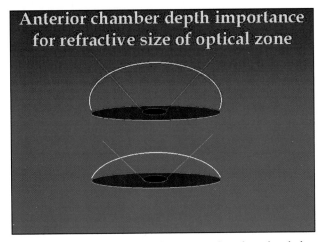

Figure 28-9. Importance of anterior chamber depth for the refractive size of the optical zone.

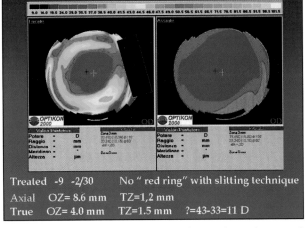

Figure 28-10. Hypercurvature in the midperiphery and "red ring" are prevented when the splitting technique is adopted.

therefore leads to effective optical zones larger than planned ablation areas. With this method, a relatively small programmed ablation area corresponds to a larger refractive effective optical zone, visible with topography and an axial algorithm (see Table 28-2).

Such a strategy has an important application in LASIK in order to avoid striae as well as glare. Effective optical zone diameter is also related to anterior chamber depth. We should program larger optical areas for eyes with deeper anterior chambers, because their refractive effective optical zone will be smaller than the planned ablation zone if not performed following our algorithm (Figure 28-9).

Creation of hypercurvature in the midperiphery is

therefore prevented (Figure 28-10). A homogeneously ablated area without a red ring can be observed on topographic maps. The axial map in Figure 28-11 shows an enlargement of the ablated area.

THE CROSS CYLINDER TECHNIQUE

Mixed astigmatism correction with two cylinder ablations of the same power and opposite signs creates a perfectly spherical OZ without modification of the spherical equivalent.

Therefore, our proposal is to correct myopic, hyperopic, and mixed astigmatism with two cross

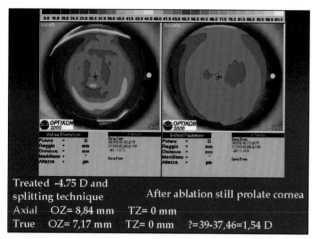

Treated -4.75 D and
splitting technique   After ablation still prolate cornea

Axial   OZ= 8,84 mm   TZ= 0 mm
True   OZ= 7,17 mm   TZ= 0 mm   ?=39-37,46=1,54 D

Figure 28-11. After ablation using the splitting technique, the cornea remains prolate. The axial map on the right shows an enlargement of the effective optical zone.

cylinder ablations (myopic and hyperopic), then correct the spherical equivalent (the sum of the spherical power and half the cylinder power).

We applied the following ablation strategy:

- Ablation of 50% of the cylinder power along the steepest meridian with 5.5-mm OZ size and 9-mm TZ size. Ablation of the remaining 50% cylinder power along the flattest meridian with OZ size split following the above-mentioned criteria. Correction of the whole spherical equivalent with an OZ size from 6.5 to 4 mm and a TZ obtained by adding 2 mm to those: from 8.5 to 6 mm.

- When the spherical equivalent is myopic, we apply the splitting technique. The total amount of negative spherical and cylindrical ablation is divided into subsequent steps with optical zones of decreasing diameters. The goal is to create a more regular dioptric gradient from the ablated area to the periphery (see Figure 28-11). The laser energy used was 120 mJ and an ablation rate of 40 Hz with a Nidek EC-5000.

CASE EXAMPLES

Case 1. Sparing tissue in a 6 D astigmatism

Usual technique: With 6.5-mm OZ and 9-mm TZ, 164 microns with an unwanted induced correction of a 2.2 D of myopia. Cross cylinder technique with 6.5-mm OZ and 9-mm TZ 62 microns in center and 34 microns in the periphery without any unwanted induced spherical correction.

Our proposal is to correct myopic, hyperopic, and mixed astigmatism with two cross cylinder ablations (myopic and hyperopic), then correct the spherical equivalent (the sum of the spherical power and half the cylinder power).

Case 2. Preoperative refraction: +1.00 D sph –4.00 D cyl (165 degrees)

Cross cylinder calculation—step 1: +2.00 D cyl (75 degrees); step 2: at -2.00 D cyl (165 degrees); step 3 at -1.00 D sph (SE) (apply splitting technique on these values).

Case 3. Preoperative refraction: +3.00 D sph –6.00 D cyl (90 degrees)

Cross-cylinder calculation—step 1: +3.00 D cyl (180 degrees); step 2: at -3.00 D cyl (90 degrees); step 3: at no SE treatment needed (apply splitting technique on these values).

Correction of the astigmatism with two cylinder ablations of equal power but opposite signs does not affect the initial spherical equivalent. Correction of the spherical equivalent must be calculated and applied thereafter.

We treat 50% of the amount of cylinder on the steepest meridian and the other 50% on the flattest meridian in order to achieve a regular and symmetrical postoperative corneal morphology. Some authors suggest different amounts of splitting between the plus and minus cylinder ablations that are related to the amount of spherical and cylindrical refractive error.[10] This was a new concept but when compared to our method, we think that it lacks in repeatability because the ablation pattern has to be different for every patient.

Moreover, with this approach and an optical point of view, the ideal symmetrical prolate physiological corneal shape cannot be achieved. We suggest splitting the cylinder symmetrically in order to avoid asymmetrical corneal shapes (Figure 28-12).

PERSONAL EXPERIENCE WITH MYOPIC ASTIGMATISM CORRECTION

We treated 44 eyes of 30 patients ranging in age from 24 to 56 years (mean age: 34.3 ± 9.3 years) with the cross-cylinder technique.

Inclusion criteria were no ocular pathology, no previous ocular surgery, and at least 1 year of refractive stability (0.50 D or less of change). An informed consent was obtained from all patients.

Table 28-3
Ablation Strategy for Case 2*

Zone	Sphere (D)	Cylinder (D)	Axis	Optical Zone Diameter (mm)	Transition Zone Diameter (mm)
1	—	+2.50	90	5.5	9
2	-1.75	-0.50	180	6.5	8.5
3	-1.75	-0.50	180	6	8
4	-1.75	-0.50	180	5.5	7.5
5	-1.75	-0.50	180	5	7
6	-1.75	-0.50	180	4.5	6.5
7	-1.75	—	—	4	6

*Preoperative refraction -8 D sph -5 D cyl (180°)

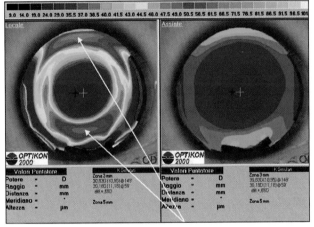

Figure 28-12. Commonly used ablation: remaining astigmatism may cause optical aberration when the pupil dilates.

The preoperative visit included uncorrected visual acuity (UCVA) and spectacle best-corrected visual acuity (SBCVA) measurement, cycloplegic refraction, videokeratography (CSO, Florence, Italy), complete anterior and posterior segment slit lamp examination, tonometry, and ultrasonic pachymetry (Mentor-Biorad Pach-Pen XL, Norwall, Mass).

Postoperative follow-up was performed daily until the epithelium healed, at day 7, and then at months 1, 2, 3, and 6. Beginning with day 7, each postoperative examination included documentation of UCVA, SBCVA, cycloplegic refraction, videokeratography, and slit lamp examination. Preoperative refraction data are reported in Table 28-4.

We used a Nidek EC-5000 excimer laser with 193-nm wavelength, 0.76 (micrometers/scan pulse) ablation rate during the myopic ablation and 0.63 during the hyperopic ablation, with 40 and 46 Hz frequency respectively, and 108 to 120 mJ/mm² energy. Active eye tracker and manual eye fixation devices were used. Follow-up was for 6 months. The data were collected with a standardized form and analyzed with a statistical program (Systat 5.01 for Windows, Systat Inc, Evanston, Ill) using a paired student's t-test ($p < 0.05$).

Postoperatively, mean UCVA improved from a preoperative value of 0.13 ± 0.2 to 0.6 ± 0.18 (p = 0.0003) at 6 months. Mean BSCVA passed from 0.75 ± 0.22 preoperatively to 0.74 ± 0.28 (p = 0.25) at 1 week after surgery to 0.8 ± 0.16 (p = 0.007) at 1 month, and to 0.86 ± 0.13 at 6 months (p = 0.001).

No eye lost two or more lines of BSCVA at the end of the follow-up, and only two eyes (9.1%) lost one line, both due to an incorrect laser setting. These eyes, with cylinder of -1.50 D, showed an axial shift of 10 and 20 degrees, respectively. Seven eyes gained two or three lines of BSCVA (31.8%) and four gained one line (18.2%). Refractive data at 6 months are reported in Table 28-5. All refractive data were statistically significant when compared to the preoperative status.

Conclusion

Visual quality is the main objective of excimer surgery, not just emmetropia. The multizone cross cylin-

Table 28-4

Preoperative Refraction

	MEAN	STANDARD DEVIATION	RANGE
Sphere (D)	-2.3	± 5.0	-12 to +3.5
Cyl (D)	-3.6	± 1.5	-1.5 to -6
Spherical equivalent (D)	-4.5	± 4.9	-13 to 1.5

Table 28-5

Final (6-Month) Refraction

	MEAN	STANDARD DEVIATION	RANGE	P
Sphere (D)	0.15	± 0.54	-0.50 to +1.00	<.0016
Cyl (D)	-0.44	± 0.36	-1.50 to +0.75	< .001
Spherical equivalent (D)	-0.07	± 0.87		< .001

der method creates a progressive transition with a low dioptric gradient between the treated and untreated cornea. When an astigmatic defect is treated, this method maintains a postoperative physiologically prolate cornea (Figure 28-13).

The spherical amount of correction is obtained by treating first the cylinder and then the spherical equivalent with the splitting technique. With the common previously used ablation strategies, postoperative topography shows an abrupt dioptric shift along the steepest meridian, while after a cross-cylinder ablation the cornea is physiologically aspherical on the whole surface.

Advantages of cross cylinder technique are:
1. Physiologically prolate symmetric corneal shape
2. Less regression
3. Better visual quality
4. Tissue sparing by splitting part of the cylinder ablation in the periphery (especially useful in LASIK)

The most important factor for a successful refractive treatment is a proper topographic study of the cornea. The splitting technique leads to a spherical and more physiological corneal surface, so the quality of patient vision is better. This kind of ablation strategy proved to be accurate and safe, with no eyes losing two or more SBCVA lines and no patient complaining of functional symptoms like halos or night glare.

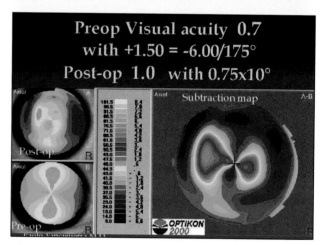

Figure 28-13. Treating an astigmatic defect with this method allows a postoperative physiologically prolate cornea. In this case, this generated a better postoperative visual acuity.

REFERENCES

1. Vinciguerra P, Sborgia M, Epstein D, Azzolini M, MacRae S. Photorefractive keratectomy to correct myopic or hyperopic astigmatism with a cross-cylinder ablation. *J Refract Surg*. 1999;15(Suppl):S183-S185.

2. Danasoury MA, Waring GO, el-Maghraby A, Mehrez K. Excimer laser in situ keratomileusis to correct compound myopic astigmatism. *J Refract Surg*. 1999;13:511-520.

3. Dierick HG, Missotten L. Is the corneal contour influenced by a tension in the superficial epithelial cells? *Refract Corneal Surg.* 1992;8:54-9.

4. Krueger RR, Binder PS, McDonnell PJ. The effects of excimer laser photoablation on the cornea. In: JJ Salz, PJ McDonnell, MB McDonald, eds. *Corneal Laser Surgery.* St. Louis, Mo: Mosby; 1995.

5. Güell J. Correction limits with LASIK. In: IG Pallikaris, DS Siganos, eds. *LASIK.* Thorofare, NJ: SLACK Incorporated; 1998.

6. Vinciguerra P, Azzolini M, Radice P. A new corneal analysis after excimer laser ablation: digitized retroillumination. In: IG Pallikaris, DS Siganos, eds. *LASIK.* Thorofare, NJ: SLACK Incorporated; 1998.

7. Vinciguerra P, Azzolini M, Airaghi P, Radice P, De Molfetta V. Effect of decreasing surface and interface irregularities after photorefractive keratectomy and laser in situ keratomileusis on optical and functional results. *J Refract Surg.* 1998;14:S199-S203.

8. Piovella M, Camesasca FI, Fattori C. Excimer laser photorefractive keratectomy for high myopia. Four-year experience with a multiple zone technique. *Ophthalmology.* 1997;104:1554-1565.

9. Vinciguerra P. The correction of astigmatism with a cross-cylinder ablation. In: L Buratto, S Brint, eds. *LASIK: Surgical Techniques and Complications.* 2nd ed. Thorofare, NJ: SLACK Incorporated; 2000.

10. Chayet AS, Magallanes R, Montes M, Chavez S, Robledo N. Laser in situ keratomileusis for simple myopic, mixed, and simple hyperopic astigmatism. *J Refract Surg.* 1998;14:S175-S176.

Chapter Twenty-Nine

Bitoric Ablation for the Treatment of Simple Myopic and Mixed Astigmatism

Arturo S. Chayet, MD

Since its clinical introduction in 1988, the excimer laser keratorefractive procedure has evolved from a central corneal ablation to treat spherical myopia to the addition of central toric ablation to selectively flatten the steep meridian, then to annular peripheral ablation to steepen the central corneal for the treatment of hyperopia. More recently, the introduction of toric paracentral ablations created a positive cylinder over the flat meridian (Figures 29-1a and 29-1b).

The initial type of ablation to treat astigmatism over the steep meridian consisted of an elliptical pattern that had the characteristic of being more selective in flattening the steep meridian but with the unplanned effect of, to some degree, flattening the flat meridian, creating a hyperopic shift on the spherical component. This toric ablation has been very effective in treating compound myopic astigmatism (Figure 29-2).

To reduce the hyperopic shift seen with the elliptical ablation, a different toric pattern was developed; this ablation profile, with a cylindrical pattern, ablates more selectively over the steep meridian and, in addition to its phototherapeutic keratectomy (PTK) profile design, allows for less hyperopic shift (Figure 29-3). This profile is still in use by many laser manufacturers (eg, Technolas 217, VisX Star) to treat simple myopic astigmatism. Our experience using this type of profile shows that the ablation pattern is too narrow; therefore, some patients complain of increased halos in scotoptic conditions. We also found a trend in cylinder undercorrection and regression, in addition to the fact that some hyperopic shift is still being induced.

Mixed astigmatism, on the other hand, has been the most difficult type of astigmatism to treat. Initial attempts consisted of using the narrow cylindrical toric profile to treat the "minus" cylinder, followed by the sequential application of the hyperopic "donut-shape" ablation to treat the "plus" sphere (Figure 29-4). Although initial positive results were published with this approach, it was basically abandoned worldwide in favor of other more advanced techniques. This approach was recently repopularized in the United States by using the so-called "double-card" approach with the VisX Star excimer laser. Our initial experience with this type of approach was far from being well accepted by our patients, and most of the time a significant undercorrection was seen in both the "positive" sphere and on the "minus" cylinder.

With the incorporation of the positive cylinder toric ablation, better results have been reported in the literature for the treatment of mixed astigmatism. Argento and coworkers, using the Bausch & Lomb Technolas 217 and converting the refraction to plus cylinder (eg, +2.00 -4.00 x 0° to –2.00 + 4.00 x 90°), treated the plus cylinder using the positive toric ablation, followed by the treatment of the minus sphere using the normal myopic ablation (Figure 29-5).

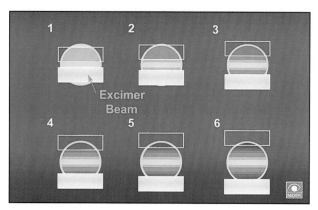

Figure 29-1a. Scanning beam of hyperopic astigmatism demonstrating scan of laser over the cornea with time. The excimer beam, shown in yellow, moves from the central cornea to the periphery as the treatment progresses. Note that the central cornea is relatively spared from treatment.

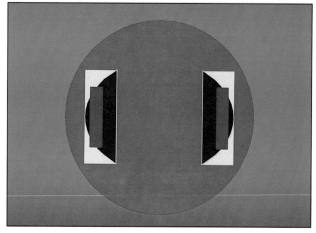

Figure 29-1b. Schematic drawing of the flat meridian ablation. The midperipheral areas at 3:00 and 9:00 are most heavily treated, as shown.

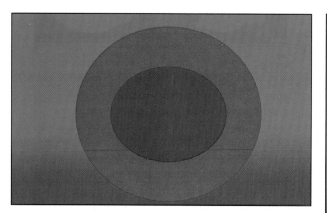

Figure 29-2. Elliptical "wide" ablation for the treatment of compound myopic astigmatism (eg, –3.00 –2.00 x 0). This ablation pattern is effective but caused a hyperopic shift.

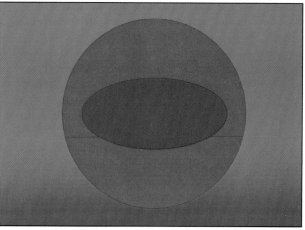

Figure 29-3. Narrow cylindrical ablation for the treatment of simple myopic astigmatism (eg, plano – 2.00 x 0). This ablation pattern tends to create a narrow effective optical zone, which may cause halos.

BITORIC ABLATION

More recently we introduced a new approach to treat mixed and simple myopic astigmatism.[1] We later named this new technique "bitoric ablation" (Figure 29-6). Ideally, when treating mixed astigmatism (spherical equivalent close to zero), it may be appropriate to flatten the steep meridian to the same extent that we steepen the flat meridian (similar to the coupling effect seen with astigmatic keratotomy). In addition, we wanted to use the "wide" elliptical ablation when treating over the steep meridian in order to achieve a larger effective optical that maintains a high quality of vision. This resulted in a formula that adjusts for the hyperopic shift, which

> We wanted to use the "wide" elliptical ablation when treating over the steep meridian in order to achieve a larger effective optical that maintains a high quality of vision.

resulted from the use of the elliptical ablation by providing the amount of cylinder to be corrected in the flat and steep meridians, respectively (Figure 29-7).

Our preliminary results with this technique were satisfactory. We subsequently conducted a clinical trial (see below) and adopted this technique as the treatment of choice for mixed and simple myopic astigmatism. As the technique evolved and other cli-

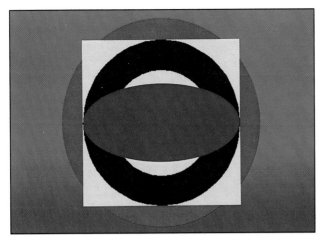

Figure 29-4. Combination of hyperopic and "narrow" cylindrical ablation for the treatment of mixed astigmatism (+2.00 –4.00 x 0). The elongated horizontal oval represents the minus cylinder treatment, and the grayish circle represents the hyperopic treatment to correct hyperopia.

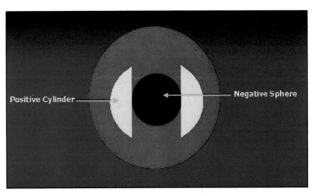

Figure 29-5. Combined use for flat meridian toric ablation and central spherical ablation for the correction of mixed astigmatism. This strategy treats the plus cylinder using the positive toric ablation, then treats the minus sphere using the normal myopic ablation.

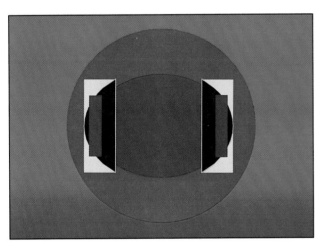

Figure 29-6. Bitoric ablation diagram demonstrating treatment of the flat meridian as represented by the grayish areas in the midperiphery at 3:00 and 9:00. The flat meridian is steepened. Note that no tissue is removed centrally with this portion of the treatment. This allows conservation of tissue. The steep meridian at 90 to 180 degrees is flattened, as represented by the dark blue oval area.

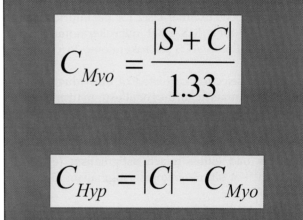

$$C_{Myo} = \frac{|S + C|}{1.33}$$

$$C_{Hyp} = |C| - C_{Myo}$$

Figure 29-7. The bitoric LASIK formula. The *C myo* (myopic cylinder machine setting) is equal to the absolute value of the sum of the preoperative sphere plus the cylinder divided by 1.33. The *C hyp* (hyperopic machine setting) is equal to the absolute value of the cylinder minus (the machine setting for the myopic cylinder setting).

nicians tried it, additional benefits were found. Vinciguerra[2,3] found that the combined use of flat and steep meridian ablation (a technique he calls "cross cylinder" ablation) not only was very effective, but was very helpful to reduce the amount of tissue removed and maintain the physiological posi-

tive asphericity of the cornea. His approach, unlike ours, is recommended for all kinds of astigmatism. He has the surgeon split, in equal proportions, the amount of cylinder to be corrected in each meridian, followed by treatment of the remaining spherical error.

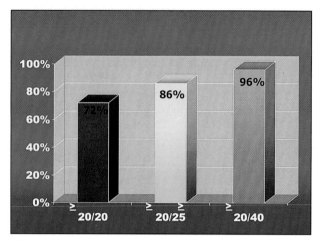

Figure 29-8. UCVA results using the bitoric ablation method.

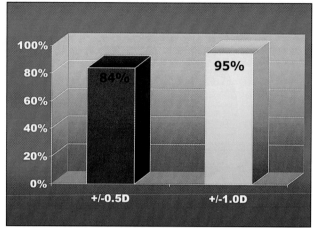

Figure 29-9. Mean percentage of cylinder correction.

SURGICAL TECHNIQUE

Our experience with bitoric excimer laser treatments is by performing bitoric LASIK. We use the Nidek EC-5000 excimer laser for the bitoric ablation and the Nidek MK-2000 microkeratome or the Bausch & Lomb ACS microkeratome to create the flap.

Patient selection consisted of individuals having regular, symmetric, orthogonal astigmatism seen on topography maps, in addition to corneas having more than 500 microns of central pachymetry without evidence of any thinner paracentral pachymetry. Patients had either mixed astigmatism (eg, +2.00 -4.00 x 0°) or simple myopic astigmatism (eg, plano -4.00 x 0°).

We use the Chayet formula to calculate the amount of cylinder to be corrected at each meridian (see Figure 29-7). We use the multistage program with the EC-5000 to sequentially treat both toric ablations.

The positive cylinder ablation is carried out first. We use the LASIK mode with the EC-5000 excimer laser, with an ablation optical zone of 5.5 mm and a transition zone of 7.5 mm. This is followed by the steep meridian cylinder ablation, also with an optical zone of 5.5 mm and a transition zone of 7.5 mm.

As shown later, the resultant correction from his approach has been found to be very stable; therefore, we have not found the need to use larger transitions zones to prevent regression of the effect.

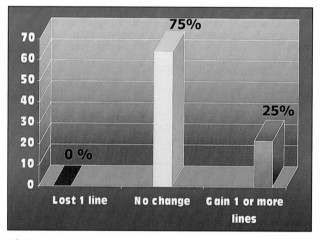

Figure 29-10. Percentage of eyes with gain or loss of BSCVA. No eyes lost one or more lines of vision.

RESULTS

Figures 29-8 through 29-11 show the results regarding uncorrected visual acuity (UCVA) (see Figure 29-8), effectiveness on cylinder correction (see Figure 29-9), changes in best spectacle-corrected visual acuity (BSCVA) (see Figure 29-10), and stability of the effect (see Figure 29-11), respectively.

As shown in these results, we are very satisfied with the results of bitoric LASIK for the treatment of simple myopic and mixed astigmatism with up to 3 years of follow-up in which 72% and 96% of the eyes achieved an UCVA of 20/20 and 20/40 or better,

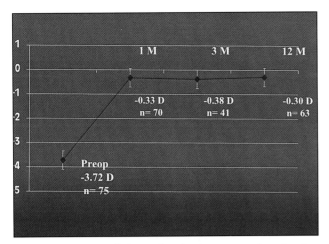

Figure 29-11. Stability of cylinder correction in the first year after surgery.

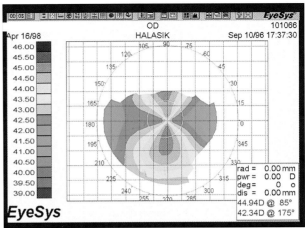

Figure 29-12a. Preoperative corneal topography of the first patient treated with bitoric LASIK. This patient had 2.5 keratometric diopters of with-the-rule astigmatism.

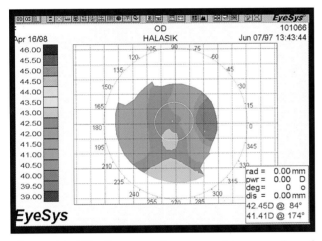

Figure 29-12b. Postoperative corneal topography of the eye shown in Figure 29-12a. There is a marked reduction in astigmatism and retention of some positive asphericity.

respectively. These results matched the percentage of eyes achieving within 0.5 D and 1.0 D of the intended cylinder correction, respectively (84% and 95%).

Possibly because of the enhanced positive asphericity resulting from this type of ablation, 25% of the eyes gained one or more lines of BSCVA.

Figures 29-12a and b show the pre- and postoperative topographies of our first patient treated with bitoric LASIK; note the excellent reduction in astigmatism, with a large effective optical zone and the simultaneous retention of the positive asphericity.

BITORIC ABLATION: A WORD OF CAUTION

Finally, I would like to stress the importance of realizing that when doing bitoric ablation, we are using two different types of cylinder correction with different signs ("minus" and "plus"). Entering the wrong axis or amount of cylinder correction can occur. We had two cases in which the axis of the positive cylinder was entered incorrectly (most often 90 degrees away). In both occasions, the amount of error was low; therefore, it was easy to correct the mistake.

FUTURE DIRECTION OF BITORIC LASIK

We are looking forward to applying the bitoric ablation technique and incorporating topography, refractive maps, and aberrometer images linked to the excimer laser. We feel that this will further increase the proportion of eyes that gain lines of best-corrected visual acuity. Meanwhile, patients and surgeons are already enjoying the benefits of bitoric LASIK for the surgical correction of mixed and simple myopic astigmatism.

REFERENCES

1. Vinciguerra P, Sborgia M, Epstein D, Azzolini M, MacRae S. Photorefractive keratectomy to correct myopic or hyperopic astigmatism with a cross-cylinder ablation. *J Refract Surg.* 1999;15(Suppl):S183-S185.

2. Vinciguerra P. The correction of astigmatism with a cross-cylinder ablation. In: L Buratto, S Brint, eds. *LASIK: Surgical Techniques and Complications.* 2nd ed. Thorofare, NJ: SLACK Incorporated; 2000.

3. Chayet AS, Magallanes R, Montes M, Chavez S, Robledo N. Laser in situ keratomileusis for simple myopic, mixed, and simple hyperopic astigmatism. *J Refract Surg.* 1998;14:S175-S176.

The Future of Customization

Chapter Thirty

The Future of Customization

Scott M. MacRae, MD
Raymond A. Applegate, OD, PhD
Ronald R. Krueger, MD, MSE

INTRODUCTION

This book is about the quest for *supervision* and the customization of ablative procedures to improve vision. In closing, we would like to address some of the challenges facing customized ablations, methods to improve outcomes, alternative strategies for achieving ideal corrections, future methods of customization, potential disadvantages of supervision, and fundamental limitations to ideal corrections.

CHALLENGES FACING CUSTOMIZED ABLATION

There are a number of challenges that need to be addressed. Wavefront sensors, as well as corneal topographic laser delivery and visual testing systems, need to be integrated and their outputs standardized to make them more time efficient and easy to use in the clinical environment. Such integration will be particularly important, if not crucial, to the investigation of the biomechanical response to therapy as well as our ability to control biomechanical responses to the patient's advantage. Each system and subcomponent needs to be optimized for quality, cost, reliability, clinical efficiency, and most importantly patient outcome. Questions include: What is the ideal laser beam profile needed to carve the ideal corneal surface? Can such a corneal profile be creat-

> There are a multitude of questions to be answered:
> 1. Can the differences in biomechanical response be predicted?
> 2. Are some aberrations necessary for proper visual function?

ed and maintained? How well do we need to track the eye? How do the biomechanical responses vary with magnitude and type of correction? To what degree are the biomechanical responses the same across individuals? Can differences in biomechanical responses be predicted? Can errors in the laser delivery system be reduced to or below the error level of the measurement system? Are some aberrations necessary for proper visual function? If so, to what extent can they be reduced without harming normal visual function? Which higher-order aberrations are the most detrimental to vision? Does PRK provide better wavefront correction than LASIK? For each patient population of interest, how good is good enough? Is it better to stage treatment to achieve an ideal wavefront correction? Do wave-guided corrections improve quality of life more than conventional treatments? Is the dream of supervision more hype than reality?

Further in our quest, it is important to remember that not all people want or desire to see perfectly. We assume that patients will benefit from supervision, but the benefit is currently unproven. Despite these challenges and unknowns, there exists many exciting opportunities to help our patients in ways that were hardly imagined a few years ago.

The questions continue in treated patients: Will supervision change with aging, and if so, how? Can these eyes be easily "tuned up" when necessary? Will the effect of cataract or progressive myopia on these patients be the same as a nontreated or conventionally treated patient? What are the long-term effects, if any?

METHODS TO IMPROVE OUTCOMES

The editors of this book believe that the future of refractive surgery is in customization of refractive surgery, with the goal of creating supervision. Customization will take many different forms in upcoming years. One objective of this chapter is to outline some of the many variations that may develop in the world of customized refractive surgery. In sharing our thoughts and beliefs, we hope to stimulate the reader to consider the possible future developments in customized refractive surgery.

Wavefront Measurement, Adaptive Optics, and Visual Simulation

Current systems use wavefront sensors to detect aberrations; however, the measurement itself (as with current autorefractors) does not include the patient's subjective preferences. One could simulate the ideal correction using adaptive optics and let the patient adjust the simulation to include the subjective preferences. Currently, state-of-the-art adaptive mirrors are very expensive (over $50,000), making them prohibitive to use in conjunction with a diagnostic wavefront sensor (see Chapter Four). Fortunately, new technologies are on the horizon that will likely bring this cost down and make it cost-effective in the clinical environment and for research. For example, Bille's group is working on adaptive optic technology, which they are calling multimicromirror-integrated active mirror matrices.[1] One of the specific goals of the technology is to show patients the desired outcome of wave-guided surgery. Other technologies are also being refined, including bimorph mirrors, membrane mirrors, and liquid crystals. For details on alternate adaptive optic technology, the reader is referred to Chapter Four, as well as Tyson[2] and Sechaud.[3]

What is unknown about technology that simulates the ideal correction is whether the patient can appreciate the full benefit without a significant adaptation period. That is, does a patient with best-corrected acuity of 20/20 prior to surgery have refractive amblyopia such that, despite a perfect retinal image, he or she will be unable to see 20/10?[4]

Ocular Anatomy

The goal of customized refractive surgery is to create the optimal ablation pattern based on the idiosyncratic anatomical needs of each eye. An -8.00 diopter (D) myope with thin corneas, a short anterior chamber depth, and small pupils may require a different treatment than an individual with the same refractive error who has thick corneas, a long anterior chamber depth, and large pupils.

Currently, there is not a preoperative whole eye scan analogous to a head MRI that would scan and screen for potential intra- or postoperative problems. Consider an individual with a high refractive error that you wish to correct with a phakic intraocular lens (IOL) followed by LASIK. Planning the surgery, as well as the surgery itself, would be improved if we could see the exact architecture of the anterior and posterior chambers, as well as the positions of all the optical elements of the eye. Such knowledge could prevent an attempted insertion of an IOL in an anatomically compromised position, as well as other surgical surprises.

ALTERNATIVE STRATEGIES FOR ACHIEVING IDEAL CORRECTIONS

Ablative customization is not the only way to achieve ideal refractive corrections. The requirements for an ideal correction include:
1. The correction must compensate for the optical aberrations of the eye over all pupil sizes.
2. The correction must maintain a fixed position with respect to the eye's optics.

Three modes of correction are currently viable: corneal refractive surgery, contact lenses, and IOLs.

Contact Lenses

An exciting area likely to capitalize on wavefront sensing and new latheing technologies is contact lenses designed to reduce the eye's higher-order aberrations. Studies done by Guirao, et al[5] indicate that slight displacements (< 0.3 mm vertical or horizontal, or rotational movement [< 5 degrees]) in contact lenses did not degrade the optical image significantly, indicating that ideal corrections in the form of contacts are likely to work better than initially anticipated. However, the advantages and disadvantages of contact lens wear will remain. The major advantage is that if it does not work, one can simply remove the lens and nothing is lost. The major disadvantage is that the patient remains aid-dependent. Aid dependency is a principal reason why patients desire refractive surgery. Nonetheless, customized contact lenses will fill a large market of those individuals who are happy with wearing contact lenses and would enjoy improving on what they already consider a good thing.

Intraocular Lenses

The use of a customized IOL based on wavefront sensing is an exciting area of future promise. At first, the precise placement of the IOL in the eye seems a formidable limitation, let alone the wavefront measurement in the presence of a cataract or the calculation of the ideal IOL from eye length and corneal topography. However, an alluring alternative is to fine-tune the IOL once in place. Imagine having a set of standard lenses from which you could select a lens using current nomograms and insert it in a typical manner. Once in place and the eye is recovered, the residual error (including higher-order aberrations) could be easily quantified and lens optical properties altered to appropriately compensate for the measured residual aberrations of the eye. These need not be ablative procedures. Biomaterials that can change their local optical index with appropriate stimulation could be optically refined once in place. If materials could be developed that would allow multiple tune-ups, then changes that occur as part of the normal aging process could easily be corrected. With the aging of the baby-boomers, we can expect to see significant effort in this area in the near future.

FUTURE METHODS OF CUSTOMIZATION

Monovision, Multifocality, and Accommodation

If we are able to improve a person's vision to the 20/10 with objects having sharper borders and higher contrast, this may open up more options in terms of a monovision strategy. Since patients would be able to see better at distance and near focus, one strategy may be to treat the patient with a monovision correction in one eye, which does not lose as much vision as with a conventional monovision ablation. Another possibility would be to make a multifocal ablation pattern on one or both corneas. Previous attempts without sophisticated tracking systems and spot lasers have demonstrated mixed results,[6,7] but they may become more feasible as the tracking systems and lasers become more precise and our understanding of how optical aberrations might be turned to our advantage.

Another important area of research will be the effect of accommodation on higher-order aberrations. As the eye accommodates, the aberration structure of the eye changes.[8] For what distance should the aberrations of the eye be minimized? It is likely that a patient's satisfaction could be improved if the treatment is adjusted based on the person's occupational and functional needs. For example, an accountant who enjoys reading for recreation may require a different wavefront customization than a person who is the same age but enjoys outdoor recreation and primarily uses his or her distance vision.

There are also lasers under development that can potentially reshape the human lens to create customized lenticular refractive surgery. Here, one uses a laser to reshape the human lens, perhaps to create a multifocal lens that would help the patient with depth of focus. However, as with multifocal contact lenses, such corrections should avoid causing large amounts of defocus and spherical aberration. Ideally, presbyopia needs to be delayed or prevented, or an accommodating lens needs to be perfected. Such strategies were unthinkable a few years ago but are now being actively explored.

Multistage Customization

A promising approach to achieve ideal waveguided custom ablations, given individual differences in response to treatment and healing, is to use a multistage procedure for customization. The waveguided "touch-up" in the near future will likely be focused on correcting all remaining ocular aberrations. This approach has logical appeal in that the individualized biomechanical response to small amounts of tissue removal is likely to be smaller than the initial treatment. Further, knowledge of the how the eye initially responded may allow the touch-up to be refined to account for individual differences in the biomechanical response.

> Multimodal customization is the use of two or more surgical procedures to correct refractive error. Example: LASIK used in combination with phakic IOL.

Multimodal Customization for High Myopia and Hyperopia

There is an increasing number of new surgical strategies that use several different modalities, such as a phakic IOL combined with laser refractive surgery. We call this area "multimodal customization." In the future, we will see many more forms of multimodal customization being developed. One possibility is the use of LASIK in conjunction with INTACS corneal inlays (KeraVision, Calif).[10] If a patient with a high degree of myopia is only slightly undercorrected with LASIK, some surgeons are now using INTACS to treat the small residual myopia. Such multimodality customization may be more common in the future.

Another interesting multimodal treatment is that of the bioptics procedure, where a phakic IOL is inserted and then the remainder of the ametropia is treated with a LASIK procedure.[11] A similar strategy could be employed with the addition of a customized ablation to enhance final vision.

Multimodal Customization for High Degrees of Irregular Astigmatism

Treatment of high degrees of astigmatism, particularly after corneal transplantation, is especially challenging. The current wavefront sensors may be too sensitive to aid us in treating eyes with 6 to 12 D of irregular astigmatism. If measurement is impossible, it may be more realistic to reduce the high degree of astigmatism using a wedge resection, a relaxing incision, or retrephination. Assuming the initial procedure reduces most of the astigmatism, then a customized ablation could be used to treat the more subtle aberrations.

Online Topometry, Topography

Another exciting area is that of online topometry[12] and topography.[13] There is one study using fringe projection that suggests using real-time feedback regarding surface changes during ablation.[12] This may potentially make laser refractive surgery even more accurate. Most of the laser companies are looking into ways to image the corneal shape changes in real-time during the laser treatments. Such devices offer the very real potential of altering the design of the procedure in real-time to correct for individualized biomechanical responses and optimizing first treatment outcomes.

POTENTIAL DISADVANTAGES OF CUSTOMIZED ABLATION AND SUPERVISION

There is an old story of the housewife who gets a long overdue new pair of glasses. When she goes home, she is appalled at the dust and dirt that have accumulated in her house while she was "visually impaired." It may be the case that some patients may not like the vision that ideal corrections can provide.

Perhaps a bigger concern is that of safety. Current safety standards in terms of light exposure assume that the eye has the typical aberrations observed in the normal population. Will near perfect imaging make treated eyes more susceptible to light toxicity? When we thin the cornea (20 to 100 microns) with LASIK or PRK, have we reduced the cornea's effectiveness in filtering ultraviolet radiation?[15]

Much of the publishing and visual arts communities have established standards based on the current limits in vision. How will this be affected by enhanced vision? Will seeing the actual dots of the imaging process be distracting?[14] Likewise, television and computer graphics rely on a raster that produces a pixel pattern that is below the resolution of the human optical system. How will this be affected when our resolution is enhanced?[14]

How will our neural visual system respond to our enhanced optics? Will there be some degree of amblyopia that precludes improvement with enhanced human optics?[16] There are many challenging questions to be addressed when we consider the future of customized ablation.

LIMITS OF CUSTOMIZATION

The first limitation is that we cannot improve beyond diffraction-limited optics. Although diffraction limits vision for small pupils (less than about 3 mm), it does not for larger pupils. For larger pupils, the Nyquest limit imposed by receptor sampling limits the accurate neural encoding of fine detail-limiting aberration-free corrections to 20/8 to 20/10 (see Chapters Two, Six, and Seven). Further, even if we do create optimal corrections, they will be optimal for only one test distance. However, despite these limitations, the benefits of increased contrast and resolution achieved by reducing the eye's aberrations (even if they are not totally eliminated) will likely far outweigh any disadvantages.[4,16]

SUMMARY

We have seen in this book how simple in concept but how complex in implementation the goal of achieving aberration-free vision can be. We have tried to give the reader a broad overview, as well as a detailed portrayal of this burgeoning field. We believe that customized ablation will help transform the way refractive surgery is performed in the future. We predict customization will be the standard of care for future generations of surgeons. Many of the creative talents of the authors in this book, as well as many others, have actually brought about this field of surgical practice. We do not need a crystal ball to mirror our excitement of what lies ahead. After being able to promise patients good odds of getting "almost as good as new" vision, we are anticipating a heady day when we can present odds favoring supervision.

REFERENCES

1. Bille JF. Preoperative simulation of outcomes using adaptive optics. *J Refract Surg.* In press.
2. Tyson RK. *Principle of Adaptive Optics.* 2nd ed. Boston, Mass: Academic Press; 1998.
3. Sechaud M. Wavefront compensation devices. In: F Roddier, ed. *Adaptive Optics in Astronomy.* New York, NY: Cambridge University Press; 1999.
4. Applegate RA. Limits to vision: can we do better than nature? *J Refract Surg.* In press.
5. Guirao A, Williams DR, Cox I. Effect of rotation and translation of the expected benefit of ideal contact lenses. *Invest Ophthalmol Vis Sci.* 2000;41(4Suppl):S429.
6. Maloney RK. Corneal topography and optical zone location in PRK. *J Refract Corneal Surg.* 1990;6:363-371.
7. Vinceguerra P, Nizzola GM, Nizzola F, Ascari A, Azzolini M, Epstein D. Zonal photorefractive keratectomy for presbyopia. *J Refract Surg.* 1998;14(2):S218-221.
8. Anschultz T. Laser correction in hyperopia and presbyopia. *Int Ophthalmol Clin.* 1994;34(4):107-137.
9. Hofer HJ, Porter J, Williams DR. Dynamic measurement of the wave aberration of the human eye. *Invest Ophthalmol Vis Sci.* 1998;39(4):S203.
10. Durrie D. The use of INTACS in LASIK undercorrections. Presented at American Academy of Ophthalmology. Orlando, Fla; October 1999.
11. Zaldivar R, Davidorf JM, Oscherow S, Ricur G, Piezzi V. Combined posterior chamber phakic intraocular lens and laser in situ keratomileusis: bioptics for extreme myopia. *J Refract Surg.* 1999;15(3):299-308.
12. Schruender. ARVO poster. Online topometry during refractive surgery by UV fringe projection. *Invest Ophthalmol Vis Sci.* 2000;41(4Suppl):S689.
13. Moser C, Kampmeier J, McDonnell P, Psaltis D. Feasibility of intraoperative corneal topography monitoring during photorefractive keratectomy. *J Refract Surg.* 2000;16:148-154.
14. Thibos LN. The prospects for perfect vision. *J Refract Surg.* In press.
15. Lerman S. *Radiant Energy and the Eye.* New York, NY: Macmillan Publishing Co, Inc; 1980:122-131.
16. Miller DT. Retinal imaging and vision at the frontiers of adaptive optics. *Physics Today.* 2000;53:31-36.

Appendices

Appendix One

Optical Society of America Wavefront Standards

Reprinted with permission from the Optical Society of America.

Standards for Reporting the Optical Aberrations of Eyes

Larry N. Thibos,[1] Raymond A. Applegate,[2] James T. Schwiegerling,[3] Robert Webb[4], and VSIA Standards Taskforce Members

[1]*School of Optometry, Indiana University, Bloomington, IN 47405,* [2]*Department of Ophthalmology, University of Texas Health Science Center at San Antonio, San Antonio, TX 78284,* [3]*Department of Ophthalmology, University of Arizona, Tucson, AZ 85721,* [4]*Schepens Research Institute, Boston, MA 02114 thibos@indiana.edu, Applegate@uthscsa.edu, jschwieg@u.arizona.edu, webb@helix.mgh.harvard.edu*

Abstract: In response to a perceived need in the vision community, an OSA taskforce was formed at the 1999 topical meeting on vision science and its applications (VSIA-99) and charged with developing consensus recommendations on definitions, conventions, and standards for reporting of optical aberrations of human eyes. Progress reports were presented at the 1999 OSA annual meeting and at VSIA-2000 by the chairs of three taskforce subcommittees on (1) reference axes, (2) describing functions, and (3) model eyes. The following summary of the committee's recommendations is available also in portable document format (PDF) on OSA Optics Net at http://www.osa.org/.
OCIS codes: (330.0330) Vision and color; (330.5370) Physiological optics

Background

The recent resurgence of activity in visual optics research and related clinical disciplines (e.g. refractive surgery, ophthalmic lens design, ametropia diagnosis) demands that the vision community establish common metrics, terminology, and other reporting standards for the specification of optical imperfections of eyes. Currently there exists a plethora of methods for analyzing and representing the aberration structure of the eye but no agreement exists within the vision community on a common, universal method for reporting results. In theory, the various methods currently in use by different groups of investigators all describe the same underlying phenomena and therefore it should be possible to reliably convert results from one representational scheme to another. However, the practical implementation of these conversion methods is computationally challenging, is subject to error, and reliable computer software is not widely available. All of these problems suggest the need for operational standards for reporting aberration data and to specify test procedures for evaluating the accuracy of data collection and data analysis methods.

Following a call for participation [1], approximately 20 people met at VSIA-99 to discuss the proposal to form a taskforce that would recommend standards for reporting optical aberrations of eyes. The group agreed to form three working parties that would take responsibility for developing consensus recommendations on definitions, conventions and standards for the following three topics: (1) reference axes, (2) describing functions, and (3) model eyes. It was decided that the strategy for Phase I of this project would be to concentrate on articulating definitions, conventions, and standards for those issues which are not empirical in nature. For example, several schemes for enumerating the Zernike polynomials have been proposed in the literature. Selecting one to be the standard is a matter of choice, not empirical investigation, and therefore was included in the charge to the taskforce. On the other hand, issues such as the maximum number of Zernike orders needed to describe ocular aberrations adequately is an empirical question which was avoided for the present, although the taskforce may choose to formulate recommendations on such issues at a later time. Phase I concluded at the VSIA-2000 meeting.

Reference Axis Selection

Summary

It is the committee's recommendation that the ophthalmic community use the line-of-sight as the reference axis for the purposes of calculating and measuring the optical aberrations of the eye. The rationale is that the line-of-sight in the normal eye is the path of the chief ray from the fixation point to the retinal fovea. Therefore, aberrations measured with respect to this axis will have the pupil center as the origin of a Cartesian reference frame. Secondary lines-of-sight may be similarly constructed for object points in the peripheral visual field. Because the exit pupil is not readily accessible in the living eye whereas the entrance pupil is, the committee recommends that calculations for specifying the optical aberration of the eye be referenced to the plane of the entrance pupil.

Background

Optical aberration measurements of the eye from various laboratories or within the same laboratory are not comparable unless they are calculated with respect to the same reference axis and expressed in the same manner. This requirement is complicated by the fact that, unlike a camera, the eye is a decentered optical system with non-rotationally symmetric components (Fig. 1). The principle elements of the eye's optical system are the cornea, pupil, and the crystalline lens. Each can be decentered and tilted with respect to other components, thus rendering an optical system that is typically dominated by coma at the foveola.

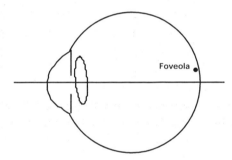

Fig. 1. The cornea, pupil, and crystalline lens are decentered and tilted with respect to each other, rendering the eye a decentered optical system that is different between individuals and eyes within the same individual.

The optics discipline has a long tradition of specifying the aberration of optical systems with respect to the center of the exit pupil. In a centered optical system (e.g., a camera, or telescope) using the center of the exit pupil as a reference for measurement of on-axis aberration is the same as measuring the optical aberrations with respect to the chief ray from an axial object point. However, because the exit pupil is not readily accessible in the living eye, it is more practical to reference aberrations to the entrance pupil. This is the natural choice for objective aberrometers which analyze light reflected from the eye.

Like a camera, the eye is an imaging device designed to form an in-focus inverted image on a screen. In the case of the eye, the imaging screen is the retina. However, unlike film, the "grain" of the retina is not uniform over its extent. Instead, the grain is finest at the foveola and falls off quickly as the distance from the foveola increases. Consequently, when viewing fine detail, we rotate our eye such that the object of regard falls on the foveola (Fig. 2). Thus, aberrations at the foveola have the greatest impact on an individual's ability to see fine details.

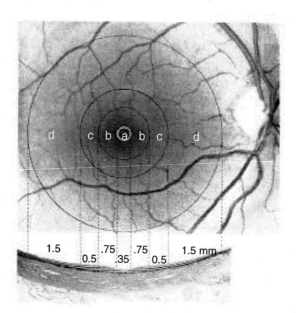

Fig. 2. An anatomical view of the macular region as viewed from the front and in cross section (below). a: foveola, b: fovea, c: parafoveal area, d: perifoveal area. From *Histology of the Human Eye* by Hogan. Alvarado Weddell, W.B. Sauders Company publishers, 1971, page 491.

Two traditional axes of the eye are centered on the foveola, the visual axis and the line-of-sight, but only the latter passes through the pupil center. In object space, the visual axis is typically defined as the line connecting the fixation object point to the eye's first nodal point. In image space, the visual axis is the parallel line connecting the second nodal point to the center of the foveola (Fig. 3, left). In contrast, the line-of-sight is defined as the (broken) line passing through the center of the eye's entrance and exit pupils connecting the object of regard to the foveola (Fig. 3, right). The line-of-sight is equivalent to the path of the foveal chief ray and therefore is the axis which conforms to optical standards. The visual axis and the line of sight are not the same and in some eyes the difference can have a large impact on retinal image quality [2]. For a review of the axes of the eye see [3]. (To avoid confusion, we note that Bennett and Rabbetts [4] re-define the visual axis to match the traditional definition of the line of sight. The Bennett and Rabbetts definition is counter to the majority of the literature and is not used here.)

When measuring the optical properties of the eye for objects which fall on the peripheral retina outside the central fovea, a secondary line-of-sight may be constructed as the broken line from object point to center of the entrance pupil and from the center of the exit pupil to the retinal location of the image. This axis represents the path of the chief ray from the object of interest and therefore is the appropriate reference for describing aberrations of the peripheral visual field.

Methods for aligning the eye during measurement.

Summary

The committee recommends that instruments designed to measure the optical properties of the eye and its aberrations be aligned co-axially with the eye's line-of-sight.

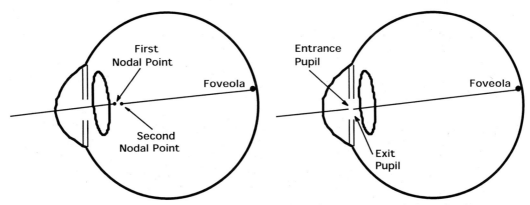

Fig. 3. Left panel illustrates the visual axis and panel right illustrates the line of sight.

Background

There are numerous ways to align the line of sight to the optical axis of the measuring instrument. Here we present simple examples of an objective method and a subjective method to achieve proper alignment.

Objective method

In the objective alignment method schematically diagramed in Fig. 4, the experimenter aligns the subject's eye (which is fixating a small distant target on the optical axis of the measurement system) to the measurement system. Alignment is achieved by centering the subject's pupil (by adjusting a bite bar) on an alignment ring (e.g., an adjustable diameter circle) which is co-axial with the optical axis of the measurement system. This strategy forces the optical axis of the measurement device to pass through the center of the entrance pupil. Since the fixation target is on the optical axis of the measurement device, once the entrance pupil is centered with respect to the alignment ring, the line-of-sight is co-axial with the optical axis of the measurement system.

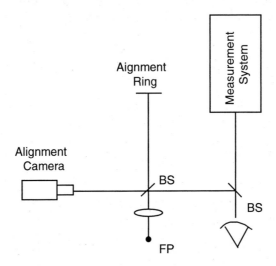

Fig. 4. Schematic of a generic objective alignment system designed to place the line of sight on the optical axis of the measurement system. BS: beam splitter, FP: on axis fixation point.

Subjective method

In the subjective alignment method schematically diagramed in Figure 5, the subject adjusts the position of their own pupil (using a bite bar) until two alignment fixation points at different optical distances along and co-axial to the optical axis of the measurement device are superimposed (similar to aligning the sights on rifle to a target). Note that one or both of the alignment targets will be defocused on the retina. Thus the subject's task is to align the centers of the blur circles. Assuming the chief ray defines the centers of the blur circles for each fixation point, this strategy forces the line of sight to be co-axial with the optical axis of the measurement system. In a system with significant amounts of asymmetric aberration (e.g., coma), the chief ray may not define the center of the blur circle. In practice, it can be useful to use the subjective strategy for preliminary alignment and the objective method for final alignment.

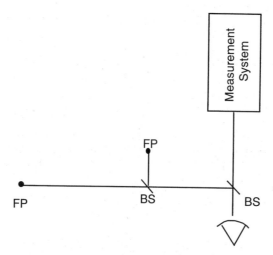

Fig. 5. Schematic of a generic subjective alignment system designed to place the line of sight on the optical axis of the measurement system. BS: beam splitter, FP: fixation point source.

Conversion between reference axes

If optical aberration measurements are made with respect to some other reference axis, the data must be converted to the standard reference axis (see the tools developed by Susana Marcos at our temporary web site: //color.eri.harvard/standardization). However, since such conversions involve measurement and/or estimation errors for two reference axes (the alignment error of the measurement and the error in estimating the new reference axis), it is preferable to have the measurement axis be the same as the line-of-sight.

Description of Zernike Polynomials

The Zernike polynomials are a set of functions that are orthogonal over the unit circle. They are useful for describing the shape of an aberrated wavefront in the pupil of an optical system. Several different normalization and numbering schemes for these polynomials are in common use. Below we describe the different schemes and make recommendations towards developing a standard for presenting Zernike data as it relates to aberration theory of the eye.

Double Indexing Scheme

The Zernike polynomials are usually defined in polar coordinates (ρ, θ), where ρ is the radial coordinate ranging from 0 to 1 and θ is the azimuthal component ranging from 0 to 2π. Each of the Zernike polynomials consists of three components: a normalization factor, a radial-dependent component and an azimuthal-dependent component. The radial component is a polynomial, whereas the azimuthal component is sinusoidal. A double indexing scheme is useful for unambiguously describing these functions, with the index n describing the highest power (order) of the radial polynomial and the index m describing the azimuthal frequency of the sinusoidal component. By this scheme the Zernike polynomials are defined as

$$Z_n^m(\rho,\theta) = \begin{cases} N_n^m R_n^{|m|}(\rho)\cos m\theta \; ; \; for \; m \geq 0 \\ -N_n^m R_n^{|m|}(\rho)\sin m\theta \; ; \; for \; m < 0 \end{cases}$$

(1)

where N_n^m is the normalization factor described in more detail below and $R_n^{|m|}(\rho)$ is given by

$$R_n^{|m|}(\rho) = \sum_{s=0}^{(n-|m|)/2} \frac{(-1)^s (n-s)!}{s! \left[0.5(n+|m|)-s\right]! \left[0.5(n-|m|)-s\right]!} \rho^{n-2s}$$

(2)

This definition uniquely describes the Zernike polynomials except for the normalization constant. The normalization is given by

$$N_n^m = \sqrt{\frac{2(n+1)}{1+\delta_{m0}}}$$

(3)

where δ_{m0} is the Kronecker delta function (i.e. $\delta_{m0} = 1$ for m = 0, and $\delta_{m0} = 0$ for m $\neq$ 0). Note that the value of n is a positive integer or zero. For a given n, m can only take on values -n, -n + 2, -n +4, ...n.

When describing individual Zernike terms, the two index scheme should always be used. Below are some examples.

Good:

"The values of $Z_3^{-1}(\rho,\theta)$ and $Z_4^2(\rho,\theta)$ are 0.041 and -0.121, respectively."

"Comparing the astigmatism terms, $Z_2^{-2}(\rho,\theta)$ and $Z_2^2(\rho,\theta)$ ..."

Bad

"The values of $Z_7(\rho,\theta)$ and $Z_{12}(\rho,\theta)$ are 0.041 and -0.121, respectively."

"Comparing the astigmatism terms, $Z_5(\rho,\theta)$ and $Z_6(\rho,\theta)$ ..."

Single Indexing Scheme

Occasionally, a single indexing scheme is useful for describing Zernike expansion coefficients. Since the polynomials actually depend on two parameters, n and m, ordering of a single indexing scheme is arbitrary. To avoid confusion, a standard single indexing scheme should be used, and this scheme should only be used for bar plots of expansion coefficients (Fig. 6). To obtain the single index, j, it is convenient to lay out the polynomials in a pyramid with row number n and column number m as shown in Table 1.

Table 1. Zernike pyramid. Row number is polynomial order n, column number is sinusoidal frequency m, table entry is the single-index j.

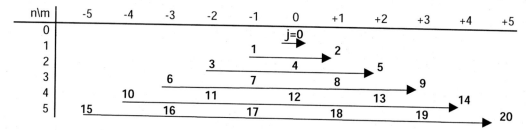

The single index, j, starts at the top of the pyramid and steps down from left to right. To convert between j and the values of n and m, the following relationships can be used:

$$j = \frac{n(n+2)+m}{2} \qquad \text{(mode number)} \tag{4}$$

$$n = roundup\left[\frac{-3+\sqrt{9+8j}}{2}\right] \qquad \text{(radial order)} \tag{5}$$

$$m = 2j - n(n+2) \qquad \text{(angular frequency)} \tag{6}$$

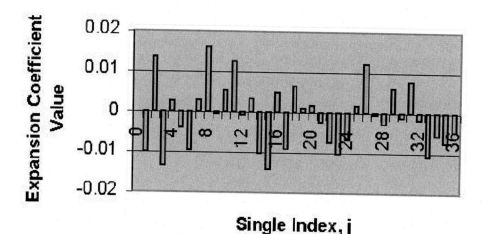

Fig. 6. Example of a bar plot using the single index scheme for Zernike coefficients.

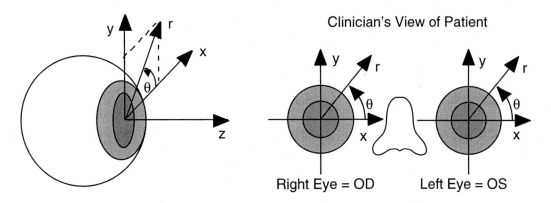

Clinician's View of Patient

Right Eye = OD   Left Eye = OS

Fig. 7. Conventional right-handed coordinate system for the eye in Cartesian and polar forms.

Coordinate System

Typically, a right-handed coordinate system is used in scientific applications as shown in Fig. 7. For the eye, the coordinate origin is at the center of the eye's entrance pupil, the +x axis is horizontal pointing to the right, the +y axis is vertical pointing up, and the +z Cartesian axis points out of the eye and coincides with the foveal line-of-sight in object space, as defined by a chief ray emitted by a fixation spot. Also shown are conventional definitions of the polar coordinates $r = \sqrt{x^2 + y^2}$ and $\theta = \tan^{-1}(y/x)$. This definition gives $x = r\cos\theta$ and $y = r\sin\theta$. We note that Malacara [5] uses a polar coordinate system in which $x = r\sin\theta$ and $y = r\cos\theta$. In other words, θ is measured clockwise from the +y axis (Figure 1b), instead of counterclockwise from the +x axis (Figure 1a). Malacara's definition stems from early (pre-computer) aberration theory and is not recommended. In ophthalmic optics, angle θ is called the "meridian" and the same coordinate system applies to both eyes.

Because of the inaccessibility of the eye's image space, the aberration function of eyes are usually defined and measured in object space. For example, objective measures of ocular aberrations use light reflected out of the eye from a point source on the retina. Light reflected out of an aberration-free eye will form a plane-wave propagating in the positive z-direction and therefore the (x,y) plane serves as a natural reference surface. In this case the wavefront aberration function $W(x,y)$ equals the z-coordinate of the reflected wavefront and may be interpreted as the shape of the reflected wavefront. By these conventions, $W > 0$ means the wavefront is phase-advanced relative to the chief ray. An example would be the wavefront reflected from a myopic eye, converging to the eye's far-point. A closely related quantity is the optical path-length difference (OPD) between a ray passing through the pupil at (x,y) and the chief ray point passing through the origin. In the case of a myopic eye, the path length is shorter for marginal rays than for the chief ray, so OPD < 0. Thus, by the recommended sign conventions, $OPD(x,y) = -W(x,y)$.

Bilateral symmetry in the aberration structure of eyes would make $W(x,y)$ for the left eye the same as $W(-x,y)$ for the right eye. If W is expressed as a Zernike series, then bilateral symmetry would cause the Zernike coefficients for the two eyes to be of opposite sign for all those modes with odd symmetry about the y-axis (e.g. mode Z_2^{-2}). Thus, to facilitate direct comparison of the two eyes, a vector R of Zernike coefficients for the right eye can be converted to a symmetric vector L for the left eye by the linear transformation L=M*R, where M is a diagonal matrix with elements +1 (no sign change) or −1 (with sign change). For example, matrix M for Zernike vectors representing the first 4 orders (15 modes) would have the diagonal elements [+1, +1, -1, -1, +1, +1, +1, +1, -1, -1, -1, -1, +1, +1, +1]

Table 2. Listing of Zernike Polynomials up to 7th order (36 terms)

j = index	n = order	m = frequency	$Z_n^m(\rho,\theta)$
0	0	0	1
1	1	-1	$2\,\rho\sin\theta$
2	1	1	$2\,\rho\cos\theta$
3	2	-2	$\sqrt{6}\,\rho^2\sin 2\theta$
4	2	0	$\sqrt{3}\,(2\rho^2-1)$
5	2	2	$\sqrt{6}\,\rho^2\cos 2\theta$
6	3	-3	$\sqrt{8}\,\rho^3\sin 3\theta$
7	3	-1	$\sqrt{8}\,(3\rho^3-2\rho)\sin\theta$
8	3	1	$\sqrt{8}\,(3\rho^3-2\rho)\cos\theta$
9	3	3	$\sqrt{8}\,\rho^3\cos 3\theta$
10	4	-4	$\sqrt{10}\,\rho^4\sin 4\theta$
11	4	-2	$\sqrt{10}\,(4\rho^4-3\rho^2)\sin 2\theta$
12	4	0	$\sqrt{5}\,(6\rho^4-6\rho^2+1)$
13	4	2	$\sqrt{10}\,(4\rho^4-3\rho^2)\cos 2\theta$
14	4	4	$\sqrt{10}\,\rho^4\cos 4\theta$
15	5	-5	$\sqrt{12}\,\rho^5\sin 5\theta$
16	5	-3	$\sqrt{12}\,(5\rho^5-4\rho^3)\sin 3\theta$
17	5	-1	$\sqrt{12}\,(10\rho^5-12\rho^3+3\rho)\sin\theta$
18	5	1	$\sqrt{12}\,(10\rho^5-12\rho^3+3\rho)\cos\theta$
19	5	3	$\sqrt{12}\,(5\rho^5-4\rho^3)\cos 3\theta$
20	5	5	$\sqrt{12}\,\rho^5\cos 5\theta$
21	6	-6	$\sqrt{14}\,\rho^6\sin 6\theta$
22	6	-4	$\sqrt{14}\,(6\rho^6-5\rho^4)\sin 4\theta$
23	6	-2	$\sqrt{14}\,(15\rho^6-20\rho^4+6\rho^2)\sin 2\theta$
24	6	0	$\sqrt{7}\,(20\rho^6-30\rho^4+12\rho^2-1)$
25	6	2	$\sqrt{14}\,(15\rho^6-20\rho^4+6\rho^2)\cos 2\theta$
26	6	4	$\sqrt{14}\,(6\rho^6-5\rho^4)\cos 4\theta$
27	6	6	$\sqrt{14}\,\rho^6\cos 6\theta$
28	7	-7	$4\,\rho^7\sin 7\theta$
29	7	-5	$4\,(7\rho^7-6\rho^5)\sin 5\theta$
30	7	-3	$4\,(21\rho^7-30\rho^5+10\rho^3)\sin 3\theta$
31	7	-1	$4\,(35\rho^7-60\rho^5+30\rho^3-4\rho)\sin\theta$

32	7	1	4 $(35\rho^7-60\rho^5+30\rho^3-4\rho)$ cos θ
33	7	3	4 $(21\rho^7-30\rho^5+10\rho^3)$ cos 3θ
34	7	5	4 $(7\rho^7-6\rho^5)$ cos 5θ
35	7	7	4 ρ^7 cos 7θ

A standard aberrator for calibration

The original goal was to design a device that could be passed around or mass-produced to calibrate aberrometers at various laboratories. We first thought of this as an aberrated model eye, but that later seemed too elaborate. One problem is that the subjective aberrometers needed a sensory retina in their model eye, while the objective ones needed a reflective retina of perhaps known reflectivity. We decided instead to design an aberrator that could be used with any current or future aberrometers, with whatever was the appropriate model eye.

The first effort was with a pair of lenses that nearly cancelled spherical power, but when displaced sideways would give a known aberration. That scheme worked, but was very sensitive to tilt, and required careful control of displacement. The second design was a trefoil phase plate (OPD = Z_3^3 = κ $r^3 \sin 3\theta$) loaned by Ed Dowski of CDM Optics, Inc. This 3rd order aberration is similar to coma, but with three lobes instead of one, hence the common name "trefoil". Simulation of the aberration function for this plate in ZEMAX® is shown in Figs. 8, 9. Figure 8 is a graph of the Zernike coefficients showing a small amount of defocus and 3rd order spherical aberration, but primarily C_3^3. Figure 9 shows the wavefront, only half a micron (one wave) peak to peak, but that value depends on κ, above.

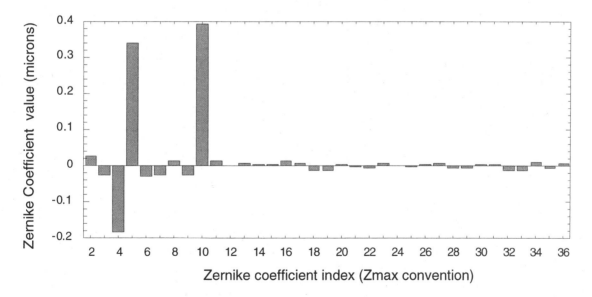

Fig. 8: Zernike coefficients of trefoil phase plate from ZEMAX® model (note different numbering convention from that recommended above for eyes).

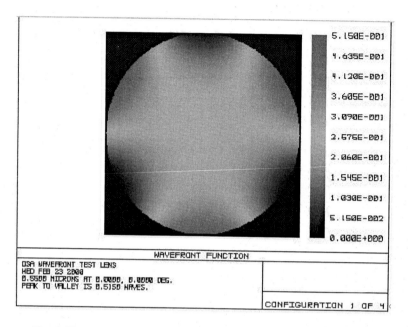

Fig. 9: Wavefront map for trefoil phase plate from the ZEMAX® model

We mounted the actual plate and found that it had even more useful qualities: As the phase plate is translated across the pupil, it adds some C_2^2, horizontal astigmatism. When the plate is perfectly centered, that coefficient is zero. Further, the slope of C_2^2 (Δx) measures the actual pupil.

$$Z_3^3(x - x_0) = \kappa\,(r - x_0)\sin 3\theta = \kappa\,(3xy^2 - x^3)$$

(7)

so

$$\frac{\partial Z_3^3(x - x_0)}{\partial x} = 3\kappa\,(3y^2 - x^2) = 3Z_2^2$$

(8)

and similarly

$$\frac{\partial Z_3^{-3}(x - x_0)}{\partial x} = -6\kappa xy = -3Z_2^{-2}$$

(9)

This means that $\Delta Z_3^3 = 3Z_2^2 \Delta x$ and then, since $W = \sum\sum C_n^m Z_n^m$, we get a new term proportional to Δx. Plotting the coefficient C_2^2 against Δx, we need to normalize to the pupil size. That could be useful as a check on whether the aberrator is really at the pupil, or whether some smoothing has changed the real pupil size, as measured. Figures 10-13 confirm this behavior and the expected variation with rotation (3θ).

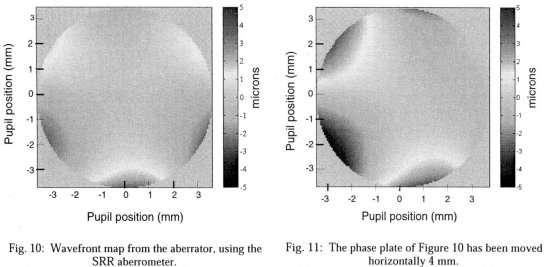

Fig. 10: Wavefront map from the aberrator, using the SRR aberrometer.

Fig. 11: The phase plate of Figure 10 has been moved horizontally 4 mm.

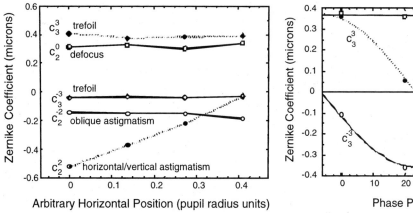

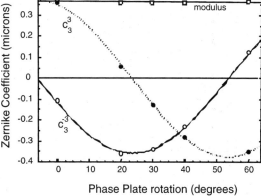

Fig. 12: Zerike coefficients are stable against horizontal displacement, except for C_3^3.

Fig. 13: Zernike coefficients C_3^3 and C_3^{-3} as a function of rotation of the phase plate about the optic axis.

Although the phase plate aberrator works independently of position in a collimated beam, some aberrometers may want to use a converging or diverging beam. Then it should be placed in a pupil conjugate plane. We have not yet built the mount for the phase plate, and would appreciate suggestions for that. Probably we need a simple barrel mount that fits into standard lens holders – say 30 mm outside diameter. We expect to use a standard pupil, but the phase plate(s) should have 10 mm clear aperture before restriction. The workshop seemed to feel that a standard pupil should be chosen. Should that be 7.5 mm?

We have tested the Z_3^3 aberrator, but it may be a good idea to have a few others. We borrowed this one, and it is somewhat fragile. Bill Plummer of Polaroid thinks he could generate this and other plates in plastic for "a few thousand dollars" for each design. Please send suggestions as to whether other designs are advisable (webb@helix.mgh.Harvard.edu), and as to whether we will want to stack them or use them independently. That has some implications for the mount design, but not severe ones. We suggest two Z_3^{3} plates like this one, and perhaps a Z_6^{0}, fifth order spherical.

At this time, then, our intent is to have one or more standard aberrators that can be inserted into any aberrometer. When centered, and with a standard pupil, all aberrometers should report the same Zernike coefficients. We do not intend to include positioners in the mount, assuming that will be different for each aberrometer.

Another parameter of the design is the value of κ. That comes from the actual physical thickness and the index of refraction. Suggestions are welcome here, but we assume we want coefficients that are robust compared to a diopter or so of defocus.

The index will be whatever it will be. We will report it, but again any chromaticity will depend on how it's used. We suggest that we report the expected coefficients at a few standard wavelengths and leave interpolation to users.

Plans for Phase II

Reference Axes Sub-committee
- develop a shareware library of software tools needed to convert data from one ocular reference axis to another (e.g., convert a wavefront aberration for the corneal surface measured by topography along the instrument's optical axis into a wavefront aberration specified in the eye's exit pupil plane along the eye's fixation axis.)
- generate test datasets for evaluating software tools

Describing functions subcommittee
- develop a shareware library of software tools for generating, manipulating, evaluating, etc. the recommended describing functions for wavefront aberrations and pupil apodizing functions.
- develop additional software tools for converting results between describing functions (e.g. converting Taylor polynomials to Zernike polynomials, or converting single-index Zernikes to double-index Zernikes, etc.)
- generate test datasets for evaluating software tools

Model eyes subcommittee
- build a physical model eye that can be used to calibrate experimental apparatus for measuring the aberrations of eyes
- circulate the physical model to all interested parties for evaluation, with results to be presented for discussion at a future VSIA meeting.

Acknowledgements

The authors wish to thank the numerous committee members who contributed to this project.

References

1. L. N. Thibos, R. A. Applegate, H. C. Howland, D. R. Williams, P. Artal, R. Navarro, M. C. Campbell, J. E. Greivenkamp, J. T. Schwiegerling, S. A. Burns, D. A. Atchison, G. Smith, and E. J. Sarver, "A VSIA-sponsored effort to develop methods and standards for the comparison of the wavefront aberration structure of the eye between devices and laboratories.," in *Vision Science and Its Applications*, (Optical Society of America, Washington, D.C., 1999) pp 236-239.
2. L. N. Thibos, A. Bradley, D. L. Still, X. Zhang, and P. A. Howarth, "Theory and measurement of ocular chromatic aberration," Vision Research **30**, 33-49 (1990).
3. A. Bradley and L. N. Thibos (Presentation 5) at http://www.opt.indiana.edu/lthibos/ABLNTOSA95
4. A. G. Bennett and R. B. Rabbetts, *Clinical Visual Optics*, 2nd ed., (Butterworth, 1989).
5. D. Malacara, *Optical Shop Testing*, 2nd ed., (John Wiley & Sons, Inc., New York, 1992).

American National Standards Institute Standards in Corneal Topography

Reprinted with permission from the American National Standard for Ophthalmics, Corneal Topography Systems—Standard Terminology, Requirements. Optical Laboratories Association; 1999.

American National Standard

Approval of an American National Standard requires review by ANSI that the requirements for due process, consensus, and other criteria for approval have been met by the standards developer.

Consensus is established when, in the judgement of the ANSI Board of Standards Review, substantial agreement has been reached by directly and materially affected interests. Substantial agreement means much more than a simple majority, but not necessarily unanimity. Consensus requires that all views and objections be considered, and that a concerted effort be made towards their resolution.

The use of American National Standards is completely voluntary; their existence does not in any respect preclude anyone, whether he has approved the standards or not, from manufacturing, marketing, purchasing, or using products, processes, or procedures not conforming to the standards.

The American National Standards Institute does not develop standards and will in no circumstances give an interpretation of any American National Standard. Moreover, no person shall have the right or authority to issue an interpretation of an American National Standard in the name of the American National Standards Institute. Requests for interpretations should be addressed to the secretariat or sponsor whose name appears on the title page of this standard.

CAUTION NOTICE: This American National Standard may be revised or withdrawn at any time. The procedures of the American National Standards Institute require that action be taken periodically to reaffirm, revise, or withdraw this standard. Purchasers of American National Standards may receive current information on all standards by calling or writing the American National Standards Institute.

Developed by

The Accredited Committee Z80 for Ophthalmic Standards -

Optical Laboratories Association
Z80 Secretariat
P. O. Box 2000
Merrifield, VA 22116-2000

Published by

Optical Laboratories Association
P. O. Box 2000
Merrifield, VA 22116-2000

Foreword   (This foreword is not part of American National Standard Z80.23-1999.)

This American National Standard was developed to address the expressed needs of those members of the ophthalmic community who use corneal topography in clinical settings, those who manufacture corneal topographers and those who teach others in the use of the information collected by corneal topographers. In particular there was a need for standardization of the terms and definitions used in the field, for standardization of the methods used for characterizing the performance of these instruments and for standardization of displays of corneal topographical information. The experts who worked together to create this standard felt that at this time there was not sufficient consensus within the ophthalmic community to set performance requirements for these instruments beyond those for minimum area measured and measurement sample density. They did feel that the method for testing these instruments, to assess their performance and for reporting and results thus obtained, could be standardized and made a part of the requirements of this standard.

This standard was created by a special working group created by the Z80 Subcommittee on Ophthalmic Instruments and included experts in the field of corneal topography from the clinical, manufacturing and academic areas of the ophthalmic community.

Suggestions for improvement of this standard will be welcome. They should be sent to the Optical Laboratories Association, P.O. Box 2000, Merrifield, VA 22116-2000, USA.

This standard was processed and approved for submittal to ANSI by the Accredited Standards Committee on Ophthalmics, Z80. Committee approval of this standard does not necessarily imply that all committee members voted for its approval. At the time it approved this standard, the Z80 Committee had the following members:

Thomas C. White, M.D., Chairman
F. Dow Smith, Ph.D., Vice-Chairman
Robert Rosenberg, O.D., Secretary

Organization Represented	*Name of Representative*
American Academy of Ophthalmology	Thomas C. White
	Paul F. Vinger (Alt)
	Dale Heuer (Alt.)
American Academy of Optometry	David M. Loshin
American Ceramic Society	Dave Kerko
	Jackson S. Stroud (Alt.)
	Herbert Hoover (Alt.)
American Optometric Association	Donald Pitts
	Robert Rosenberg (Alt.)
	William "Joe" Benjamin (Alt.)
	Gregory L. Stephens (Alt.)
	Jeffrey L. Weaver (Alt.)
American Society of Cataract & Refractive Surgery	John J. Alpar
	Jack T. Holladay (Alt.)
	Stephen H. Johnson (Alt.)
Contact Lens Institute	Ed Schilling
Contact Lens Manufacturers Association	Quido Cappelli
Food and Drug Administration	David Whipple
	Robert Landry (Alt.)
Health Industry Manufacturers Association	Douglas Fortunato
	Dennis Hahn (Alt.)
	Susan Zagame (Alt.)
	Stanley Rogaski (Alt.)
Industrial Safety Equipment Association	Arthur J. Salce
	Janice Bradley (Alt.)

Organization Represented	Name of Representative
National Academy of Opticianry	Jeffrey C. Snodgrass
	Floyd H. Holmgrain (Alt.)
National Association of Optometrists and Opticians	Arthur Newman
National Institute of Standards and Technology	Thomas Lettieri
Prevent Blindness America	Tod Turriff
Opticians Association of America	C. Richard Sanders
	David A. Digby (Alt.)
Optical Laboratories Association	Daniel Torgersen
	Jeffrey Kosh (Alt.)
	Henry Hart (Alt.)
OMA The Optical Industry Association	William C. Thomas
	Ken Wood (Alt.)
	Richard Whitney (Alt.)
	Darryl Meister (Alt.)
Optical Society of America	F. Dow Smith
	Richard A. Phillips (Alt.)
Sunglass Association of America	Ken Frederick
	David Elliott (Alt.)
	James Pritts (Alt.)
	Renee Kluzniak (Alt.)
Veterans Health Administration	Sharon Atkin
	Bill Monaco (Alt.)
US Leader to ISO TC172/SC7	Charles Campbell
(Liaison between ISO & Z80)	

The Working Group for Topography, which falls under the Instrument Subcommittee, had the following members who worked on the writing of this Standard:

Charles E. Campbell, WG Chair
David Loshin, Subcommittee Chair

Raymond A. Applegate
Douglas Brenner
Robert Buckingham
Quido Cappelli
John E. Greivenkamp
Howard C. Howland
Stanley Klein
Steve Klyce
David D. Liu
Scott M. MacRae
Robert K. Maloney
Robert Mandell
Cynthia Roberts
Robert Rosenberg
Edward J. Sarver
Michael K. Smolek
Nancy K. Tripoli
Tim N. Turner
Sidney Wittenberg

AMERICAN NATIONAL STANDARD   ANSI Z80.23-1999

American National Standard
for Ophthalmics –

Corneal Topography Systems –
Standard Terminology, Requirements

1   Scope and purpose

1.1   Scope

This American National Standard applies to instruments, systems and methods which are intended to measure the shape of the cornea of the human eye over a majority of its anterior surface. The measurements may be of the curvature of the surface in local areas, three dimensional topographical measurements of the surface or other more global parameters used to characterize the surface. Instruments classified as ophthalmometers or keratometers are not covered by this standard.

1.2   Purpose

This standard defines certain terms which are peculiar to the characterization of the corneal shape so that they may be standardized throughout the field of vision care and have common meaning for all those who have occasion to participate in this area.

This standard sets forth minimum requirements for instruments and systems which fall into the class of corneal topographers.

This standard sets forth tests and verification procedures which will verify that a system or instrument complies with the standard and so qualifies as a corneal topographer in the meaning of this standard.

This standard sets forth certain tests and verification procedures which will allow the verification of capabilities of systems which are beyond the minimum required for corneal topographers.

2 Normative references

The following standard contains provisions that, through reference in this text, constitute provisions of this American National Standard. At the time of publication, the edition indicated was valid. All standards are subject to revision, and parties to agreements based on this American National Standard are encouraged to investigate the possibility of applying the most recent editions of the standards indicated below.

ANSI Z80.20-1998, *Ophthalmics - Contact Lenses - Standard terminology, tolerances, measurements and physicochemical properties*[1]

ISO 8429:1986, *Optics and optical instruments - Ophthalmology - Gradual dial scale*[1]

ISO 10110-12:1997, *Optics and optical instruments - Preparation of drawings for optical elements andsystems - Part 2: Aspheric surfaces*[1]

---

[1] For electronic copies of some standards, visit ANSI's Electronic Standards Store (ESS) at www.ansi.org. For printed versions of all these standards, contact Global Engineering Documents, 15 Inverness Way East, Englewood, CO 80112-5704, (800) 854-7179.

ISO 15004 :1998, *Optics and Optical Instruments - Ophthalmic instruments - Fundamental requirements and test methods*[1]

ISO 60601-1:1988, *Medical electrical equipment - Part 1: General requirements for safety*[1]

Foley JD, van Dam A, Finer SK, et.al. *Fundamentals of Interactive Computer Graphics.* Addison-Wesley, Reading 1990

3 Terminology

3.1   Corneal apex: The location on the corneal surface, of a normal cornea, where the mean of the local principal curvatures is greatest.

3.2   Corneal eccentricity (e): The eccentricity (e) of the ellipse which best fits the corneal meridian of interest (see 3.9). If the meridian is not specified, the corneal eccentricity is that of the flattest corneal meridian (see Table 1 and Annex A).

3.3   Corneal meridian (θ): The curve created by the intersection of corneal surface and a plane which contains the CT axis. A meridian is identified by the angle, θ, that the plane creating it makes to the horizontal as described by ISO 8429. The value of θ, for a full meridian, takes values from 0 to 180 degrees.

3.3.1   Corneal semi-meridian: The portion of a full meridian extending from the CT axis toward the periphery in one direction. The value of θ for a semi-meridian takes values from 0 to 360 degrees.

3.4   Corneal shape factor (E): A value which specifies the asphericity and type (prolate or oblate) of conic section which best fits a corneal meridian. Unless otherwise specified, it refers to the meridian with least curvature (flattest meridian) (see Table 1 and Annex A).

$$E = 1-p$$

NOTE - The negative of E is defined by ISO 10110-12, Part 12: Aspheric surfaces, as the conic constant designated by symbol K. The negative of E has also been called asphericity and given the symbol Q.

3.5   Corneal topographer: An instrument or system which measures features of the corneal surface of living human eyes in a noninvasive manner.

A corneal topographer which uses a video camera system and video image processing to measure the corneal surface by analyzing the reflected image created by the corneal surface of a luminous target is also referred to as a videokeratograph.

3.5.1   Optical sectioning corneal topographer: A corneal topographer which measures the corneal surface by analyzing multiple optical sections of that surface.

3.5.2   Placido ring corneal topographer: A corneal topographer which measures the corneal surface by analyzing the reflected image of a Placido ring target created by the corneal surface.

3.5.3   Reflection based corneal topographer: A corneal topographer which measures the corneal surface using light reflected from the air - precorneal tear film interface.

3.5.4   Luminous surface corneal topographer: A corneal topographer which measures the corneal surface using light back scattered from a target projected onto the precorneal tear film or the corneal anterior tissue surface. Back scattering is usually introduced in these optically clear substances by the addition of a fluorescent material into the precorneal tear film.

3.6   Corneal topographer axis (CT axis): A line parallel to the instrument optical axis and often coincident with it, which serves as one of the coordinate axes used to describe and define the corneal shape.

3.7   Corneal vertex: The point of tangency of a plane perpendicular to the CT axis with the corneal surface (see Figure 2).

3.8   Curvature

   NOTE - For the purposes of this standard the units of curvature are mm^{-1}.

3.8.1   Axial curvature (K_a): The reciprocal of the distance from a surface point to the CT axis along the corneal meridian normal at the point (see Figure 1). K_a is defined by the equation:

$$K_a = \frac{1}{r_a}$$

K_a is also, and equivalently, defined as the average of the value of the meridional curvature from the corneal vertex to the meridional point and given by the equation:

$$K_a = \frac{\int_0^{x_p} K_m(x)dx}{x_p}$$

where

   x   is the radial position variable on the meridian

   x_p is the radial position at which K_a is evaluated

3.8.2   Gaussian curvature: The product of the two principal normal curvature values at a surface location.

   NOTE - Gaussian curvature has units of inverse millimeters squared.

3.8.3   Meridional curvature (K_m): Local surface curvature measured in the meridional plane. Meridional curvature is in general a nonnormal or oblique curvature. It is the curvature of the corneal meridian at a surface point. K_m is also defined by the equation:

$$K_m = \frac{\partial^2 M(x)/\partial x^2}{\left(1 + (\partial M(x)/\partial x)^2\right)^{3/2}}$$

where

   M(x) is a function giving the elevation of the meridian at any perpendicular distance, x, from the CT axis (see Figure 1).

3.8.4   Normal curvature: The curvature at a surface location of the curve created by the intersection of the surface with any plane containing the local surface normal.

3.8.4.1 Mean curvature: The arithmetic average of the principal curvatures at a surface location.

3.8.4.2 Principal curvature: The maximum or minimum normal curvature at a surface location.

3.9   Eccentricity (e): A value descriptive of a conic section and the rate of curvature change away from the apex of the curve, i.e. how quickly the curvature flattens or steepens away from the apex of the surface. Eccentricity ranges from zero to positive infinity for the group of conic sections:

Circle (e=0); ellipse(0<e<1); parabola (e=1); and hyperbola (e>1).

In order to signify use of an oblate curve of the ellipse, e is sometimes given a negative sign that is not used in computations. Otherwise, use of the prolate curve of the ellipse is assumed.

3.10   Elevation: The distance between the corneal surface and a defined reference surface, measured in a defined direction from a specified position.

3.10.1   Axial elevation: The elevation as measured from a selected point on the corneal surface in a direction parallel to the CT axis.

3.10.2   Normal elevation: The elevation as measured from a selected point on the corneal surface in a direction along the normal to the corneal surface at the point.

3.10.3   Reference normal elevation: The elevation as measured from a selected point on the corneal surface in a direction along the normal to the reference surface.

3.11   Keratometric constant: The value 337.5 used to convert corneal curvature from inverse millimeters (mm -1) to kerametric diopters.

3.12   Keratometric diopters: Curvature, in inverse millimeters (mm -1), multiplied by the keratometric constant, 337.5.

3.13   Meridional plane: The plane which includes the surface point and the chosen axis.

3.14   Normal

3.14.1   Surface normal: A line passing through a surface location perpendicular to the plane tangent to the surface at that location.

3.14.2   Meridian normal: A line passing through a surface location, perpendicular to the tangent to the meridian curve at the location and lying in the plane creating the meridian.

3.15   p-value: A number that specifies a conic section such as an ellipse, a hyperbola or a parabola. (See Table 1.) With a conic section given in the form:

$$\frac{z^2}{b^2} + \frac{x^2}{a^2} = 1$$

the p-value is defined by:

$$p = \pm\frac{a^2}{b^2}$$

where

    a and b are constants
    + indicates an ellipse
    - indicates a hyperbola

3.16 Placido ring target: A target used in corneal topographers consisting of multiple concentric rings. Each individual ring lies in a plane; however, the rings are not in general coplanar.

3.17 Radius of curvature: The inverse of the curvature. The units of radius of curvature, for the purpose of this standard, are millimeters.

3.17.1 Axial radius of curvature (r_a): The distance from a surface point, P, to the axis along the corneal meridian normal at the point (see Figure 1). r_a is also defined by the equation:

$$r_a = \frac{x}{\sin\phi(x)}$$

where

   x is the perpendicular distance from the axis to the meridian location millimeters

   $\phi(x)$ is the angle between the axis and the meridian normal at location x

3.17.2 Meridional radius of curvature (r_m): $r_m = 1/K_m$ (see Figure 1).

3.18 Surface

3.18.1 Aspheric surface: A nonspherical surface. For corneal topography, a surface with at least one principal meridian that is a noncircular section. For ophthalmic lenses, an axisymmetrical surface.

3.18.2 Atoric surface: A surface having mutually perpendicular principal meridians of unequal curvature where at least one principal meridian is a noncircular section. These surfaces are symmetrical with respect to both principal meridians.

3.18.3 Oblate surface: A surface whose curvature increases as the location on the surface moves from a central position to a peripheral position in all meridians.

3.18.4 Prolate surface: A surface whose curvature decreases as the location on the surface moves from a central position to a peripheral position in all meridians.

3.18.5 Reference surface: A surface, which can be described in an exact, preferably mathematical fashion, used as a reference from which distance measurements are made to the measured corneal surface. In addition to its mathematical description, the positional relationship of the reference surface to the corneal surface shall be specified. For instance, a reference surface might be described as the sphere which is the best least squares fit to the measured corneal surface. Likewise, a plane could serve as a reference surface.

3.18.6 Toric surface: A surface for which the principal curvatures are unequal and for which principle meridians are circular sections. Such surfaces are said to exhibit central astigmatism.

3.19 Toricity: The difference in principal curvatures at a specified point or local area on a surface.

3.20 Transverse plane: The plane perpendicular to the meridional plane which includes the normal to the surface point.

4 Requirements

Corneal topographers complying with this standard shall meet the requirements of 4.1 and 4.2.

4.1 Area measured

When measuring an 8 mm spherical surface, a corneal topographer shall directly measure locations on the surface whose radial perpendicular distance from the corneal vertex is at least 3.75 mm. If the maximum area covered by a corneal topographer is reported, it shall be reported as the maximum radial perpendicular distance from the corneal vertex sampled on this 8 mm spherical surface.

4.2 Measurement sample density

Within the area bounded by the requirement of 4.1, the surface shall be directly sampled in sufficient locations so that any surface location within the area has a sample taken within 0.5 mm of it.

4.3 Measurement and report of performance

When the performance of a corneal topographer for the measurement of either curvature or elevation is assessed and reported, the testing shall be done in accordance with 5.1, 5.2 and 5.3 and the analysis and reporting of results shall be done in accordance with 5.4.

5 Test methods and test devices

Corneal measurements made with corneal topography systems collect data from a major portion of the corneal surface and consist of thousands of individual measurements. Each measurement is associated with a surface location and, when repeated measurements are made, some alignment variability will always exist. This is especially true for human corneas as opposed to test surfaces. While this does not affect the overall validity of measurements, it does mean that the same identical points are not measured from one measurement to the next. Therefore it is best to use a method of analysis which will not overly penalize local, random error but will give an overall measure of system performance. It is possible and practical to align the system as identically as possible between repeated measurements and then treat the entire measurement (or specified parts of it) as an ensemble and find measures of mean error and standard deviation for the ensemble. Such measures will be used herein to assess corneal topography system performance.

5.1 Types of test

5.1.1 Accuracy

An accuracy test shall be conducted by measuring a test surface specified in 5.2 using the method specified in 5.3.1 and analyzing the measured data using the method specified in 5.4. An accuracy test tests the ability of a corneal topography system to measure the absolute surface value of a known surface at known locations.

5.1.2 Repeatability

A repeatability test shall be conducted by measuring human corneas as specified by 5.3.2 and analyzing the measured values using the method specified in 5.4. A repeatability test tests the ability of corneal topography system to report the same measured values at similar locations for a human cornea when these measurements are taken close together in time.

5.2 Test surfaces

5.2.1 Reflection based systems

The test surfaces shall be constructed of glass or of optical grade plastic, such as polymethylmethacrylate. The surfaces shall be optically smooth. The back of the surfaces shall be blackened to remove unwanted reflections.

5.2.2 Luminous surface systems

The test surfaces shall be constructed of optical grade plastic, such as polymethylmethacrylate, impregnated with fluorescent molecules. The surfaces shall be optically smooth. The back of the surfaces shall be blackened to remove unwanted reflections.

5.2.3 Optical sectioning systems

The test surfaces shall be constructed of glass or of optical grade plastic, such as polymethylmethacrylate. If desired, the bulk material of which the surface is formed may be altered to produce a limited amount of bulk optical scattering to assist in the measurement process. The surfaces shall be optically smooth. The back of the surfaces shall be blackened to remove unwanted reflections.

> NOTE - If necessary, test surfaces for use in establishing the repeatability of measurements may be constructed as meniscus shells.

5.2.4 Specification of test surfaces

The curvature and elevation values of a test surface shall be given in the form of continuous mathematical expressions along with the specification of the appropriate coordinate system for these expressions. This ensures that the values for curvature or elevation can be obtained for any given position on the surface and that this can be done if there is a specified translation or rotation of the given coordinate system. This requirement is necessary as in use, in accordance with the requirements of 5.3.1 and 5.4, the position coordinates needed to find the parameter values will result from measurements by the corneal topography system under test and so can take any value within the range of the instrument.

The specification of test surface shall include tolerance limits on curvature, expressed as a tolerance on radius of curvature given in millimeters and tolerance limits on elevation given in micrometers.

> NOTE - Specifications for various test surfaces which have been judged to be useful for the assessment of the performance of cornea topographers are given in Annex A.

5.2.5 Verification of test surfaces

Test surfaces used in accordance with 5.3.1 shall be verified to conform to their specification given in accordance with 5.2.4 within the limits specified in accordance with 5.2.4. Verification of elevation may be done either (a) by direct measure of the surface using profilimetry of precision at least twice that of the tolerance at a sample density at least that specified for the instrument by 4.2, or (b) by transference methods using a verified master surface and a measurement device of sufficient precision so that measurement differences of the master surface may be used to correct measured values of tested surface. Verification of curvature may be done either (a) by mathematical calculation from verified elevation values or (b) by direct physical measurement of curvature with a method of precision twice that of the specified tolerance limits.

5.3 Data collection

5.3.1 Test surfaces: Align the test surface to the instrument in the manner specified by the manufacturer of the system for measuring human eyes. Measure the surface and save the measured data. At each measured point, the data set consists of the value of the measured variable and the two-dimensional position of the measurement.

5.3.2 Human corneas: Align the instrument to the eye in the manner specified by the manufacturer of the system. Measure the corneal surface and save the measured data. At each measured point, the data set consists of the value of the measured variable and the two-dimensional position of the measurement. Move corneal topographer with respect to the eye and then recenter it. Take a second measurement and save the measured data.

5.4 Analysis of the data

The treatment of the corneal topographic data consists of a comparison between the measured values of two data sets. The structure of the data sets is slightly different for the analysis of accuracy and the analysis of repeatability, so they will be given separately.

5.4.1 Structure of the accuracy data set

For the purpose of accuracy determination, one data set consists of the measured values and measurement locations from a measurement of a known test surface. The other data set consists of the known values of the test surface at the locations measured by the instrument and reported as part of the data set. The analysis of the paired sets of data is done in accordance with 5.4.3.

5.4.2 Structure of the repeatability data set

For the purpose of repeatability determination, a sample population of human corneas is chosen. Two measurements are taken on each cornea in the sample population, in close proximity in time, forming paired measurements. The ensemble of these paired measurements for the entire sample population comprise the data set. The measurement positions for a given cornea will generally not be identical and comparison is made between points which have the same nominal locations. The analysis of the paired sets of data is done in accordance with 5.4.3.

5.4.3 Analysis of the paired data sets

For each data set pair, a difference in measured values is taken. This gives rise to a data set of difference values, designated dD_{ijk}, for each measured point on the corneal surface. The indices i and j label the two data sets used. The index k labels the position of the individual points. The position is specified by two coordinate values which may be, for instance, the meridian (θ) and radial position (x) on which the point lies. The known values for the test surface are calculated from knowledge of its surface shape and the measured position.

The difference values, dD_{ijk}, are next grouped into subsets based on their position values. Each subset is associated with one of the measurement zones specified in Table 2 and comprised of those data points whose positions are within that measurement zone.

Each subset of difference values is then treated as an ensemble. The mean values, M_{ij}, and standard deviations, SD_{ij}, are taken for the ensemble, where

$$dD_{ijk} = w_k\left(D_{ik} - D_{jk}\right)$$

$$M_j = \frac{1}{n}\sum_{k=1}^{n} dD_{ijk}$$

$$SD_{ij} = \sqrt{\frac{\sum_{k=1}^{n}\left(dD_{ijk} - M_{ij}\right)}{n - 1}}$$

where

   n is the number of measured points

   i,j are the indices specifying the two data sets

   k is the index specifying the point location

   D_{ik} is data value at point k, it can be a curvature value, a power value or a n elevation value

   M_{ij} is the ensemble difference mean for the data sets i and j

   SD_{ij} is the standard deviation of the ensemble differences for the data sets i and j

   w_k is the area weighting value for position k as found using the method given in Annex C

5.4.4 Report of performance

The performance of a corneal topography system shall be described by reporting the following information;

5.4.4.1 Accuracy

   a) specifications of test surface used

   b) orientation of test surface with respect to the CT axis

   c) mean difference for each zone per Table 2

   d) standard deviation of differences for each zone per Table 2

5.4.4.2 Repeatability

   a) number of eyes in the sample population

   b) mean difference for the sample population for each zone per Table 2

   c) standard deviation of the differences for the sample population for each zone per Table 2

6 Accompanying documents

The corneal topographer shall be accompanied by documents containing instructions for use together with maintenance procedures and their frequency of application. In particular this information shall contain:

a) name and address of manufacturer

b) a list of accessories suitable for use with the corneal topographer

c) a reference to this American National Standard if the manufacturer claims compliance

d) any additional documents as specified in 6.8 of IEC 60601-1:1988

7 Marking

The corneal topographer shall be permanently marked with a least the following information:

a) name and address of manufacturer or supplier;

b) name and model of the corneal topographer

c) additional marking as required by IEC 601-1:1988

Table 1 - Conic section descriptors

conic section	value of p	value of E	value of e
hyperbola	p<0	E>1	e>1
parabola	0.0	1.0	1.0
prolate ellipse	1>p>0	0<E<1	*0<e<1
sphere	1.0	0.0	0.0
oblate ellipse	p>1	E<0	*0<e<1

* The eccentricity (e) does not distinguish between prolate and oblate orientations of an ellipse (see 3.11 and Annex A)

Table 2 - Analysis zones for accuracy and repeatability testing

Area
Central diameter =<3 mm
Middle 3 mm<diameter<= 6 mm
Outer diameter> 6 mm

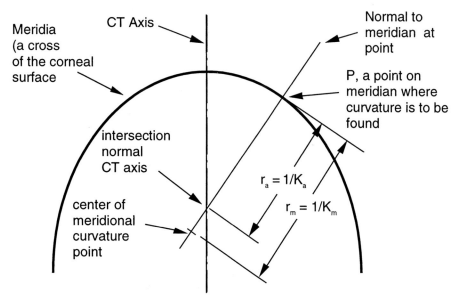

Figure 1 - Illustration of axial curvature, K_a, axial radius of curvature, r_a, meridional curvature, K_m, and meridional radius of curvature, r_m

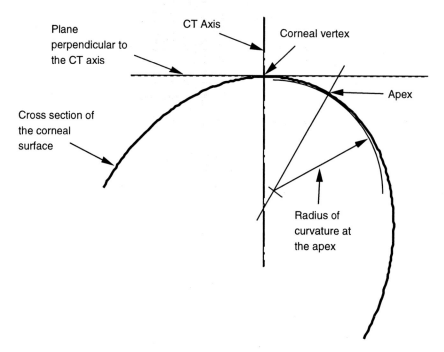

Figure 2 - Illustration of the corneal vertex and the apex

Annex A
(informative)

Test surfaces for corneal topographers

A.1   General

This annex gives various test surfaces which have been judged to be useful for assessing the performance of corneal topographers. For each type of surface a brief description is given along with its special applicability.

A.2   Spherical surfaces

Spherical surfaces are useful test objects for a variety of reasons. They have traditionally been used as test surfaces for keratometers and corneal topographers because they can be made and verified to extremely high precision. Their sphericity can be verified interferometrically and their absolute radius of curvature can be directly measured to submicron accuracy. They are useful for verifying the absolute scaling of a corneal topography system, for providing a standardized surface to measure system area coverage and for testing the sensitivity of a system to axial position (or defocus errors).

Spherical surfaces are easy to specify as they are defined by a single parameter, their radius of curvature. On the other hand, the lack of variables means that they cannot adequately assess all aspects of the performance of a corneal topography system and so must always be augmented by other more complex surfaces.

The three surfaces specified in Table A.1 are chosen to be representative of the middle and the two extremes of the curvature of cornea found in the human population and hence the range expected for a corneal topography system.

A.3   Surfaces of revolution

Surfaces of revolution in which the generating arc is more complex than a circle are useful in that they can offer surfaces which present the corneal topography system with topographical situations more like those found in the human population than can spherical surfaces, yet they can be very precisely produced using high precision, numerically controlled lathes of the type used to manufacture contact lenses.

While these surfaces possess an axial symmetry which is seldom found in the human cornea, this symmetry can easily be broken in a controlled fashion by tipping the surface by a specified amount and in a specified direction from the CT axis of the instrument under test. As the surface can be completely described analytically with respect to its axis of symmetry, the values of either curvature or elevation can easily be found in the tipped coordinate system so that comparison can be directly made to measured values.

A.3.1   Ellipsoids of revolution

When the generating arc of a surface of revolution is an ellipse, an ellipsoid of revolution is the resulting surface. Such a surface is quite like many normal corneas and so is a useful surface to test the performance of a corneal topography system for this important case. In addition, such a surface has a continuous and exactly known rate of change of curvature with respect to position.

Hence it is very useful to assess the ability of a corneal topography system to accurately map a surface with such behavior. When an ellipsoid of revolution is tipped, any axial symmetry which the system may have relied on to assist in the analysis of surfaces is broken and a fair test is given to the corneal topographer to measure a general, yet not too complex surface. Ellipsoids of revolution are not as easy to verify as are spheres, yet, because of the axial symmetry forced upon them by their method of generation, a limited number of meridians may be verified by pro-filimetry to ensure that the surface is indeed made as specified.

Ellipsoids of revolution are in the class of conics of revolution. They may be generated as either prolate or oblate surfaces. Both are useful test surfaces because while most human corneas are prolate surfaces, some corneas are found to be oblate.

Other members of this class are hyperboloids of revolution and parabolas of revolution. The hyperbola of revolution can be useful as a simulation of a keratoconic cornea in that such surfaces can be produced with a high apical curvature and with a proper choice of a conic constant, low curvature values in the periphery. When such a surface is presented to a corneal topographer in a tipped and rotated orientation, a situation simulating keratoconus is created with a surface whose surface parameters can be exactly calculated.

A.3.2   Higher order polynomial surfaces of revolution

Corneas which have undergone refractive surgery procedures are left with surface characteristics which cannot be adequately modeled by conics of revolution because they exhibit localized high variations in curvature in those areas known as transition zones. To test the ability of a corneal topographer to faithfully map such surfaces, surfaces of revolution with generating arcs consisting of higher order polynomial curves are useful. They can be manufactured using the same type of high precision numerically controlled lathes mentioned in 3.1. Because the generating arc is a polynomial function of order higher than 2, the second derivatives of the surface and hence the curvature is a continuous function of position which can be exactly calculated. The verification of such surfaces by profilimetry is no more complex a task than is that task of verifying a conic surface of revolution.

A.3.3   Multicurve composite surfaces with continuous first derivative

While higher order polynomial surfaces of revolution can be designed to test some of the special characteristics of refractive surgical cases, it is difficult to create annular bands with localized curvature quite different from surrounding areas using a single polynomial function for the entire generating arc. It is easier to create a surface of revolution comprised of sections of arc, with a smooth mathematical function, in which the sections are joined so that the first derivative of the composite generating arc is always a continuous function of position. Such surfaces do not exhibit continuous curvature at points where the sections of the arcs join.

If the sections of the composite generating arc are chosen to be circles, and the centers of some those circles lie on the axis of revolution, the resulting surface has associated areas which are spherical. This opens the possibility of verifying these areas interferometrically, a highly precise method which is not easily used for surfaces of revolution other than spheres.

Tricurve 1 from Table A1 is designed to simulate a cornea which has been flattened surgically in its central area to correct for myopia and has a narrow high curvature transition zone which joins the central area with the peripheral area which has unaltered curvature. Both the central and peripheral areas are spherical, so that they may be easily verified, while the transition zone takes the form of a circular torus with high constant curvature along the meridian. By tipping this surface by a specified and controlled amount the effect of a decentered ablation can be simulated and ability of the corneal topographer to adequately map such a condition assessed.

Tricurve 2 from Table A.1 is designed to simulate a keratoconic cornea. A spherical central area of high curvature and minimal area is joined to a transition circular torus with low, constant curvature along the meridian. This torus is then joined on its out boundary to a spherical peripheral area whose curvature is in the range of the normal cornea. When this surface is presented to the corneal topographer tipped in a specified and controlled fashion, it simulates the changing and asymmetrical surface conditions of the keratoconic cornea.

Multicurve from Table A.1 is designed to simulate the refractive surgical case of a hyperopic ablation. A spherical central area of moderately high curvature is joined to a spherical peripheral area of lower curvature via a transition area. The transition area is a surface of revolution, the generating arc of which consists of two circular segments designed to join the inner and outer spherical surfaces and one another with no discontinuity in the first derivative in the combined generating arc. The innermost circular arc of the transition is concave whereas the outermost is convex so that the transition area takes the form of a circular torus whose meridional curvature changes from negative to positive. This is the important special feature of this surface because it is a necessary geometric feature of any cornea that has had tissue removed centrally in order to steepen the central area while leaving the periphery untouched. This surface tests the ability of a corneal topographer to measure such a surface feature.

Table A.1 - Test surfaces

Surface type	Radius of curvature (mm)	Eccentricity	Zone width (mm)	Diameter (mm)
sphere	6.50	0.0		12.7
sphere	8.00	0.0		12.7
sphere	9.00	0.0		12.7
ellipsoid of revolution	7.80 (apical)	0.5		12.7
tricurve 1	9.38 (central) 6.03 (transition torus) 8.23 (peripheral)	0.0 central N/A 0.0 peripheral	diameter <= 6 mm 6 mm < diameter <8 mm diameter >= 8 mm	12.7
tricurve 2	5.00 (central) 11.50 (transition torus) 8.04 (peripheral)	0.0 central N/A 0.0 peripheral	diameter <= 2 mm 2 mm < diameter <6 mm diameter >= 6 mm	12.7
multicurve	7.34 (central) transition (see Fig A.1) 8.04 (peripheral)	0.0 central N/A 0.0 peripheral	diameter <= 6 mm 6 mm<diameter<9 mm diameter >= 9 mm	12.7

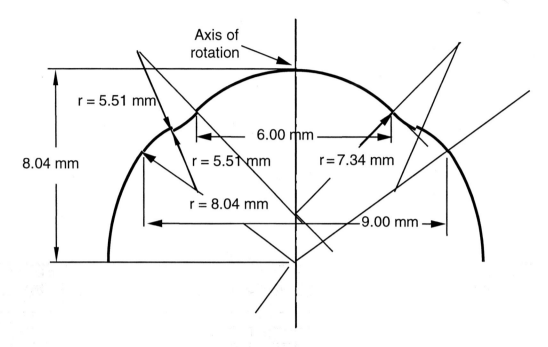

**Figure A.1 - Illustration of a multicurve test surface
designed to simulate a hyperopic ablation**

Annex B

(normative)

Standardized displays for corneal topographers

B.1   General

To facilitate the interpretation and comparison of corneal topographical results taken with different corneal topographer systems, this annex sets forth standardized displays which may be used by any corneal topographer. Specified are scale intervals, scale center value and color convention. There is nothing in this standard to imply that displays using parameters different from these standardized ones may not be used by corneal topographers complying with this standard. However, if compliance with this standard is claimed, a corneal topographer shall make these displays available to the user and shall designate them as displays conforming to ANSI Z80.23.

B.2   Presentation

The following information shall be included in standardized maps;

- Step size (units)
- Color legend
- Map type
- Reference to ANSI Z80.23

B.3   Standardized scale and scale intervals

Standardized curvature maps shall use one of the three following corneal diopter intervals:

0.5 D

1.0 D

1.5 D

There shall be at least 21 but not more than 25 displayed intervals differentiated by color. Central interval shall have a curvature value of 44 D.

Should the choice of dioptric interval and curvature found result in areas of the cornea where the value of curvature is greater than the highest interval or smaller than the lowest interval, those areas shall be displayed with the color assigned to highest interval or the lowest interval as appropriate.

Standardized elevation maps shall use one of the four following corneal diopter intervals:

2 microns

5 microns

10 microns

20 microns

There shall be at least 21 but not more than 25 displayed intervals differentiated by color. Central interval shall have an elevation value of 0.0 microns.

Should the choice of elevation interval and elevation found result in areas of the corneal where the value of elevation is greater than the highest interval or smaller than the lowest interval, those areas shall be displayed with the color assigned to highest interval or the lowest interval as appropriate.

B.4   Standardized color scale

Standardized curvature maps shall use the following color pallet.

Scale interval (D)	0.5	1.0	1.5
Red	49	54	59
Green	44	44	44
Blue	39	34	29

The hue shall be monotonically decreasing from green to red and shall be monotonically increasing from green to blue. (See Foley and van Dam for definition of hue, see clause 2.)

Standardized elevation maps shall use the following color pallet.

Scale interval (microns)	2	5	10	20
Red	20	50	100	200
Green	0	0	0	0
Blue	-20	-50	-100	-200

The hue shall be monotonically decreasing from green to red and shall be monotonically increasing from green to blue. (See Foley and van Dam for definition of hue, see clause 2.)

Annex C

(normative)

Calculation of area weighting values

C.1   General

Area weighting of the data is used to ensure that the specific sampling distribution is equivalent to a uniform sampling distribution. If the data is collected over a square grid positional distribution, the area weighting values shall all be set equal to 1.0.

C.2   Area weighting values for polar coordinate distributions (Placido ring systems)

The area weighting value for each data point within a subset, w_k, shall be calculated as follows:

$$w_k = \frac{nr_k}{\sum\limits_{k=1}^{n} r_k}$$

where

k is an index specifying measurement in the subset

n is the number of measurements in the subset area

r_k is the radial position of measurement k

C.3   Derivation of area weighting factor for polar coordinate distributions

To give measured values a weighting based on their area, a ratio is formed between the area associated with the measurement, dA_k, and the average area of measurement in the subset of measurements under consideration, $<dA_k>$. Figure C.1 shows the geometry of the area associated with a measurement taken at radial position value r_k on a given meridian. It is assumed that the angle between meridians is constant so that the angle between the dotted meridians (dθ) associated with point k is the same for all measured points. These meridians form two of the boundaries of the area, dA_k. The other two boundaries are approximated by the radial positions midway between the mean radial positions, $<r_1>$ and $<r_3>$, for the rings on either side of the measured point. The distance between these two boundaries, dr, is the value;

$$dr = \frac{\langle r_3 \rangle - \langle r_1 \rangle}{2}$$

It is assumed that this value is essentially constant throughout the subset area.

The distance between the other two boundaries is given by the value $r_k d\theta$. So the value of dA_k is given by:

$$dA_k = r_k d\theta dr$$

Since the value dθdr is taken to be a constant over the subset area, the mean value of an area associated with a measured point, $<dA_k>$, is given by:

$$\langle dA \rangle = \frac{\sum_{k=1}^{n} dA_k}{n} = \frac{\sum_{k=1}^{n} r_k \, d\theta dr}{n} = d\theta dr \frac{\sum_{k=1}^{n} r_k}{n}$$

Therefore the ratios between the area associated with measurement k and the average area for the subset area, w_k, is:

$$w_k = \frac{dA_k}{\langle dA_k \rangle} = \frac{r_k \, d\theta dr}{d\theta dr \dfrac{\sum_{k=1}^{n} r_k}{n}} = \frac{n r_k}{\sum_{k=1}^{n} r_k}$$

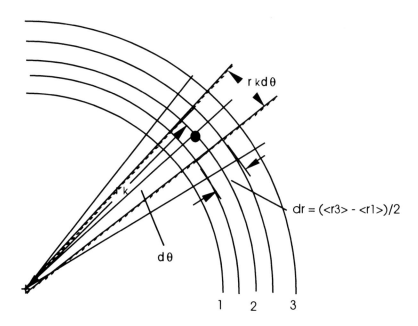

Figure C.1 - Geometry used to find area weighting factors for polar coordinate distributions

Index